ALSO BY JOHN BATESON

*The Last and Greatest Battle: Finding the Will,
Commitment, and Strategy to End Military Suicides*

The Final Leap: Suicide on the Golden Gate Bridge

Building Hope: Leadership in the Nonprofit World

THE EDUCATION OF A CORONER

LESSONS IN INVESTIGATING DEATH

JOHN BATESON

SCRIBNER NEW YORK LONDON TORONTO SYDNEY NEW DELHI

Scribner
An Imprint of Simon & Schuster, Inc.
1230 Avenue of the Americas
New York, NY 10020

First Scribner hardcover edition August 2017

SCRIBNER and design are registered trademarks of The Gale Group, Inc.,
used under license by Simon & Schuster, Inc., the publisher of this work.

For information about special discounts for bulk purchases,
please contact Simon & Schuster Special Sales at 1-866-506-1949
or business@simonandschuster.com.

The Simon & Schuster Speakers Bureau can bring authors to
your live event. For more information or to book an event,
contact the Simon & Schuster Speakers Bureau at 1-866-248-3049
or visit our website at www.simonspeakers.com.

Interior design by Kyle Kabel

Manufactured in the United States of America

1   3   5   7   9   10   8   6   4   2

Library of Congress Control Number: 2016059878

ISBN 978-1-5011-6822-2
ISBN 978-1-5011-6824-6 (ebook)

To Suzan, as always

CONTENTS

PROLOGUE

Ana Valiente was twenty-three and working as a housekeeper at a senior center in San Rafael, California, when she disappeared. Originally from El Salvador, where her family still lived, she was hardworking, upbeat, and dependable. After she failed to show up for her job on December 6, 2006, coworkers reported her missing.

Two weeks later, she was still missing. Police had zeroed in on a suspect, though, thirty-nine-year-old Gregorio Mendez-Deleon. He was born in Guatemala, married with three children, and worked as a driver at the Marin County Sanitary District's recycling center. According to other people at the center, he was in a sexual relationship with Ana, who had become pregnant.

The recycling center had a camera that filmed cars as they drove in and out, and Mendez-Deleon's car, with Ana visible in the passenger seat, was captured leaving the center on Tuesday, December 5, at 4:30 P.M. That made Mendez-Deleon the last person to be seen with her. Later, a backhoe operator at the center, knowing that Ana had disappeared and Mendez-Deleon was considered a "person of interest," came forward and told police that he had dug a hole one night at Mendez-Deleon's request in a remote area of the recycling center grounds.

"That was when things started to get interesting," Ken Holmes tells me.

Holmes was the coroner of Marin County. He had been in the job eight years at that point, but had worked in the coroner's office nearly thirty years altogether, first as an investigator, then as the assistant coroner. By 2006 he had handled hundreds of homicides and thousands of other deaths.

Police brought Mendez-Deleon in for questioning, and in short order induced a confession. Mendez-Deleon said that he and Ana were sitting in his Toyota sedan after dark on December 5 in front of a Wendy's restaurant in downtown San Rafael. They had an argument, then Mendez-Deleon took out a pocketknife and started stabbing Ana in the neck. She was a big woman, more than two hundred pounds, and wedged into the small car. She couldn't get away, and Mendez-Deleon continued to attack her. Within minutes she was dead.

Holmes pauses, shakes his head, then says, "As often happens in cases like this, one problem quickly became two. The first problem was what to do with Ana's body. Her killer knew that he had to get rid of it, but how? The second problem was what to do with his car. The interior, especially on the passenger side, was drenched with her blood. It became even bloodier when he decided to cut off her legs. She was too big for him to move otherwise."

The recycling center wasn't far away, and Mendez-Deleon decided to go there. Although it was after hours, the backhoe operator was still around and Mendez-Deleon convinced him to dig a hole at the rear of the property. The backhoe operator didn't know what the hole was for, but he was willing to do Mendez-Deleon a favor. After he left, Mendez-Deleon put Ana's legs in one plastic bag and the rest of her in another bag, maneuvered both bags into the hole, and pushed all of the dirt back into place to cover up everything. Then he got a truck and drove it over the site several times to compact the soil, after which he erased the tire marks.

Now he just needed to get rid of his car. That was relatively easy; he took it to a friend's wrecking yard and had it crushed. He told the friend that he couldn't get it smogged, so rather than pay a junkyard to come and get it, he wanted it flattened, then he would borrow a pickup truck and take his flattened car to a metal scrapper.

In his confession, Mendez-Deleon indicated the general area where Ana's body had been buried. It was dark at the time, though, and he didn't know the exact location. The backhoe operator didn't know, either, or how deep the hole was. He thought it was about five feet, but he wasn't really sure.

That was when the coroner's office was summoned. Holmes was briefed by police, then he and his staff went to work.

"We knew we were going to have to go digging," he says, "and we were going to have to do an archaeological dig. If you know that there's a body, you have to be forensically perfect from the get-go, which means using small paintbrushes and soup spoons and small garden trowels because we don't know how deep it is to the body."

Over the years, Holmes had worked with the Federal Bureau of Investigation on numerous cases, and maintained good relations. FBI agents were involved anytime a death occurred on federal property, or a federal employee was killed, or a crime was committed that crossed state lines. Other times, though, if local agents weren't busy and Holmes could use help on a case, the FBI provided it. In this instance, Holmes received a call offering the assistance of the FBI's special response unit—four agents with expertise in archaeological digs. He had never worked with this particular team before, which was based out of the area but accepted immediately.

The team showed up towing a box trailer that was sixteen to eighteen feet long. When they opened up the back, Holmes stared in amazement.

"It was like Costco for forensics. There was every conceivable thing you could use or need, including Tyvek suits for all of us, little wire flags in various colors to mark locations, and pop-up tents to hide the dig from news helicopters, which were hovering all around us after reporters got wind of the case."

Without knowing the exact location, the FBI team marked off the area in six-foot squares, then used flat shovels to scrape away at the soil, which was full of shale and rocks. Whenever they got deep enough to realize that soil hadn't been disturbed, they moved on to another square of the grid.

The dig went on for two days before they found the spot and dug down five feet to the bags. One of Holmes's investigators, Darrell Harris, was there the first day, and another investigator, Pam Carter, was present the second day. Holmes dropped by several times as well. Both days, throughout the process, federal agents deferred to the coroner's office.

"It wasn't like you see on TV," Holmes says, "where the FBI comes in and pushes everybody out of the way. They didn't do that; they absolutely didn't do that. They were our best friends, and loved doing this kind of stuff because they didn't get to do it very often. It wasn't their jurisdiction and they knew it; they were just lending their resources and expertise. Someone even came around at lunchtime and took our orders for sandwiches and coffee or soft drinks. They never sent us a bill for anything."

While the dig was taking place, police located Mendez-Deleon's crushed car. Holmes had it taken to a large training center at the Novato Fire Department so that firefighters could open it up.

"They had never worked on anything so compacted before," he says, "and considered it great practice. They also weren't used to participating in a homicide investigation, which added a thrill factor."

The Jaws of Life is a big, compressed-air separator. Its hydraulic ram uses pneumatic pressure to pull apart smashed objects piece by piece. In two and a half hours, firefighters separated the door panels, seats, and carpets, all of which were covered with blood.

Holmes was able to confirm Ana's identity through a fingerprint check with the Department of Homeland Security. She didn't have a driver's license but possessed a valid passport, so her fingerprints were in the DHS database. Holmes also had the blood in Mendez-Deleon's car analyzed and it matched that of Ana Valiente.

With that information, Mendez-Deleon was charged with the murder of Ana and also the six-week-old child she was carrying. Since double homicides are subject to the death penalty in California, it was a potential capital punishment case. During legal proceedings, however, the second murder charge was dropped because the unborn child wasn't far enough along to meet the definition of a fetus, according to state law.

In his trial, which Holmes testified at, Mendez-Deleon recanted his confession and said that an unidentified third party was to blame. According to his public defender, Mendez-Deleon was afraid that he would be targeted and killed at San Quentin Prison. The prison is in Marin County and is where all male death row inmates in California are incarcerated. Like many prisons, it is controlled by gangs, and Mendez-Deleon would be at their mercy. That was of little concern to the prosecution, however. In a plea bargain, Mendez-Deleon was sentenced to sixteen years.

Looking back on the case, Holmes says, with a bemused smile, "Just another day at the office," knowing that it was anything but. Then again, there weren't many days that were routine.

CHAPTER 01

FIRST BLUSH

I first met Ken Holmes in 2010 when I interviewed him for my book *The Final Leap*, about suicides from the Golden Gate Bridge. I was executive director of a nationally certified crisis intervention and suicide prevention center in the San Francisco Bay Area at the time, and Ken's office was responsible for conducting the autopsies of most Golden Gate Bridge jumpers, as well as for notifying their families of the death. After the book came out, I was recruited to serve on the board of the Bridge Rail Foundation, an all-volunteer, nonprofit organization dedicated to ending suicides on the bridge. Ken was on the board also, and we had numerous opportunities to talk further. It didn't take long for me to realize that his experiences over nearly forty years in the Marin County Coroner's Office and the cases he'd handled would make a riveting subject for a book.

I had another reason for writing *The Education of a Coroner*: I didn't know much about the workings of a coroner's office, and wanted to learn more. How do coroners approach a death scene and what do they look for? How are families notified of a death, and what psychological techniques are employed? How has the world of forensic pathology changed with advances in technology?

The first time Ken and I met to discuss it was in a brew pub in Larkspur, in central Marin County. He had been retired three years by that time, although he still had—and continues to have—frequent contact with many of his former colleagues, and also attends annual conferences of the California State Coroners Association, where he once was president. We had communicated by email before then and I had run my general idea by him. I would review eight hundred case files that he had preselected and copied onto electronic disks, then we would schedule a series of days when we would meet and discuss the cases that I thought were the most interesting. Along the way we also would talk about his background, training, responsibilities, lessons learned, and people he worked with. First, though, I said I needed to get a sense of whether the stories he told were compelling and had universal appeal.

"Sure," he said, and with no further prompting he launched into a thumbnail sketch of one case, then another and another until after only a few minutes my head was spinning. He apologized and said that once he started talking about his work, it was hard for him to stop.

Holmes is a natural storyteller, and his deep, melodic voice is both authoritative and soothing. A barrel-chested man with sharp eyes—even in his seventies—strong hands from having spent years outdoors, and a handsome face framed by a trimmed gray beard, he is someone who makes friends easily and holds on to them because at the end of the day, and especially at this stage in his life, friends and family are what matter most. He is quick to laugh—especially at himself—and has a range of knowledge that is impressive. Whether it is medicine, politics, hunting, guns, home repair, sports, food, wine, or cars, he can hold his own in a conversation with anyone.

"Let's back up," I said, "and focus on one case for now. You pick."

"Okay," he said, and he proceeded to tell me some of the highlights of the Carol Filipelli case, which is described a little later in this book.

At the end, all I could say was, "How many more stories do you have like that?"

He shrugged and said, "Dozens?"

* * *

Some of the cases cast Holmes in the national spotlight because of who they involved—rock legend Jerry Garcia, rapper Tupac Shakur, porn kings Jim and Artie Mitchell, and the infamous Trailside Killer. It was the deaths of people who weren't well known, however, that remain the most vivid and noteworthy in his mind.

Several cases took nearly a decade to close, two took twenty years, one took thirty, and one took forty-four years. It might seem like a luxury for a coroner to be able to pursue cases so doggedly—certainly that's not possible in large cities and statewide coroner's offices. In some respects it was, but Holmes's belief—then and now—is that family and friends of the deceased deserve to know what happened no matter how long it takes. Coroners deal with death, but their purpose is to find answers for the living.

If the work of coroners were less dramatic, we wouldn't have so many TV shows about it. Holmes watches some of them and says that they get most—though not all—of the details right. Even so, inevitably he comes away thinking that real life is more moving than any fictionalized treatment can be. Nothing beats a story that happens to be true.

It helps to have a glamorous setting, which is why the original *CSI* TV show was set in Las Vegas and there is now *CSI: Miami*, *CSI: New York*, and *NCIS: Los Angeles*. If the emphasis were on gritty, then we would have *CSI: Camden*, *CSI: Detroit*, and *NCIS: Compton*.

The setting where Holmes worked is every bit as enthralling as the biggest cities with the brightest lights. I say that not because I was raised in Marin—as an adolescent it didn't seem all that exciting—but because the county has a national reputation, despite its small size. Part of that is due to its physical beauty. Situated just north of San Francisco, Marin is surrounded by water. The Pacific Ocean lies to the west, and the eastern and southern borders end at San Francisco Bay. Only the northern portion abuts land—the beginning of California's legendary wine country. Otherwise, access is across the Golden Gate Bridge to the south or the Richmond–San Rafael Bridge to the east.

There are no large urban centers, processing plants, factories, or notable industries in Marin. Mostly the county consists of coastline, rolling hills, dairy farms, and small towns. Hundreds of thousands of people come every year to visit Point Reyes National Seashore, Golden Gate National Recreation Area, Muir Woods, Mount Tamalpais, Stinson Beach, Tomales Bay, and Samuel P. Taylor State Park.

The other reason why Marin is well known is its affluence. It ranks among the top twenty counties in the United States in terms of household income, and is home to rock stars, movie stars, professional athletes, and wealthy business executives. The median price of homes is just under $1 million, and in many communities it's considerably more.

This doesn't mean that all is rosy, however. In 2014, the Robert Wood Johnson Foundation reported that nearly 25 percent of adults in Marin engage in binge drinking during any given month—one of the highest averages in the state. More than thirty residents die per year from drug overdoses, a large number in a small county. In addition, Marin is second to San Francisco when it comes to suicides from the Golden Gate Bridge.

Marin also has pockets of poverty. In the Canal District of San Rafael, people from dozens of cultures, speaking a multitude of languages, live close together in low-income housing. In Marin City, built during World War II to house shipyard workers and immigrants, local residents—predominately African-American—lived for years in crowded tenements until gentrification started pushing them out, creating new sources of tension.

Then there is San Quentin Prison, the oldest prison in California and one of the largest penitentiaries in the United States. Built in 1852 on 432 acres of shoreline property in Marin, San Quentin is, almost certainly, the most expensive piece of real estate in America—and perhaps the world—that is devoted to housing convicted felons. In 2009 the land was estimated to be worth $2 billion, and it has only increased in value since then. All of California's 750 male death row inmates are locked up there, as well as more than four thousand other hardened criminals, male and female. To a motorist approaching Marin County from the Richmond–San Rafael Bridge, the prison looks, at first glance, like a huge sand-colored hotel on the waterfront. As one gets closer, however, one sees the twelve-foot-high concrete walls that are topped by coils of electrified barbed wire, notices that all of the window openings are mere slits even though the view outside them is spectacular, and knows that San Quentin was built with a much different purpose in mind.

THE CORONER'S OFFICE

It's in this setting that the coroner's office in Marin County operates. Throughout Holmes's career, it was on the second floor of the Marin Civic Center in San Rafael, the county seat. The building was the last one designed by famed architect Frank Lloyd Wright and features a roof the color of the sky, scalloped balconies, and pink stucco walls, all intended to blend into the surrounding environment.

The office, which has since moved, isn't what one might expect. Before I interviewed Holmes the first time, in 2010, I envisioned it to be part morgue with shrouded bodies laid out on stainless steel tables, waiting to be autopsied, and part laboratory with slides being inspected under microscopes. Like many small counties, however, Marin doesn't have a morgue because it's too expensive. Instead the coroner's office contracts with local mortuaries and private physicians to receive the bodies of dead people and conduct autopsies when warranted. The county also doesn't have a lab for analyzing specimens that are collected at a death scene. Fingernail scrapings, pubic hair samples, vaginal swabs, and the like are sent to outside labs. There are only a handful in California that specialize in this kind of analysis, with the primary one operated by the state Department of Justice. Samples from any case that might go to court—particularly homicide cases—are sent there. The DOJ lab doesn't handle body fluids, though, so blood, urine, and gastric samples are sent elsewhere.

Employee offices look the same as the offices of any other business with a modest budget—older desks and chairs, older computers and phones, and bookcases crammed with special texts, trade journals, binders, and miscellaneous papers. For all of Holmes's thirty-six years, there was a staff of seven. Six employees—the coroner, assistant coroner, three death investigators, and a secretary—were full-time. One position—the medical transcriber—was part-time. He or she took the voice recordings of forensic pathologists during autopsies and turned them into written summaries.

The common areas are more distinctive. There are evidence lockers, an old bank safe to store money that is collected at a death scene, refrigeration units to store specimen samples, and dozens of four-drawer metal file cabinets that are filled with case files, some of which date back more than 150 years, to the time when California became a state.

The role of the coroner originated in twelfth-century England. "Crowners," as they were known at the time, conducted inquests on behalf of King Richard I to identify the deceased, determine how they died, and—most important—collect death taxes on their estates. It was the height of the Crusades, the Catholic Church was trying to restore Christianity in and around the Holy Lands, and money was needed to finance numerous campaigns.

Coroner's offices today are vestiges of this royal system. Coroners are either elected by the populace or appointed by designated entities, with the requirements varying state by state and oftentimes county by county. In the highest form, coroners are medical examiners, meaning they are licensed physicians who are trained and certified in forensic pathology. Most people assume that all coroners are MEs, but this isn't the case. Many coroners are licensed physicians who have no training in forensics, while in hundreds of communities across the country—including Marin County—the coroner isn't required to have any medical training at all, much less a medical degree. He or she just needs to have a clean record, meaning no felony convictions, be twenty-one or older, and have a high school diploma. Some counties don't even require that, however. One county in Indiana elected a coroner who was eighteen and still in high school.

A 2015 review by the National Academies of Sciences, Engineering, and Medicine compared county coroners and medical examiners. The biggest benefit of county coroners, according to the review, is that they reflect the will of the people. In American political culture, elected officials represent a community's needs and values better than anyone else because they are chosen by voters. In addition, county coroners have equal footing with other locally elected officials—members of the board of supervisors, sheriffs, judges, and district attorneys—which enables them to operate independently from these entities. The main drawback is that the coroner may not be medically proficient since it's not a requirement of the job.

On the medical examiner side, the major advantage, according to the review, is that the overall quality of death investigations is better. In addition, there is more uniformity. For statewide medical examiner offices, there are the added benefits of centralized administration, which is expensive to start but less expensive to sustain, and improved service to rural areas, which often don't have the capacity to operate coroner offices on their own.

Nineteen states—in general, the smallest ones—have a state medical examiner system. The largest states, including California, Texas, New York, Illinois, Pennsylvania, Ohio, and Georgia, have a mix of medical examiner and county coroner offices.

As the most populous state, California is unusual—but not unique—in that the coroner's office is combined with the sheriff's department in forty-nine of fifty-eight counties. In these areas the sheriff serves as coroner, too—despite having little or no medical training—and appoints another law enforcement person to oversee the day-to-day duties who, in all likelihood, has no medical training, either. The result is that the work of the coroner's office is controlled by the sheriff, which can create problems. Because sheriffs focus on criminal activity, the emphasis of the coroner's office in these counties is to support homicide investigations. Less time is spent delving into deaths by accident, suicide, or natural causes, and frequently in these instances autopsies aren't conducted, in order to save money. Cases in which the manner of death is undetermined, but clearly isn't homicide, also get short shrift, leaving families in the dark as to what caused their loved one to die.

The lack of national standards for coroners is hard to understand inasmuch as a death certificate is one of our most important documents. It is used by families to collect life insurance, file for payment from special funds for certain types of deaths, such as mesothelioma, and change names on deeds, trusts, and other valuable assets. Death certificates also are used by the government to stop Social Security payments, by businesses to change or eliminate pension payouts and health care coverage, by various public and private agencies to inform current funding decisions and future policies, and by researchers to track how society is changing.

In *Working Stiff: Two Years, 262 Bodies, and the Making of a Medical Examiner*, author Judy Melinek talks about the value of a death certificate. "It's no big deal if you don't have a birth certificate," she says. "Other forms of identification will suffice to secure a job, open a bank account, even file for Social Security. However, if your survivors cannot produce a death certificate after your demise, they will descend into bureaucratic purgatory. They can't bury your body, transport it across state lines, liquidate your investments, or inherit anything you have willed them."

Coroners aren't the only people who are authorized to sign death certificates. Depending on the state, a primary care physician, attending physician, nonattending physician, or nurse practitioner can sign. Most of the time, these signatories confirm a death by natural causes where no investigation is needed. In homicides, suicides, and accidents, coroners typically sign the certificate after an autopsy has been performed.

CAUSE AND MANNER

The results from an autopsy and the findings of toxicology tests help the coroner determine the cause and manner of someone's death. Although cause and manner seem like the same thing, they are, in fact, different. Cause refers to the physical reason why a person died. A gunshot to the head, an overdose of drugs, blunt-force traumatic injuries such as those resulting from a vehicle accident or a fall, sharp-force injuries like stabbings, inhaling a deadly gas like carbon monoxide, and asphyxiation due to drowning, hanging, or strangulation are examples of cause. Deaths from heart attacks, strokes, seizures, and other diseases also are examples of cause.

Manner refers to the way in which a person dies. There are five recognized categories in the United States: homicide, suicide, accident, natural, and undetermined. Each one has legal implications for law enforcement and can have financial consequences as well.

A ruling of homicide means that there is likely to be a police investigation. Detectives collect evidence of criminal activity and present it to a district attorney, who decides whether or not to prosecute. If the case goes to trial, the coroner is called to testify, but only to the extent of explaining how a determination of cause was reached. Inasmuch as coroners' rulings are fact-based and unbiased, there are occasions when the explanation is as helpful to the defense—mainly by discouraging the district attorney from trying the case—as it is to the prosecution.

A ruling of suicide usually ends any police involvement. In some instances, this is welcome news for family members who otherwise might be implicated for murder. Other times, a determination of suicide can end up voiding a decedent's life insurance policy if it was taken out or renewed within two years of the person's death (beyond two years, the policy can't be nullified). In addition to the possible financial impact, a death by suicide can be stigmatizing and cause family members to feel guilty, embarrassed, or angry on top of the other emotions that a loved one's death tends to generate, such as sadness, depression, loneliness, and despair. For this reason, family members may push hard for the coroner to rule that the death was accidental rather than a suicide.

If a death is determined to be accidental, it means that there was little if anything the decedent could have done in the moment to prevent it. A woman falls off her horse, lands on her head, and fractures her skull. A boat capsizes and someone drowns. An apartment building catches on fire and one of the tenants dies from smoke inhalation. Sometimes blame may be placed on another person, such as the driver in a fatal vehicle collision whose inattentiveness, recklessness, or drunkenness caused the accident. Alternatively, the victim's own ignorance or carelessness may play a major role. A man is swept off a rock while fishing and is washed out to sea. A homeowner who is trimming trees on his property touches a high-voltage wire with his saw and is electrocuted. A farmhand loading bales of hay into an auger feeding wagon falls into the wagon and is mutilated. Each of these is among the many deaths that Holmes investigated in his career, and each was avoidable, but not in the instant that it happened. At that moment it was too late.

As for natural deaths, which typically comprise about 60 percent of the deaths a coroner's office handles, these are the result of a disease rather than an injury. This doesn't mean that the person died of "old age," since young people can have a known or unknown health problem that isn't treated or ends up being mistreated. Rather, it means that the person suffered from a heart condition, tumor, seizure, or aneurism that proved to be fatal.

Sometimes it's impossible to determine the manner in which someone died. When a car goes off the road and hits a tree or catapults off a cliff, did the driver fall asleep at the wheel, swerve to avoid an animal, lose control, or intend to die? If the person had a stroke or heart attack there will be forensic evidence, but otherwise, in the absence of skid marks, it may not be possible to tell. Similarly, if someone is found dead in bed due to a drug overdose, was it accidental or intentional? A suicide note might provide the answer, but only 20 percent of suicide victims leave a note, so oftentimes the coroner has little to go on. Is a patient's death during surgery merely unfortunate or is there evidence of medical malpractice? Every medical procedure has risks; the question is whether doctors bear any responsibility for the outcome.

In cases where the coroner doesn't have enough information to make a definitive ruling, the official manner of death is "undetermined." This can be altered if new evidence comes to light; however, it can only be altered once. The last thing anyone wants is for the manner of someone's death to be perpetually changing. That would wreak havoc with law enforcement, the courts, health care providers, insurance companies, and families.

Marin County has an average of 1,500 to 1,800 deaths per year. Roughly 300 of these require autopsies because the cause and manner of death aren't clear. Trauma cases, accident cases, and other cases that are out of the ordinary or unusual end up in a pathologist's hands.

"On TV and in the movies they use the word 'suspicious,'" Holmes says, "but that's not a word we ever used. We said it was 'out of the ordinary' or 'unusual.' Not that it's wrong to use 'suspicious'—it might be part of the vernacular in other coroners' offices—it just wasn't part of ours. To say that a death is suspicious is to offer an opinion; something doesn't seem right. Instead, we presented the facts and left the interpretation to others."

THE ROAD TAKEN

Holmes was raised by his paternal grandparents in the Central Valley town of Fresno, California. His grandfather was the fire chief of Fresno and a huge influence on Holmes's life.

"He taught me morals, integrity, and work ethic," Holmes says. "He also was a guiding light when it came to life in politics, which I didn't fully appreciate until years later, when I entered the political arena."

Most boys Holmes's age were passionate about three things: sports, guns, and the outdoors. Holmes was, too, but he also was transfixed by something that his friends had no interest in—anatomy.

"I was the kid who tried to figure out how that bird died, or what happened to the jackrabbit," he says. "When I first started hunting, at age eight, I was as interested in what happened to the bullet as I was in getting the animal ready to eat."

He remembers the first jackrabbit he ever skinned. "Once I skinned it I could see the shoulder and the foreleg, and I could work the shoulder and I could see the shoulder bone rotating in the socket because the muscle there is thin. I said to my granddad, 'Gee, look at that.' He said it was called a ball-and-socket joint. I kept working it, and in my mind I was struck by the fact that it was so simple yet worked so well."

Early on, Holmes's grandmother determined that if an animal was wounded, her grandson was the one who would tend to it. One time someone's collie got hit by a bus in front of Holmes's house. Holmes was playing with three of his friends and witnessed the accident. He didn't know whose dog it was, but he got a stick and two handkerchiefs and splinted the dog's broken leg.

In middle school, Holmes had to write a report describing three occupations he was interested in pursuing. Two choices—being a physician and being a veterinarian—seemed obvious. Both had a significant drawback, though—all of the additional years of study that were necessary. Holmes liked school, but not that much. Even so, he listed doctor and vet as two of his choices. He had no idea for a third choice, however.

"You know, the coroner does autopsies," his grandfather said. "That's medicine."

Holmes perked up. "What are autopsies?"

His grandfather explained that autopsies are postmortem examinations to determine how and why someone died. Usually they are done in a morgue, he said, but because Fresno County didn't have one at the time, they were conducted at a local mortuary instead.

"Do you want me to set up a meeting with the funeral director there?" he asked.

Holmes nodded, instantly intrigued. He was even more interested when he saw the funeral director drive up in a big black late-model Cadillac. The man was wearing an expensive suit and equally expensive shoes. In addition, the funeral home was plush and quiet, the sort of place where Holmes could imagine himself working.

The funeral director affirmed that all autopsies for the coroner's office were done at his mortuary, and he explained the process and what the job entailed. By now Holmes sensed that he might have found his calling. There was just one more thing he needed to know.

"How long does it take to be a funeral director?"

"Three years after high school," the man said. "One year of mortuary college and two years of apprenticeship."

That clinched it. Holmes wrote in his report that his third career choice was funeral director.

From the outset, he knew that his real goal was to be a coroner, not a funeral director. "I just didn't know how to get there," he says.

In school, his favorite subject was science. He also was enamored with mysteries, especially those that featured his namesake detective, Sherlock Holmes.

After he graduated from high school, Holmes attended Fresno City College for two years and started an apprenticeship at the funeral home he had visited with his grandfather. In those days, a person didn't have to go to mortuary college first. During the apprenticeship, Holmes learned two important things about himself.

The first was that he had no qualms about death. On the contrary, when he watched his first autopsy, he was so enthralled that eventually his boss had to ask him to leave the doctor alone because he was asking too many questions. The person's chest had been cut open, exposing all of the internal organs, and Holmes would point to various body parts and ask, "What's that?" The doctor would explain, then remove the deceased's heart, kidneys, and other organs and place them in Holmes's hands.

"It was a mesmerizing experience," he says, "and I couldn't get enough of it. Throughout my apprenticeship, whenever there was an autopsy I went and watched, even if I didn't have to be there. I continued to ask questions and listen to the doctor as he recorded his findings into a Dictaphone. The result was that I began to develop a good grasp of medical terminology when I was still in my teens."

The other thing Holmes learned about himself was that he had a lot of compassion. "I didn't know it," he says, "but I did. From the beginning, I enjoyed working with families. I felt comfortable around them, and they, in turn, were grateful for my help in making funeral arrangements."

San Francisco College of Mortuary Science emphasized the physical sciences—anatomy, pathology, bacteriology, and chemistry. One of the skills that was taught was embalming. It involves withdrawing blood and waste matter from human organs, reshaping or reconstructing disfigured or maimed bodies using clay, cotton, plaster of Paris, and wax, injecting embalming fluid with a pump into arms and legs, closing incisions using needles and sutures, joining lips with a needle and thread, and applying cosmetics to give a dead body a lifelike appearance. Holmes didn't know it at the time, but the fact that he became a licensed embalmer proved to be a critical stepping-stone to his future career.

After he graduated, he applied to coroners' offices around the Bay Area, but there weren't any openings. Needing to work, he took a job at a mortuary in Sonoma County, just north of Marin. At that time, Sonoma County had only one coroner's investigator. He was retired from the California Highway Patrol and responded to homicides and accidental deaths, but not to traffic accidents because the police could take care of those. Even so, there were more cases than he could handle so he commissioned every licensed embalmer in the county to be a deputy coroner. This meant that Holmes and other embalmers were responsible for writing a brief report—only a few lines—following suicides and other types of deaths that weren't being investigated, leaving the investigator to focus on trauma cases.

One day the investigator was at the mortuary where Holmes worked. He wasn't there to see Holmes, but he couldn't help but pull him aside.

"Damn, Holmes," he said. "You wrote a report the other day; I wouldn't write one that long. You went into all sorts of detail you didn't need to. I certainly got a great picture of what you saw, though."

FORTUNE INTERVENES

Holmes was married and had a son and daughter by this time. In coaching his son's Little League team, he became friends with another coach, named Henry. One Friday morning Holmes was at the mortuary and it was quiet. No one else was around and there wasn't anything in particular that he needed to do. Although it was a hot day, Holmes decided it would be a good time to see if he could get the big fountain in front to work properly. He had always liked to tinker, and the fact that it sprayed water sporadically bothered him. Still wearing his standard uniform—black slacks and a white shirt—he rolled up his sleeves and was working on the fountain when Henry drove by. Henry honked and waved, and Holmes waved in return. Because he wasn't in a hurry, Henry turned around, came back, and the two of them moved to the shade and got to talking. At first they talked about Little League, then Holmes asked Henry what he was doing there. Henry said he had stopped to see a man named Tom who worked at another mortuary nearby. After that Henry mentioned, offhand, something that would change Holmes's life. He said that Tom told him the Marin County Coroner's Office was adding a new position, a third death investigator, and Tom had applied for it.

Holmes was floored. He knew the two current investigators in Marin and the assistant coroner. Despite making repeated inquiries, however, Holmes had never been told that a job was opening up.

As soon as Henry left, Holmes called the coroner's office. It was one o'clock. He said he had just heard that another investigator was going to be hired, and asked what the process was for applying. A secretary told him that interested candidates had to fill out an application from the Human Resources Office, and the filing deadline was five o'clock that afternoon.

Holmes closed the mortuary, told the answering service that he had an emergency, and raced ten miles to the Marin County Civic Center, where all county offices were based. The Human Resources Office was on the top floor of the four-story building, tucked so far in back that it seemed like Siberia. Holmes tried to remain calm as he asked for an application. It turned out to be six pages long, and a woman told him that he needed to attach copies of his high school and college transcripts. Holmes filled out the application as neatly as he could by hand, and said that he could provide the attachments but couldn't get them that day. The woman said that since it was Friday, it probably would take a couple of days for applications to be processed, so if he could get them to her by the first part of the following week she would add them to his application. She didn't need to be so accommodating, but she was.

On Monday, Holmes called his high school and college to get the transcripts. Faxes didn't exist in those days so he paid to have them mailed overnight. Tuesday afternoon he delivered the documents to Human Resources, and the woman included them.

It turned out that there were sixty-eight applicants for the one position. As with most government jobs, people in the HR office did the initial screening. One of the requirements listed by the coroner, Dr. Ervin Jindrich, was that the person have a California embalmer's

license. Jindrich himself was a certified forensic pathologist, but he knew the value of an embalmer's license.

"It meant you're not afraid of death," Holmes says, "and you're used to people crying."

Being unafraid of death is an obvious requisite for a coroner. Doctors, soldiers, cops, and firefighters become habituated to death the more they witness it, but coroners have to start out undaunted by dead people in all their forms. As for being used to people who are crying, this might sound cold or insensitive, but in fact it was practical and relevant. Coroners' investigators have to be able to function in an environment where people are feeling enormous pain and grieving a significant loss.

"It's easy to get sucked into someone's grief and want to comfort them," Holmes says, "but you also have to be able to step back and focus on other aspects of the job."

As it turned out, half the candidates lacked an embalmer's license and were eliminated from further consideration. Tom, the man who had told Holmes's friend Henry about the opening, was still in the running, however. Moreover, he knew everyone in the Marin coroner's office even better than Holmes. Tom had worked with them longer and more closely. In a moment of ill-advised and inappropriate candor, Keith Craig, the assistant coroner, told Holmes that Tom had the inside track and almost certainly would be hired. Hearing this, Holmes was despondent. His dream job was going to someone else.

Tom was so confident of his standing, however, that he hadn't submitted all the information that HR required. As a result, his application was thrown out. Craig, among others, was flabbergasted to learn that Tom hadn't made it past the first step. He had seemed like a sure thing.

That was the opening Holmes needed. He went through the interview process, which culminated in oral boards before a panel of five coroners from neighboring counties, and ended up being ranked the top candidate.

Looking back to that period of time, Holmes still marvels at the confluence of events that ended with his hiring. The fact that it was a quiet day, that he was outside the mortuary fiddling with the fountain, that Henry not only waved but stopped and came back because he wasn't pressed for time, that Henry mentioned the position not knowing that Holmes would be interested in it, that Holmes had enough time to get to the civic center and fill out an application, that HR allowed him to add grade transcripts after the filing deadline, and that Tom's application was thrown out because it was incomplete, seemed nothing short of miraculous.

After he started, Holmes asked Jindrich why he hired him. After all, Holmes had no investigative experience.

Jindrich was thirty-five at the time—only three years older than Holmes—and had been elected coroner a year earlier after working as an autopsy specialist for the coroner's office in San Francisco. In appearance he resembled a young Abraham Lincoln with a narrow face, full beard, sharp eyes, and a sweep of dark hair.

Jindrich said, "Your understanding of medical terminology and medical situations was much higher than anybody else's. You can learn fairly quickly to be a good death investigator if you have a natural tendency to ask questions. I can teach you what you need to know. It takes years and years to learn medicine, however, and I don't have time to teach you that because in two weeks you're going to need to hit the street."

Clearly, all of the time that Holmes had spent standing next to doctors during autopsies and asking questions had paid off. When he succeeded Jindrich as coroner, Holmes emphasized the same qualities in hiring investigators as Jindrich had—that is, familiarity and comfort with death, extensive knowledge of medicine, an innate inquisitiveness and willingness to ask questions, plus compassion for grieving families.

This last is as important for investigative reasons as it is a requisite of human kindness. Investigators who relate poorly to families can't

always obtain the information needed to make an accurate determination regarding someone's death. When they ask a question, they often get yes-or-no answers because most individuals are cautious. If an investigator can convince people that he or she is on their side, however, family members and friends answer at greater length, sometimes providing important details with little or no prompting.

This was the part of the job that Holmes found particularly rewarding, and some of the people he came to know after notifying them of a death continue to send him emails periodically and greeting cards during the holidays. Either they want him to know that they are well, or they just want to stay in touch.

At the time Holmes was hired, however, the day when he would be responsible for hiring other investigators was far off in the future. He was thirty-two years old, fresh-faced, with keen eyes and a receding hairline that he compensated for by growing long sideburns, and there was much that he needed to learn first. He was about to enter a different world than the one he knew.

CHAPTER 02

BAPTISM BY FIRE

During his first two weeks, Holmes shadowed the assistant coroner, Keith Craig. Craig was the person responsible for training and managing the three investigators. His widow's peak of steel-gray hair was slicked back, his mustache was groomed, and he wore aviator-style glasses. For the most part humor was wasted on him, and he was happiest when there was little to do. Five years earlier he had retired from the California Highway Patrol, collecting a good pension, but he wasn't ready to retire altogether yet.

"He was a holdover from the previous coroner," Holmes says, "because Dr. Jindrich thought he needed to keep someone who was familiar with administrative details."

The two death investigators were holdovers, too, and Jindrich had no hesitation when it came to retaining them. Both men were experienced, having started four years before Holmes, competent, and dedicated. Like Holmes they were former morticians and embalmers.

Bill Thomas was twenty-seven, single, five foot nine, and originally from the Midwest. He had a full head of dark hair, a handsome face, and a captivating personality.

"In addition to being funny and engaging," Holmes says, "Bill told the most outrageous stories without ever cracking a smile. His charisma and humor made him a hit with everyone, especially women.

Most of the nurses in most of the emergency rooms in Marin dated Bill at some point, and many of them, I think, would have jumped at the chance to marry him if he had proposed. He was somebody who everyone gravitated to."

Don Cornish was the opposite. Tall and somewhat portly, with just a fringe of hair, he was forty years old and reserved. He also was devout in his Christian faith, although he never preached it. For many years, Holmes didn't know he had any faith at all. Cornish was happily married and had four daughters, none of whom he ever referred to—at least in Holmes's presence—by name. Instead, he called them Daughter #1, #2, #3, and #4. He and his family owned twenty acres of land in Calistoga where they raised livestock and harvested fruit trees. Calistoga is in Napa County, more than an hour's drive north of Marin County. All during his tenure as a death investigator, which lasted twenty-seven years, Cornish maintained a small apartment close to work in order to avoid commuting.

Bill Thomas and Don Cornish were the ones who ended up primarily training Holmes, but it was Craig whom Holmes followed his first two weeks. The first week, Craig handled each case while Holmes observed. The second week, Holmes handled cases with Craig looking over his shoulder. Starting his third day, Holmes wrote the case report even though Craig did the work. Afterward, Craig reviewed it.

Holmes's first report concerned a suicide from the Golden Gate Bridge. A California Highway Patrol officer called the coroner's office after the body of a fifty-five-year-old woman was found on Lime Point, a pinprick of land below the north tower of the bridge. Craig and Holmes responded, and Holmes noted their findings with terse objectivity, as instructed.

> Arrived at Lime Point at 1330 [1:30 P.M.]. Deceased was lying face down among the rocks on shoreline on east side of Golden Gate Bridge north of north tower. Clothing consisted of white bra, yellow blouse, and maroon with white polka-dotted slacks and vest. An ob-

vious fracture of the right leg was apparent at the scene. Officer Lee of the CHP gave Assistant Coroner Craig a pair of tan sandals and two pairs of glasses that he stated were found on the bridge above the deceased. An apparently abandoned vehicle was found at Vista Point by Officer Lee, registered to the husband of deceased. Identification was made through this registration. Marin County Sheriff's Office checked the address, found no one at home, and in conversation with neighbors was given the husband's telephone number at work. Telephone notification made after physical description given by husband and identification of old scars. Husband stated that his wife had been ill for about five weeks with a cold-like illness. He had made an appointment for her tomorrow to see her physician. Autopsy pending.

Craig read the report and had one comment. "You forgot to mention that no note was found."

The death of a twenty-nine-year-old woman ended up involving Craig and all three investigators in the coroner's office, mainly because a number of people needed to be interviewed and none of them was particularly cooperative. The woman, a nurse, died at the home of a psychologist in Bolinas following what was described by participants as an encounter group session but more likely was a drug party.

The night before she died, she and a dozen other people were at the house. According to the psychologist, stated through his attorney, the decedent "acted out," was angry, and yelled frequently. The next morning, someone noticed that she wasn't moving. A local physician was called to the residence, and he pronounced her dead.

Everyone who was present maintained that the get-together was therapeutic in nature and participants paid several hundred dollars to attend. This was contradicted, however, by physical evidence Holmes and other investigators found that a smorgasbord of narcotics had been consumed.

It appeared likely that the woman died from an overdose of a psychiatric, hallucinogenic drug known as MDA. She had fifty-milligram capsules in her possession, and a substantial quantity was found in her system. The coroner's office urged the district attorney to file manslaughter charges against the psychologist, but the DA decided that there wasn't enough evidence. The manner would remain undetermined.

A week later, Craig and Holmes were called to the scene of a warehouse fire in Novato. Two youths—Alan Pariani, age seventeen, and Robert Lomanson, eighteen—were working at the back of the warehouse when a drum of Scotchgard exploded in the front. The wall of flames prevented their exit, so they tried to escape through metal doors in the rear. These doors were padlocked from the outside, however. When Craig and Holmes arrived, they found a heartbreaking scene. The boys' dead bodies were near the rear doors, victims of burns and smoke inhalation. It turned out that a month earlier the warehouse had been cited by fire marshals for unsafe conditions, including the padlocked doors; however, no corrective action had been taken yet.

FIRST HOMICIDE

After two weeks of training, Holmes began his first shift alone. It was a Wednesday night, supposedly the quietest night of the week. At 12:28 A.M., he was notified by the county's Communications Center that the body of a young woman had been found in a Novato trailer park, the victim of an apparent homicide.

The Communications Center handled most of the emergency calls in the county. Dispatchers relayed information to the coroner's office, as well as to local fire departments, paramedics, the Public Works Department, animal control, and police in all but four Marin cities (those four cities had their own police dispatch centers).

Despite the late hour, there were half a dozen police cars parked in the area, motors off but blue lights flashing, when Holmes arrived. He could see cops in uniforms and shiny badges milling around, talking in small groups and waiting for him. All were at least four trailers from the actual site, a mobile home with a detached metal storage shed in the rear. As soon as Holmes exited his car, he understood why they were keeping their distance. It was an unusually hot night, and the malodorous smell of decomposing flesh was one that Holmes knew well.

Decomposition begins as soon as someone dies. Internal chemicals and bacteria break down a body's tissues and initiate the decaying process. In the first stage, flies and ants arrive. After that the body becomes bloated as other insects—maggots and beetles—feed on tissues under the skin and lay larvae. The beginning of active decay is marked by the body deflating as larvae hatch, pierce the skin, and release the body's gases, which are the source of the putrid odor. Once most of the flesh has been removed, the odor dissipates and many of the insects that were feeding on the body leave. In the last phase of decomposition, other scavengers—centipedes, millipedes, snails, and cockroaches—consume what is left until only bones remain.

Dealing with the smell is one of the biggest challenges for coroners. "It hits you," Dr. Melinek says in her book, as "an assault, not a scent. You flinch, heave back in revulsion. It invades your throat, assails your taste buds, even stings your eyes."

Says Holmes, "The odor stays with you for days no matter how many times you shower. When you burp, you smell it. If you fart, you smell it. Sometimes I had to throw away the sports coat and slacks I wore to a death scene. Other times I took them to be professionally cleaned, and the woman at the counter made a face and said, 'Ew! What's that smell?' There's no escaping it."

As a onetime mortician, Holmes was familiar with decomposition. What he learned after he started working in the coroner's office was that decomposition is an important element of forensic science because it helps coroners estimate the time of death. The kinds of insects found in a body, the sequence in which they appear, and where they are in the life cycle offer clues that narrow the window between the time that a person died and when his or her body was discovered.

The surrounding temperature and humidity influence how fast a body decomposes. Warm temperatures and high humidity accelerate the process while cooler temperatures and lower humidity slow it down. This is why coroner's investigators note the ambient temperature at a death scene, so that they can gauge how long decomposition has been taking place.

Near the mobile home Holmes was met by two other officers and a civilian named Orrell. All of them were covering their noses and mouths with handkerchiefs to try to combat the smell. Orrell told Holmes what he had already told the officers, namely that he was a teacher at San Quentin Prison, and the mobile home was owned by a paroled felon he knew named James McQueary.

McQueary told Orrell earlier that day that he had picked up a female hitchhiker and brought her to his mobile home before he went off to work. When he returned, she was dead. Her neck had been slashed, and she was clothed only in panties. McQueary said he didn't know who killed her, but because people would think he did, he called Orrell, whom he thought he could confide in. Orrell told him that he was obligated to notify the police, and McQueary asked him to wait twenty-four hours until McQueary could, in his words, "square it with his wife." Orrell said he couldn't do that, that he needed to call the police as soon as he got off the phone with McQueary.

Behind McQueary's residence was the shed, and the odor emanated from there. The officers told Holmes that the shed had been padlocked, and they had to use bolt cutters to gain access. The floor was covered with heavy cardboard, and a mattress box spring was standing on edge to one side. Outside the shed, near a chain-link fence, was a freshly dug hole five feet long, two feet wide, and two feet deep—apparently intended as a grave.

The decedent was in the rear of the shed, wrapped in two blankets and small sections of shag carpet. On top of her battered and slashed body were the clothes she had been wearing when she disappeared—a dark jacket, floral-print dress, and high-heeled shoes—plus a tan purse.

Inside the purse was identification. The clothes and identification matched the information in a missing-persons report that had been filed a week earlier for nineteen-year-old Terry Ann Listman. Holmes confirmed her identity through a subsequent comparison of Terry's dental records.

The air inside the shed was like a furnace, even at midnight, and the smell of decomposition was overwhelming. As Holmes peeled back the carpet and blankets, the temperature got even hotter because Terry's body was generating heat. The odor also intensified, almost forcing Holmes out of the shed because it was so pungent.

After noting the condition of the body, plus the circumstances in which it was found, Holmes and one of the police officers drove to Terry's house. It was Holmes's first death notification on his own, and he tried to be factual without sounding officious. He told Terry's parents that their daughter had been found, that she was the apparent victim of a murder, and that her body had been taken to a funeral home for autopsy. He spared them the details, only telling them that she wasn't recognizable and they shouldn't try to view her remains.

"Instead, remember her the way she was when you last saw her," he said.

Terry's mother had driven her to a bus stop in Novato at 7:30 A.M. the day she disappeared, never knowing that it would be the last time she would see her daughter. Terry was taking public transit to a job she started two weeks earlier as a clerk in a San Rafael office, but she never made it. At 9 A.M. she called her employer "in a shaky voice," he said, and said she was delayed by personal problems. In all likelihood, she already had been abducted and was forced to make the call.

Later, her parents pushed to see the photos that police officers and Holmes had taken at the scene. This isn't unusual. Until they see the photos, family members often hold on to the slim hope that the deceased is someone else and their loved one is still alive. The photos usually aren't released to families, however, mainly because they tend to be graphic and unsparing in their depiction of what happened.

Legally, families can't be prevented from seeing them, but in this instance the coroner's office refused.

"The photos looked nothing like Terry because of the brutality of her murder and because her body was badly decomposed," Holmes says. "It would have been awful for her parents to have that final memory of her."

Terry's parents could have taken the coroner's office to court to access the photos, but they didn't have the fight in them to do that. As a result, the photos stayed hidden.

"So what happened to McQueary?" I asked.

Holmes didn't remember, but he retrieved a large black binder of newspaper clippings that the coroner's office maintained in his early years. Every day the secretary pored through articles and notices in the *Independent Journal*—Marin County's primary newspaper—and clipped any news story or obituary that pertained to a case that the coroner's office handled. The clippings were dated with a black pen and Scotch-taped onto twenty-by-twenty-four-inch sheets of paper in more or less chronological order. They ended in 1981 because people lost interest in them, and when Holmes retired thirty years later, he heard that the new coroner was going to throw the binder away.

"I'll take it if no one else wants it," Holmes said.

The articles had yellowed with age but proved to be an important resource in compiling this book because they added details that weren't in the coroner's files or available pre-Internet. Chief among them was what happened to the killer in homicide cases. Typically, these cases take several years to play out, by which time the coroner's office has moved on to other cases.

Now Holmes leafed through pages until he found several articles with follow-ups to Terry Listman's death. It turned out that McQueary had been released from San Quentin the previous year after serving four years for kidnapping, assault, and attempted rape. On parole, and required to have a job, he was employed as a barber in a convalescent hospital. People there knew him as a smooth talker, and he was able to convince his wife that he was innocent. The two of them fled to Washington State, where he was arrested a year later and convicted of Terry's murder.

In the coming months and years, Holmes would be called to the scene of many grisly deaths. None would match this first one, though.

"More police officers were moved that night by the condition of Terry's body than I ever witnessed again," he says. "Even longtime cops were visibly affected."

The experience would stay with Holmes forever.

A BUSY FIRST MONTH

Two days after Terry Listman's death, Holmes was investigating another murder. This time a thirty-nine-year-old real estate agent named Donald Moore was found dead in a vacant one-story house in Mill Valley. Holmes learned that Moore had had an appointment to show the house the previous evening to a man who said that he wanted to see vacant homes only. The following morning, when Moore didn't return to his own home, his wife called the police and said that her husband was missing.

The same day, another realtor went to the house to show it to a client. He discovered that the lockbox had been broken and the front door key was missing. When he looked through the window, he saw Moore lying lifeless on the dining room floor.

It was clearly a homicide. Moore's throat had been cut and some of his blood had splattered fifteen feet. Holmes measured the distance, as he had been instructed to do, and took photos. Moore didn't have a wallet on him, but he did have business cards. A woman from his office came to the morgue and identified his body so that Moore's wife wouldn't have to do it. Holmes was left with telling Mrs. Moore that her husband had been murdered. After she recovered from the shock, she told Holmes that she had a six-year-old son from a previous marriage that had been a disaster, and married Moore just recently.

It didn't take long for police to solve the case. Mrs. Moore's first husband, a forty-one-year-old contractor named Darrell Gardner, was spotted the next day, "grinning from ear to ear," according to a witness. It turned out he paid four thousand dollars to two men to kill his ex-wife's new spouse. All three men were convicted and sent to prison.

Moore's death was followed by the death of a twenty-five-year-old secretary. She died from carbon monoxide poisoning and thermal burns resulting from a fire in her split-level, wood-frame home in Inverness, where she and her husband lived.

The husband told Holmes that at 1 A.M. his wife woke him and yelled, "Get out of the house, it's burning!" She even pushed him out of the building. As he exited, he turned to grab her, but she had gone back inside. The last he saw of her, she was outlined in a sheet of flames.

The Marin County Fire Department responded, and firefighters called the coroner's office after finding the woman's remains on top of a bed and beneath fallen roof beams. The fire was still burning in sections of the building when Holmes arrived, wearing a helmet, turnout, heavy coat, and gloves. The woman's body was completely charred, her abdominal organs were exposed, and both of her legs and one arm were missing. Holmes lifted what was left of her out of hot cinders so that she could be delivered to a funeral home for autopsy. The results, when they came back, were negative; no drugs or alcohol were found in her system. The woman's husband told Holmes that she must have gone back inside to retrieve something, although he didn't know what it was.

Holmes investigated two other homicides his first month, making a total of four—more than the whole office handled in a typical month. In addition, he investigated five suicides, four accidental deaths, two undetermined deaths, and several natural deaths. It was just the luck of the draw as to which investigator was on duty at the time the call came in. When Dr. Jindrich told Holmes that he would need to hit the ground running, it was truer than Holmes knew.

CHAPTER 03

THE BARBECUE MURDERS

Ken Holmes had been on the job only two months when the coroner's office was called in to investigate a case in Terra Linda that received national attention as it unfolded and was compared to Truman Capote's *In Cold Blood* and Vincent Bugliosi's *Helter Skelter*. The *Washington Post* called it a "close-up of a deadly family explosion," while the *Philadelphia Inquirer* said it was a "grim tale of love, hate, sex, drugs, and murder." The *Los Angeles Times* described it as a "round robin of drugs, shoplifting, [and] sexual kinkiness that transcended mere promiscuity, pop mysticism, demonology, and total rebellion." Holmes just calls it "the Olive case."

Terra Linda is a sleepy bedroom community in Marin County that is annexed to San Rafael. My parents moved there when I was four, and stayed there long past the time when I and my younger siblings attended Terra Linda High School. Violent crimes were virtually nonexistent, and when two sets of human bones were found in a barbecue pit in a park, it set off a wave of local interest that culminated in a courtroom trial that was spellbinding.

In *Bad Blood: A Family Murder in Marin County*, author Richard Levine recounts the initial meeting between Charles "Chuck" Riley and Marlene Olive. It was in front of Terra Linda High School, six years after I graduated. Marlene was sitting cross-legged on the ground, "her downcast face hidden from onlookers by the curtain of her long dark hair." She was sixteen years old and stifling sobs, not because she had been hurt but because she was on her first acid trip and it wasn't a good one.

Riley, age nineteen, got the crowd to back off, then knelt beside her. He offered her a marijuana joint to "level her out," but she refused it, as well as his overtures to learn her name or have a conversation. Several minutes later a female friend came and led her inside the school to a restroom.

Marlene and Riley would never forget the day, but for different reasons. Riley had never had a girlfriend, and felt that he had met the love of his life. Overweight, sexually naïve, and lacking confidence, he was struck by Marlene's apparent innocence and hypnotized by her penetrating eyes. She, in turn, believed that after dropping LSD she had undergone a personality change. She started hanging out with a different crowd and began cultivating a wild streak that resulted in frequent fights with her parents, especially her mother.

Up to that time, Marlene and Riley had led considerably different lives. Neither smart nor athletic, Riley gained a measure of popularity by selling drugs to fellow students. After he graduated, he continued to be their supplier. That was what he was doing at the high school that day, dealing marijuana. Marlene was adopted as an infant by James and Naomi Olive, and she felt perpetually abandoned, first by her birth mother, then by her adoptive parents—her father who always seemed busy with work and her mother who was withdrawn and alcoholic. The family had moved to Ecuador when Marlene was young because of a business opportunity for James, and Marlene—who learned Spanish and English simultaneously—spent a lot of time on her own. She idolized her father, who was tolerant and loving, but resented her mother, whose emotional and psychological problems led to frequent shouting matches between the two. As Marlene grew into adolescence, and especially after the family moved to Marin County, the hostility she felt for her mother escalated. Her mother was too restrictive, too overbearing, and too helpless as far as Marlene was concerned. The world—and certainly Marlene herself—would be better off without her.

At the beginning of his relationship with her, Riley fawned over Marlene while she paid him scant attention. After a while, though, his puppy-dog devotion began to have an effect and she realized that he would do anything for her. Around this time she developed a strong affinity for the occult, believing that she had mystical powers and was capable of controlling people with her eyes. She also read and believed in *The Satanic Bible*.

The Satanic Bible instructs witches in training to manipulate people by attracting and holding their attention. In Chuck Riley, Marlene Olive found a willing subject for her spells.

The Olives welcomed Riley into their home early on, believing that he was a better influence on their daughter than her other friends. After all, he was working—first selling vacuum cleaners, then water beds. Moreover, he was polite, respectful, and dressed conservatively, buttoning his shirts all the way to the neck until Marlene chided him about it. Meanwhile, Marlene's mother thought that her daughter dressed "like a whore" in low-cut tops, an opinion that led Marlene to wear even more provocative clothing to annoy her.

Riley's parents saw the hold that Marlene had on their son and in one way were pleased; Riley started exercising more, shedding pounds and improving his physique. In another way, though, they were alarmed. He submitted to her demands so willingly that it was as if he no longer was able to make decisions on his own.

On numerous occasions, Marlene told her friends that she wished her mother was dead. Her friends shrugged it off; after all, many adolescents don't get along with their parents. Even when Marlene asked if anyone knew someone who would kill for money, her friends didn't take it seriously. By this time she and Riley were lovers— monogamously on his part, less so on hers—and she felt that she couldn't tolerate her mother any longer. Moreover, when she saw some of her father's papers accidentally, she realized that she was the sole beneficiary of her parents' life insurance policy and stood to inherit between $30,000 and $50,000 if her parents died. She told Riley that it would be enough for the two of them to start a new life in South America.

Riley was mesmerized by the promise of spending the rest of his life with her. Already she had convinced him to shoplift clothes, jewelry, purses, and perfume from local department stores, going so far as to tell him in advance which items she wanted.

Realizing that Riley wasn't nearly the positive influence they had thought, James and Naomi Olive forbade their daughter from seeing him. Riley was horrified by the thought that the two of them might be separated. When Marlene told him to get a gun in order to kill her mother, he did.

What happened next became the subject of newspaper headlines around the country. While James and Marlene were out, Riley went to the Olives' one-story, ranch-style house in Terra Linda. Marlene had made sure that the front door was unlocked, and Riley stepped inside. Mrs. Olive was in a bedroom napping, and Riley had the gun in a paper bag. He didn't shoot her, though. Instead, Naomi Olive was bludgeoned with a claw hammer. The hammer became lodged in her head, and Riley was about to pull it out when he heard a car in the driveway. The sudden return of Marlene and her father surprised him, and Riley hid behind a large dresser. When James Olive walked in, he saw the open door and his wife lying on the bed with blood all around her and the hammer buried in her skull. Then he saw Riley.

James Olive grabbed a knife that was on a nightstand by the bed and came toward Riley, who fired four shots through the paper bag. The bullets exploded in James Olive's body and he went down in a heap, mortally wounded.

In the moment, both teens were numb to what had just happened. In his testimony, Riley said that afterward he walked into the living room and stared at the fireplace for a long time. Then Marlene brought him a beer, and shortly thereafter she began undressing him and they had sex. After that they went out to dinner with several friends, following it with a drive-in movie by themselves. During the movie they talked about burning the bodies and decided that the large concrete cistern at China Camp, which served as a fire pit, was the best place to do it.

China Camp State Park is a historic site on the shore of San Pablo Bay in San Rafael. A onetime Chinese-American shrimp-fishing village, it was a popular hangout for teens, and Marlene and Riley had been there on occasion, getting drunk and doing drugs with friends. They struggled to put the bodies of Marlene's parents into plastic garbage bags and load them in the family's station wagon. To get rid of some of the evidence and also cover the bodies in case anyone happened to look in, they threw the mattress from Naomi Olive's bed over the remains of her and her husband.

When they arrived at China Camp, it was dark and deserted. They dumped the bodies of James Olive, fifty-nine, and Naomi Olive, fifty-two, out of the bags and into the cistern after discarding the mattress in the surrounding woods. At one time the cistern had stored rainwater for a now abandoned dairy farm. Since then it had been filled with crushed rock except for the top two feet. After they splashed kerosene on the Olives, they set them on fire. Too scared to stay and watch for fear of being caught, they raced out of the park and returned to the Olives' house. Early the next morning, Marlene made Riley drive back alone to the cistern to see whether both bodies had burned completely. A portion of James Olive's body hadn't, and Riley doused it with more kerosene and lit it again.

The following week, Marlene and Riley acted as if nothing had happened. They continued to live in the Olives' house and socialize with friends, one of whom came to the house and helped Marlene clean up the mess. To anyone who called and asked to speak with Mr. or Mrs. Olive, Marlene made up stories about her parents being away and not knowing when they would return. As far as she was concerned, the worst was over. Her parents were now just bones and ashes, and she and Riley were free. It wouldn't be long, she thought, before she received her inheritance.

A GOLD CROWN

Shortly after Riley had burned the final remains of James Olive, a San Rafael firefighter who was in the area noticed a plume of smoke coming from China Camp. When he went to investigate, he saw charred bones in the cistern and assumed that local hunters had been roasting a deer in the pit. Upon closer examination, though, he saw a piece of jawbone with a tooth that had a gold crown. That's when the coroner's office entered the picture.

Keith Craig responded, along with Rodger Heglar, a physical anthropologist who was on contract with the coroner's office. They began sifting through the cistern, finding more human bones and pieces of burned clothing and charred flesh. Every item that was recovered was taken back to the office to be studied in order to learn who had died.

The following day, Dr. Heglar examined the bones and fragments. There were portions of the cranial vault and face, vertebrae, ribs, scapula (shoulder bone), ulna (elbow bone), talus (ankle bone), and assorted long bones (that is, bones such as the femur and tibia—the thigh bone and shinbone—that are longer than they are wide). Heglar determined that the fragments of cranial and long bones differed somewhat in size, suggesting that the bones were from two people, with one person being larger than the other. He noted that there weren't parallel examples of the same bone to prove that the remains comprised two people, but it seemed likely. Moreover, the size of the bones from the lower jaw and shoulder were consistent with those of a female age forty-five to fifty-five, he said.

Meanwhile, James Olive's business partner, a man named Phillip Royce, became increasingly concerned when Olive didn't show up for work or call. Royce phoned the Olive residence multiple times, always talking to Marlene. She gave him cryptic answers regarding the whereabouts of her father, and after a week Royce contacted the police.

The first officer who went to the house questioned Marlene at length. Even though she provided rambling and contradictory stories about her parents, as well as a fabricated tale about visiting a friend in the Lake Tahoe area and coming home to find her parents gone with no note or explanation, the officer accepted what she told him. Her ability to tell detailed lies with seeming innocence and absolute conviction was persuasive.

Then Bart Stinson, a forty-nine-year-old police investigator, took charge of the case. Holmes worked with him numerous times over the next decade, before Stinson retired, and was in awe.

"Bart was the best interrogator I ever saw," Holmes says, "mainly because he never seemed to interrogate anyone."

Soft around the middle, balding on top, with oversized glasses, Stinson cut a fatherly figure. He would sit down next to someone as if he had all the time in the world and just have a conversation. By the end of it, though, the person had revealed far more than he or she ever intended.

Marlene told Stinson different stories of where she'd been and how long she'd been gone. Each story seemed plausible until Stinson asked a telltale question that caused it to fall apart. That produced a new story, which caused Stinson to press harder. She was good at invention, but he wasn't deceived.

Eventually she told him the truth—or something close to it. She said that Chuck Riley killed her parents and the two of them burned the bodies in the cistern at China Camp.

Police arrested Riley at the water bed company where he worked and read him his rights. Bart Stinson knew from experience that people who are guilty usually waive their right to remain silent because they are eager to learn how much the police already know. Riley was no exception. Without the benefit of legal counsel, he answered Stinson's questions until he had backed himself into a corner.

"I did it! I did it!" he said finally, burying his face in his hands. "I didn't want to do it. Marlene made me do it. She kept asking me and asking me, begging me and begging me for months. Telling me to do it or she wouldn't love me anymore."

Now that the coroner's office had a good idea whom the charred remains in the cistern at China Camp belonged to, the three investigators—Bill Thomas, Don Cornish, and Holmes—began tracking down dental records and X-rays for James and Naomi Olive. They found a dentist in San Rafael who was able to provide records and X-rays for Mr. Olive, and a dentist in Coral Gables, Florida, who provided records and X-rays for Mrs. Olive. This information was given to a dentist in Mill Valley, who compared it with the gold crowns and fragments of jawbones found at the site. He concluded that there was "incontrovertible" proof that the remains were those of Naomi Olive. The crowns and bone fragments matched her dental structure exactly. Fewer remains were found of James Olive, none of which provided certain identification, although "the similarities were reasonably conclusive," the dentist said.

RILEY'S TRIAL

Because she was a minor, Marlene Olive was tried as a juvenile for her role in the murders. After she was convicted, she was sentenced to the California Youth Authority, where she could be released anytime that officials there felt she was rehabilitated. Release was automatic on her twenty-first birthday unless she was considered unreformed, in which case she could be held to age twenty-three. As a juvenile, she wasn't convicted of aiding and abetting in two homicides because California's Welfare and Institutions Code stipulated that the crimes of incarcerated minors weren't specified. Chuck Riley's fate was much different. His parents were able to scrape together enough money to hire William "Bill" Weissich as his defense attorney. Weissich was highly respected and had successfully argued several capital punishment cases. The challenge he faced was that Riley already had confessed to both murders, which made him eligible for the death penalty if convicted. Weissich was convinced that his client wasn't in his right mind at the time of the murders, though, that he was under Marlene's spell. In addition, Riley said he was "spaced out" the entire day, having taken LSD before the murders and smoking marijuana, snorting cocaine, and drinking beer afterward.

To prove how easily Riley could be manipulated, Weissich hired three hypnotists. Each one put Riley under and testified that Riley was among the most hypnotizable people he had ever encountered. Under hypnosis, Riley said he didn't kill Naomi Olive—Marlene did. Riley said that he found the hammer embedded in Mrs. Olive's skull and was going to take it out when he was surprised by James Olive, whom he shot in self-defense.

The case went to a grand jury first to determine whether there was sufficient evidence to try Chuck Riley. In her grand jury testimony, Deanna Krieger, seventeen, the friend who helped Marlene and Riley clean up after the Olives were killed, said that Riley told her he bludgeoned Naomi and shot James, then he and Marlene cremated the bodies in the cistern at China Camp.

During the trial, however, Krieger told a different story. She said that Marlene told her she killed her mother. "She just told me that when she hit her mom over the head with a hammer," Krieger said, "blood and stuff went all over the place."

Krieger also testified that Marlene considered herself a "high priestess" who could command Riley to do anything she wanted. Krieger told jurors about the shoplifting episodes, about Riley supplying Marlene with cocaine and other drugs to take on dates with other men, about Marlene instructing Riley to take nude photos of her that she planned to submit to various men's magazines, and about Marlene carrying a tarot card that she said symbolized her dominance over Riley.

Tapes of Riley's two confessions were played for jurors, which Bill Weissich, his attorney, tried to counterbalance with testimony from Riley's parents in which they said their son wasn't rational after his arrest. He was sobbing heavily, apologizing and telling them, "She made me do it."

During the trial, the Marin County Superior Court room was packed. People listened with rapt attention as scenes of debauchery, deceit, and alienation were recounted. When Riley took the stand, interest ratcheted even higher and his testimony was riveting.

"I saw Mrs. Olive with a hammer protruding from her forehead. . . . It had a paralyzing effect. I was hurt and frightened. I started to freak out . . . started to leave the house, but I couldn't leave until I removed that hammer. . . . It took all my strength. I got blood all over my hands. The blood felt like it was burning my hands. . . . I slung it off."

Earlier that day, Riley said, Marlene had asked him how hard you have to hit someone in order to kill the person. Afterward, he told her that he would take the blame for both murders.

Other youths testified at Riley's trial. Two boys said that they had had sexual relations with Marlene, and she had asked each of them if he would kill her mother or find someone who would. Another teenage boy said he had talked with Marlene while both of them were in Marin Juvenile Hall, and "she said she killed her mom with some kind of mallet."

In his closing argument, Assistant District Attorney Joshua Thomas rebutted the version of events that Riley stated initially under hypnosis and then in his courtroom testimony. Although a Stanford psychologist had testified that highly hypnotizable people are "prone to suspend their own judgments and take other people's suggestions," adding that "[t]his desire to please could influence a confession," the prosecution presented its own expert witness to refute it. He said that people under hypnosis usually speak in the present tense, while

Riley often spoke in the past tense. This discrepancy was evidence, the prosecution said, that Riley was lying.

As for the defense's contention that Riley was under the influence of drugs at the time he committed murder, the prosecution's position was that this wasn't unusual. Riley was a heavy drug user, and his state of mind was no different on the day that the Olives were killed than on any other day. In regards to the theory put forth by the defense that Riley was bewitched by Marlene, it was "almost ridiculous," according to the district attorney. Thomas also argued that Riley's use of a stolen gun to kill James Olive was evidence of premeditation since stolen weapons can't be traced.

The jury deliberated for four days and ultimately sided with the prosecution. Riley "personally committed" both first-degree murders, jurors said.

If Marlene Olive had confessed to killing her mother, her sentence wouldn't have changed. She would have been remanded to the California Youth Authority and released within six years. Chuck Riley's sentence would have been different, however. He would have been imprisoned fifteen years to life with the possibility of parole after seven years. Instead, because he was convicted of killing two people rather than one, he received the death penalty. When capital punishment was ruled unconstitutional in California in 1978, his sentence became life in prison without parole.

AFTERMATH

In 1978, three months before she was scheduled to be paroled, Marlene escaped from a California Youth Authority facility in Southern California. Ten months later she was picked up by police in New York City because she "looked young" and was evasive when they asked her questions. She was hooking, didn't have proper ID, and wouldn't tell officers her name, how old she was, or where she came from. At the police station she gave the phone number of her public guardian in Marin County. The guardian told officers that Marlene had escaped from the CYA facility in Ventura and there was a no-bail warrant out for her arrest.

Marlene was returned to California but incarcerated only briefly. Upon release, she was arrested for being part of a large forgery and counterfeiting ring in Southern California. She was convicted as an adult and sentenced to five years in prison. That was followed by other prison terms for check forgery, making false statements to authorities, and possession of drugs. Her current whereabouts are unknown.

In contrast, Chuck Riley has spent the last forty years behind bars. He has applied for parole more than a dozen times, and been denied each time.

"I can attest from firsthand experience that many death row inmates are truly evil," Holmes says. "However, I don't believe Chuck is one of them. He was this young, baby-faced cherub of a kid, not particularly attractive, absolutely virginal, not only physically but mentally, and she sucked him in."

Holmes's opinion then as well as now is that justice was poorly served. "I understand the community witch hunt," he says, "but they let her skate and jammed this kid badly. It was so obvious. Why he's in there for life without the possibility of parole is beyond me. He should have done seven years, then been released. Okay, he killed somebody, but he truly wasn't in his right frame of mind."

Many of the newspapers that reported the case referred to it as "the barbecue murders." When Riley was first incarcerated, other inmates nicknamed him "Barbecue." Eventually it was shortened to just "Q." After capital punishment was abolished, he was one of the last death row inmates to be transferred from San Quentin to the California Men's Colony in San Luis Obispo. A year later he was moved back to San Quentin, though, and he has been there ever since.

In 1981, Levine drove Marlene from Los Angeles, where she was living, to San Luis Obispo, where Riley was incarcerated. He and Marlene hadn't seen each other in five years, and the meeting was awkward. During his time in prison, Riley had slimmed down, no longer a cherub, while Marlene's physical appearance had deteriorated due to drug use, jail terms, and time spent on the street.

At one point Riley asked Marlene what she was thinking. Her response, according to Levine, was "I was just thinking about what had gone down. We just lost our marbles."

It was as close as she came to expressing remorse.

Over the years, Holmes went to San Quentin Prison numerous times. Usually it was to investigate an inmate's death. Every once in a while he would see Riley in passing. When he did, he would stop and say, "Hey, Chuck. How are you doing?"

Riley didn't seem to know what to say other than, "Okay."

Only once did they have a conversation. It was no more than two minutes and consisted mainly of Holmes asking Riley how he spent his time. Riley said that he read a lot.

"Good," Holmes said. "Reading is good."

Reading not only gives inmates a purpose—the chance to further their limited educations—but tends to keep them out of trouble. In Riley's instance, however, whatever he learned through books was offset by a general cluelessness that hadn't changed much since youth.

"The last time I saw you, I was here, too," Riley said to Holmes one time, as if he could go anywhere and it were merely coincidental that they happened to meet again at San Quentin.

Holmes could only shrug and wonder if more years in prison would make any difference. Probably not.

Things didn't turn out well for Bill Weissich, Riley's attorney, either. Ten years after the trial, Holmes responded to a shooting in a San Rafael law office. When he arrived, he saw Weissich sitting at his desk with a bullet hole in the middle of his forehead and an empty .45-caliber casing on the floor nearby. A onetime prosecutor, Weissich had been killed by a seventy-two-year-old man named Malcolm Schlette, whom he had sent to prison for arson and attempted murder many years earlier. After he was released, Schlette sought revenge.

Weissich's secretary was an eyewitness to the shooting, and after Schlette fled she called the police and described Schlette's getaway vehicle, a blue van. A cop stopped it several blocks away and ordered Schlette to get out. Schlette did, but only after he swallowed cyanide. He collapsed in the street, unconscious, with foam dribbling out of his mouth.

Holmes responded to that death, too, but had to wait to examine Schlette's body until a bomb squad arrived. Schlette had taped a grenade to his throat and strapped what appeared to be dynamite to his waist (it turned out to be road flares).

Looking back on Weissich's murder Holmes says, "It never ceased to amaze me how some cases were rewoven with the same people appearing multiple times and, on occasion, in different ways. That certainly was the case with Bill."

CHAPTER 04

14K3, 10-49, 10-55

Shortly after the Olive murders, another investigator in the office, Bill Thomas, told Holmes that there was an investigators club. It was a select group that met in a special meeting place whose location was a secret.

"You have to earn your way into it," Thomas said. "Once you do, you'll receive a key to the clubhouse. Until then, though, neither Don nor I can even tell you where it is."

Holmes had never been an investigator before and didn't know that there were any perks to the job beyond his salary and county benefits. Dr. Jindrich hadn't mentioned any to him when Holmes was hired.

"What do I have to do?" Holmes asked.

"From time to time I'll give you a question," Thomas said, "and you'll need to give me a detailed, written response."

Holmes knew that he had a lot to learn, and he was eager to prove himself to his peers, Thomas and Don Cornish. "Okay," he said.

"The quality of your answers, the depth of thought behind them, will determine whether you get a clubhouse key or not," Thomas said. His voice was grave and forboding. "Don and I earned our keys, and if you don't earn yours, you won't be able to go there with us."

As a boy, Holmes had been active in Scouting and worked through the levels to Star Scout. Many of the life skills he had acquired, from surviving in the wilderness to tying knots, he learned in Scouts. Because of this experience, he appreciated the value of group membership.

"This will get you started," Thomas said. "Which came first, the chicken or the egg? Support your answer with appropriate documentation."

It never occurred to Holmes that Thomas was pulling his leg. Holmes didn't know Thomas well yet, and he sounded so serious that even though it was an age-old question, Holmes accepted it as the first step in securing a clubhouse key. He wrote out an answer, stating that the chicken came first, and gave it to Thomas. Thomas looked it over, grunted without offering an opinion or betraying the slightest emotion, then said that Holmes would receive another question soon.

Every few weeks for the next several months, Thomas gave Holmes a question, which Holmes responded to in writing. All the while Thomas talked about the fabled benefits of this select group who shared a secret meeting place. At Thanksgiving, Thomas presented Holmes with a key on a metal ring that had a tag reading "Investigators Clubhouse." He also gave him a specially made T-shirt that featured a large turkey with its tail feathers spread wide. Only then did Holmes realize that he was the turkey. There was no clubhouse and no group. Bill Thomas and Don Cornish had found an easy mark.

THE ACADEMY

Every successful coroner must have a good understanding of medicine and forensics, be compassionate in dealing with grieving family members, and be a skilled investigator. The first trait is acquired and takes years of study to learn. The second trait is largely innate; either you have a lot of compassion for people—including strangers—or you don't. The last trait is developed, and in California it starts at a police academy.

Coroners in the Golden State don't have to be physicians—and many aren't—but they do have to complete the same twenty-two-week course that police officers take to qualify for work in the field of law enforcement. This might seem like an odd requirement for coroners, but it is at the heart of how their job is viewed. Coroners—even ones whose office is independent from the sheriff's office—are seen as extensions of the police. Not only do their investigations often support police activities, but in emergencies they are expected to provide backup protection to officers. If there is a shoot-out, manhunt, or hostage situation in which the police are understaffed and an investigator from the coroner's office is present, he or she is counted on to assist. This means that all death investigators must be armed while on duty, and test annually at a gun range to maintain their proficiency.

The academy covers all aspects of police work—basic powers of arrest, major sections of the Penal Code, motor vehicle law, community policing, conflict management, investigative procedures, and first aid. It also includes physical training, firearms training, and a week of pursuit driving and safe driving. One of the skills that is taught is how to lift latent fingerprints off various kinds of surfaces.

Patent prints are fingerprints left in blood, grease, ink, and sometimes dirt, which clearly are visible to the human eye. Latent prints are deposits of human oils left on an object that aren't visible. An investigator brushes white, black, or bichromatic powder on the surface, then uses lifting tape to pull off a fingerprint. White powder is used on dark surfaces, dark powder is used on light-colored surfaces, and bichromatic powder, which is a combination of white and black powder, is used on either.

When Holmes began in 1975, investigators used a brush made from camel hair or squirrel hair. Later he transitioned to a fiberglass brush because it distributes the powder more evenly, which is critical. The two biggest mistakes that inexperienced people make when dusting something for fingerprints are using too much powder and brushing it on too thickly. A heavy stroke can wipe away latent print residue, so the key is to spread the powder gently with as few strokes as possible.

Holmes learned that smooth surfaces like glass, tile, porcelain, lacquered furniture, and shiny metal are the easiest to lift prints from. Paper, cardboard, drywall, leather, and most dashboards are harder. Organic surfaces—tree leaves, fruit peels, and feathers—are formidable. Most difficult are fabrics, human skin, and rough or textured surfaces such as checkered handgun grips.

Transparent adhesive tape is used to lift the print. It is unrolled a little at a time, and folded over slightly into a tab for handling so that the person doesn't get his or her own fingerprints on the tape. Then it's laid on the powder and rubbed to make sure that contact is complete and there are no bubbles underneath the tape. After the tape is firmly in place, it's pulled up gently and evenly, and pressed onto the blank side of an eight-inch-by-eight-inch fingerprint card. The other side of the card is preprinted with fill-in boxes for the date, time, case number, and related information, which the investigator completes.

Another important skill, especially for coroner's investigators, is how to manage people at a death scene. "You get a sergeant who is full of himself," Holmes says, "and a patrol deputy who has been on the street only six or seven months and has never seen a dead body, and there is a widow or widower and three crying kids, all in the same room at the same time, and you're in charge. The sergeant wants to be in charge, but can't be, and the deputy doesn't know what the hell to do but the sergeant is telling him what to do, and may be telling him the wrong things. The coroner's investigator needs to take charge and manage the situation."

When someone from the coroner's office arrives at a death scene, he or she is the senior authority, outranking everyone, including police chiefs. More than once in Holmes's career, a police chief didn't want to leave a scene that Holmes was working. One time it was the chief's first murder in his small town and he had a prurient interest. His captain took him aside.

"Come on, Chief," he said. "The reporters are here and they're listening to this, and there's no reason for you to be inside because you're not doing the investigation."

The chief refused, and Holmes decided to let him stay, only because it would look bad if he cuffed him. Later, though, Holmes had a word with the mayor, who reminded the chief that at a death scene the coroner has jurisdiction over the police, not the other way around.

Usually, coroner's investigators go to the academy first, before they start handling cases. It's not a prerequisite, but some of the skills that are taught have particular relevance to new investigators in a coroner's office. These include how to secure a scene, manage bystanders and reporters, collect evidence, interview witnesses, and write a report that summarizes the findings in a way that can be used in court if necessary.

The first course that was offered shortly after Holmes was hired was full, though. The next course was four months away, and Dr. Jindrich couldn't wait that long; Holmes needed to start investigating cases immediately.

As a lifelong hunter, Holmes was familiar with many kinds of handguns and shotguns. He also was a World War II buff and knew a lot about machine guns, bazookas, and the like. At the academy he learned about other types of weapons, from small derringers to rapid-fire assault rifles. What he didn't learn at the academy he learned on the job and in continuing education classes over the years. Of paramount importance was knowing how to unload a weapon so that it could be transported safely to the coroner's office. Beyond that, he had to be able to identify the caliber and type of weapon found at a death scene, as well as calculate the number of shots that had been fired based on the gun's bullet capacity and the number of empty casings in the chamber and on the ground.

From the start, Holmes made a point of learning about each new weapon he encountered. Later, when he became the assistant coroner, responsible for training others, he instructed his investigators on each weapon's characteristics, noting differences between a pump-action shotgun and an automatic shotgun, for instance, or between a break-open pistol and a semiautomatic one.

COMM CENTER

Each of the three investigators worked a twenty-four-hour shift. They were on duty one full day, then off the next two days. Shifts started at 8 A.M., when they were expected to be in the office. At 5 P.M. they went home and were on call until the shift change at 8 A.M. the following day.

Most death notifications came from the county's Communications Center. They were relayed by phone if the investigator was in the office or at home, and by radio if he was in the field.

If the call came by phone, the dispatcher said something like, "Hey, Ken. We just got a call from San Rafael PD. They responded to a house fire at 35 Canal Street and found a body in the back room. It's an elderly woman and they think it's the owner or the person who lived in the house. When you get there, contact Battalion Chief Smith." Or the notification might be, "There's a two-car accident on Highway 101 southbound near the Mill Valley exit. One person is dead at the scene and three others are being taken to Marin General with injuries. Talk to Officer Brown."

Investigators would get as much information as possible from the dispatcher over the phone because it was a private conversation. Nobody was listening in. If the call came by radio, though, the notification was brief and codes were used.

"14K3, 10-49 Canal Street, 10-55, 904." Or, "14K3, 10-49 to 101 south, 10-55, 11-80."

14 was the code for the coroner's office, K was the code for the investigator on duty, and 3 was Holmes's number. Bill Thomas was K1 and Don Cornish was K2, while Dr. Jindrich was 14A (for

administration) and Assistant Coroner Keith Craig was 14A2. 10-49 meant go to the following location. 10-55 was the code for a dead body, 904 the code for a fire, and 11-80 the code for a traffic accident with injuries. A confirmed suicide was 10-56 while an attempted suicide was 10-56A.

"That's all I would get on the radio if I was mobile," Holmes says. "Many people—mainly shut-ins and reporters—listen to police and fire calls all day long, and dispatchers don't want to light up the air. When I got to the scene, it could be almost anything if the call came over the radio."

Dispatchers knew how to reach him at any given moment. As soon as he started his shift, Holmes phoned the Communications Center and said, "10-88," meaning he was now on duty. When he got in his car, he radioed in and said, "10-8," meaning he was mobile. Every time he got out of the car, he used other codes—10-7 if he was stopping for a meal, which meant he was off the radio but could be reached on his pager, or 10-10 if he was home and on call, which meant he could be reached by phone.

"When you're on duty, it's like being umbilically tied to the center," he says. "Dispatchers always know where you are."

An electronic tote board at the center displayed up-to-the-second information for all key people in the county who were on duty—everyone in the sheriff's office, fire department, public works, animal control, coroner's office, and ambulance companies, public and private. All any dispatcher had to do was look at the board to see how to reach anyone. This also included how to reach individuals in the California Highway Patrol, FBI, state and national park services, and Coast Guard. The latter had its own dispatch system, but people in the Communications Center had radio access to the actual boats.

The 10 code—so named because most of the numbers start with 10—is common to most municipal police agencies. For a variety of reasons, San Francisco and the California Highway Patrol use different codes (9 code and 11 code, respectively). A dead body in Marin is 10-55, for instance, while in San Francisco it's 9-80. The FBI has a different numbering system, which is classified. Everything should be uniform, but it's not.

"It's up to dispatchers at Comm Center to translate," Holmes says, "and up to everyone who's connected to know what the codes mean. It was another thing I had to learn."

The Communications Center is the nerve center for all emergency services in Marin County. For most of Holmes's tenure, it was in the basement of the Civic Center. It was sheltered with reinforced concrete, hardwired, and without windows because no one wanted to risk someone throwing a bomb inside. Eventually the center moved to the second floor of a three-story building across the highway from the Civic Center. The new space is huge, open, and has windows that are unbreakable. Whereas five to seven dispatchers used to work in the center at any given time, today it's twice that number because of everything that is being managed there.

As one might expect, action inside the center is frenzied and intense, no matter the time of day. In all but two instances, dispatchers juggle multiple emergency calls simultaneously, coordinating people and equipment like air traffic controllers. The two exceptions are police pursuits and hostage situations. In these instances the dispatcher who answers the call when it comes in handles it exclusively and everyone else relieves him or her of other responsibilities. The Communications Center manages everything, including getting the hostage negotiator to the scene, because not every police department has one. The dispatcher tells the person next to him or her, "Get San Rafael's hostage negotiator on my line," and takes it from there. The same is true for police pursuits, although these tend to be short, usually lasting three to five minutes. The dispatcher talks to the lead car and the cars behind it, letting everyone know what's going on.

"We have a car coming in two miles ahead, east off of Sir Francis Drake Boulevard."

Communications Center dispatchers are 911 operators as well.

"Is he breathing? Get him off that soft surface, get him down on the floor, and start compressions. I'll help you count." If a caller doesn't know CPR, the dispatcher teaches the person on the phone, kids included. Dispatchers have to maintain their poise, be calm and reassuring, and also assert authority when necessary.

"Be quiet and listen to me. Stop asking questions; do your compressions."

Sometimes, if Holmes was in the office at night and it was quiet, he would go down to the basement and hang out in the center. It was a way for him to get to know the system and the people, and for them to get to know him. In addition, the action was riveting.

"Sometimes I'd be there an hour and a half," he says, "and just watch in awe. They handled so many things at once, and did it so well. Every single shift the people were balls to the wall."

SHARING A CAR

County government couldn't or wouldn't pay for each investigator to have his own car so the three investigators shared one. Most of the time it was a Rambler station wagon.

"Ugliest cars on the planet," Holmes says, "because the county always bought what was cheapest. It had amazing get-up-and-go, though."

The cars were traded in between 75,000 and 100,000 miles because county administrators decided that the cost of maintaining and repairing them after that wasn't worth it. The county would buy a fleet of cars, and the next time the investigators' car was due for service, it would be replaced.

"The only question we were asked," Holmes says, "was whether we wanted the blue one or the green one."

Early on the car had a big-whip antenna for the sheriff's radio system, but some police cars had the antenna wired inside the rear fender well, out of sight, and the investigators were able to get this, too. There was a siren inside the grille and an outside speaker that could be switched on if they were outside the car but nearby.

"The car didn't have Christmas tree lights on top or anything like that," Holmes says. "We just had a bulb with a red light that we would drop down from inside."

It also didn't have a decal with the county seal on it. Dr. Jindrich didn't want families to be forewarned by the sight of a county car pulling up in front of their home.

During the early 1980s, the investigators had a Chevy Chevette that happened to be dark red. Mechanics at the county garage nicknamed it the Blood Clot.

"One time I had to go to a wreck in the middle of the night in west Marin," Holmes says. "I've got this silly red bulb, and I'm trying to get people to move out of the way; wrecks invariably draw a crowd. They looked in the rearview mirror and saw this toy car behind them with a red light and a siren, and didn't move. So I got on the loudspeaker—it was one of the few times I ever used it—and told them to pull over or be arrested. They did, but made sure to give me dirty looks as I passed."

With one car between them, the investigators had to work out a system for handoffs. Around 7:30 A.M., the person whose shift was ending drove to the house of the next person on duty. That person got behind the wheel and drove the first person home. Along the way, the first person briefed the second person on everything that had happened in the last twenty-four hours. Then the second person drove to work in order to be in the office by 8 A.M. It was a somewhat cumbersome routine, but this way the car was always available and each investigator was apprised of recent developments.

The car itself had two big toolboxes with everything they might need—camera equipment, fingerprint kits, report booklets, collection bottles and bags (zip-lock plastic bags for liquids; sandwich-sized paper bags for biological specimens), tape measures, temperature gauges, digging tools, flashlight, blunt scissors to cut off clothing, body bags of various sizes, evidence seals, insect collection kits, and more. One of the most important items was a magnifying glass, referred to as "the clue finder."

Investigators carried both toolboxes whenever they approached a possible crime scene because they didn't want to be going back and forth, contaminating possible evidence. At the front door, they put on booties before going inside. If they had to go back out to the car, they took the booties off, went to the car, came back, and put the booties on again so that they weren't transferring anything. Just picking up a leaf or sand and bringing it inside a house could change things. It was a practice that developed over time. When Holmes started, they didn't have booties. Instead he was told, "Watch where you walk."

Holmes remembers an incident that makes him chuckle today. "The sheriff's office had a really good crime scene investigator named Ed. One time I walked into a double homicide in Kentfield, and Ed was filling me in on what happened. We were standing just inside the front door, and I said, 'So, where did this whole thing go down?' He said, 'Well, it started here at the door and went all the way down the hall. The first woman is in there and the second one is in there.'"

Two women, ages thirty-seven and forty, had been shot. Plastic bags of heroin were near their bodies, and drug paraphernalia was in the bathroom.

"It turned out they were pretty high up in the drug world," Holmes says, "and were killed in separate rooms. I happened to be looking down when Ed shuffled his feet, and I saw that he was standing on a nine-millimeter casing. I said, 'So, the shooting started around here?'"

Ed said, "Yeah, we think it was right here."

Holmes said, "Would that be the nine-millimeter casing you were just standing on?"

Ed looked down, saw the casing, and rolled his eyes. "Oh my God, I can't believe I just did that."

He went outside and walked around the house a couple of times, muttering to himself. "In that particular instance it didn't matter," Holmes says, "but it could have."

Each investigator had a foot locker in the car to hold his own fire gear—turnout, boots, gloves, coat, and helmet—because they were different sizes. They kept hiking boots and mountain gear in the locker, too, for times when they had to climb up a hillside or down an embankment to get to a dead body.

The expectation was that investigators would be on the scene within a half hour of receiving the call unless they were on another case already or the scene was a remote area of the county. It wasn't a state or county mandate; rather, it was something Dr. Jindrich required.

"It seemed like the right thing to do," Holmes says. "In San Francisco, cops wait two hours or more for the coroner to arrive. They're busier and have a bigger population, so it's understandable."

Law enforcement appreciated the fast response. If the scene was a house, though, and no one else was present, the coroner's investigator made the cop stay because he didn't want to be there alone due to the liability. A family member could claim later that something valuable was missing and imply that the investigator took it.

CHAPTER 05

AT THE SCENE

Whenever Holmes arrived at a death scene, the police officer who responded to the initial call from the county's Communications Center met him outside, away from anyone else who happened to be present. Then, in private, the officer told Holmes what he had learned.

"It's a ninety-two-year-old woman named Bertha," the cop might say. "She hadn't seen her doctor in four months. Meals on Wheels came by yesterday and dropped off a meal, and when the volunteer came today the meal was still on the front porch. He knocked, but didn't get an answer, so he went around the back, looked in the window, saw her in bed, unmoving and not breathing, and called us. We jimmied the door, went in, and confirmed that she's 10-55."

With that brief rundown, Holmes knew what the police knew even before he entered the house. From the minute he went inside, however, he was looking around. She was probably in the back bedroom, but he scanned each room anyway. If he saw her walker lying on its side, or that her cane had slid in dust on the floor, he took note of it because he could never back up. It might be that the caretaker kicked the cane out from under her, and she fell and hit her head and the caretaker lifted her and put her in bed. Holmes would never know it if he didn't notice the cane. Or he might notice the cane, think nothing of it, step in the dust to pick it up, and ruin the evidence.

This scenario was one Holmes actually used at the police academy when it was his responsibility to lay out a death scene for a training session. New recruits who didn't see the cane or ignored it failed to uncover the truth.

Investigators try to take note of everything, not necessarily writing it down unless it's a lot to remember, but not ignoring anything, either. There might be a will on a table that police failed to see. Maybe Bertha planned her death. Maybe she deliberately stopped taking her medication, or she took too much of it.

This is why investigators count all of the decedent's pills, every pill in every bottle that is at least six months or newer. Many people don't throw away medication for years, which is why only newer medications are counted. The quantity of pills oftentimes is staggering.

"Three cases out of five," Holmes says, "we came back to the office with shopping bags—literally—full of bottles of meds."

Every case other than a natural death was treated as a homicide. Even if there was a suicide note, the coroner's office considered it a homicide until the investigator knew for a fact that it wasn't. Murders draw the most attention, mainly because there is a good chance that the case will end up in court, and this way it was less likely that something would be overlooked or wrongly assumed.

After talking with the responding officer, Holmes sought out anyone who was present at the scene and knew the deceased—family members, neighbors, caretakers, friends, apartment managers, janitors—whoever. He sat down with them if it was appropriate, or remained standing if that was more proper, and asked them to tell him everything he needed to know. He didn't say, "All I want are the facts, ma'am." Instead, he said, "Tell me about Bertha."

He gleaned what he could, and always went to these individuals first, before examining the deceased. For one thing, Bertha was dead and not going anywhere until Holmes okayed it, so she could wait.

More important, though he couldn't help Bertha he might be able to help the people around her, even if it was nothing more than helping them understand why he was in their house.

Until *Quincy* and other TV shows, coroners were foreign to most people, thrust into their lives without them knowing or comprehending why. Even today, many people have misperceptions about the role of the coroner. Fictional characterizations emphasize the detective and doctor sides of the job because these are what interest readers and viewers the most, while other facets—consoler, advocate, educator, mentor, teacher, and bureaucrat—are largely ignored. Yet all are important.

Holmes might tell family members and others that the reason he was there was that Bertha's doctor wasn't available and police officers thought it would be best for the coroner to come out and take a look. If everything was as it should be, Holmes told them that he would leave soon and Bertha's doctor could complete the death certificate when he or she had the chance.

If the surviving family member was an elderly woman, Holmes sat next to her on the couch—"I wouldn't sit across from her or stand over her, I would sit next to her on the couch"—and if it was appropriate he'd take her hand before he told her why the coroner was involved. It might be because a doctor wasn't present and the decedent could have an infectious disease, so it was a safeguard for her to have the coroner make sure that that wasn't the case. If it wasn't a natural death, then the reason he was there might be more obvious, but he always explained it anyway.

After that, he went to the room or place where the body was. Sometimes family members followed, and he never asked them not to, because it was their home and their loved one. From a few feet away, he tried to match what he was seeing with what he already knew. The cop said this and the family said that. Did it jibe with what he observed? Next, he did the TV thing, putting two fingers on the side of the person's neck to see if there was a pulse. If loved ones were present, Holmes nodded for their benefit, confirming that the person was indeed dead. He didn't say, "Yeah, the fireman was right." He just nodded.

At the police academy, and as part of his initial training, Holmes learned to look for indications of foul play even if that didn't seem likely. He learned to pull down the decedent's lower lip and raise the eyelids because if a person suffocates, his or her lower lip might be chewed up. Even a frail, elderly woman who died because someone put a pillow over her head might have a chewed-up lip. He also examined the little fold of tissue at the front of the mouth, before the teeth, called the frenulum. If it was torn, or if the tongue was bitten, those were signs that the person might have been strangled or had a seizure. Broken fingernails were another clue. They indicated a struggle and a possible homicide.

Next, Holmes looked at the decedent's eyes using a magnifying glass if necessary to check for petechia hemorrhages. These are little dots from broken blood vessels in the whites of the eye. Oftentimes the dots are no bigger than pinpricks, but if they are present it means the decedent ran out of oxygen or his or her blood supply returning to the heart was cut off.

"In a manual strangulation," Holmes explains, "if you close down over somebody's neck, you stop the blood from getting back to the heart so it starts backing up. The pressure from the heart pumping blood ruptures all of the tiny arteries, and these little petechia hemorrhages start to appear. You see them all over in the white of the eye, and it's an indication that there was some restriction to the blood flow back to the heart. It could be caused by several things, but the most likely one is someone had his hands around the decedent's neck, or a sheet around the neck, or a whole pillow over the face. The killer thinks he's restricting the person's airway, and he is, to a point, but he's also restricting the blood flow. He sees the decedent's eyes go wide, but he doesn't see the tiny dots. We do."

If somebody was dead and a witness said the person had a heart attack, Holmes lifted up the decedent's shirt. This was because in a typical heart attack, a person's skin color is normal from the heart down and berry-colored from the heart up. The heart has stopped working while everything else is still functioning.

"The person's neck, cheeks, and all around the mouth might be deep red or purple—not so much the lips," Holmes says. "The change isn't due to strangulation or to being inverted and hung by the heels; it's the result of a heart attack. Thus, if someone said that the deceased had multiple heart attacks in the past and this was just one more, and I didn't see lividity to prove it, then I had to ask more questions. It still could be a heart attack; it just wasn't a typical heart attack."

There were other signs that he learned to look for. Were the hands relaxed or were the fingers stretched? Were the toes curled under or were they stretched? Were the legs crossed?

If the hands were relaxed and the person's legs were crossed, it meant that at the moment of death, he or she wasn't afraid and didn't know that anything bad was going to happen. If appendages were stretched, however, it meant the person had a heavy muscular contraction and may have experienced pain before dying.

"Somebody who is suffocated with a pillow, for instance, won't have his or her feet crossed, and the typical killer won't think afterward to position them that way," Holmes says.

All of these were part of the picture that he was looking at. The picture was a puzzle and the pieces needed to fit together.

"If I didn't see any of these things," he says, "that was good because it matched the story I was told when I got there. Even if I saw some of these things, however, it didn't necessarily mean that there was anything wild or crazy going on. It just meant that I needed to ask more questions in order to better understand what I was seeing."

LIVIDITY, RIGOR, AND TEMPERATURE

After taking a stand-back look, then doing "the little run-through," as Holmes calls it—checking the lip, examining the eyes, looking at the tongue, seeing whether the fingernails were broken or blanched (turning red or purple or white), and noting the position of fingers, legs, and toes—he checked for lividity, rigor mortis, and body temperature. These are the big three when it comes to estimating the time that has elapsed since the person died. Each one provides part of the answer, and Holmes tried to get the three of them to converge until the window of time was narrowed as much as possible.

Lividity refers to the coloration of a person's skin after death. The heart stops pumping, and blood begins to settle in response to gravity, turning the skin dark red or purple. For example, if a dead man is lying on his back, the backs of his ears and the back of his neck will be red, but his cheeks won't be. If he's lying on his stomach, then his chest and the front of his legs will be red. It's a little harder to tell if the person has dark skin, but still discernible.

Lividity usually starts within thirty minutes of death. After eight hours it is fairly fixed because blood congeals and vessels begin to break down. There are exceptions, though.

"Lividity happens rapidly when people have been lying for days, dying slowly," Holmes says. "Their blood is getting sluggish, and when their heart finally stops, their blood gravitates within minutes. Conversely, if someone is riding a bicycle, pumping hard, right before dying, his or her blood might not even start to coagulate for an hour."

Lividity is important for another reason besides helping to determine the time of death. If Holmes saw that the decedent was lying on his right side, for example, but his left side was red, then the person had been moved. Maybe paramedics changed the person's position to put a monitor on. If he knew this, Holmes didn't need to ask any more questions about lividity. If no one claimed to have moved the decedent, though, more investigation was needed.

Rigor mortis, from the Latin words for "stiffness" and "of death," refers to the condition of a body when limbs become rigid and hard to move due to chemical changes in muscles after someone dies. It begins about eight hours after death in most cases, and always starts in the jaw, regardless of the person's position or the ambient temperature. This is because the jaw is the strongest muscle in the human body. With the onset of rigor mortis, the jaw begins to clamp down or lock shut. Then rigor mortis works its way down, affecting the elbows before the wrists and the wrists before the fingers, the legs before the ankles and the ankles before the toes. After twenty-four to forty-eight hours, depending on the temperature, rigor mortis starts to dissolve on its own. The order is the same. The jaw starts to loosen, then the arms and fingers, followed by the legs and toes. Thus someone with a rigid jaw but flaccid legs is in the early stages of rigor mortis, meaning that he or she has been dead roughly eight hours. If it's the reverse, if the jaw is loose but the feet are tense, then the person is in a later stage and probably has been dead a day or more.

Again, though, there are exceptions. In one case, Holmes observed rigor mortis start in only twenty minutes.

"He was a professional body builder who was in the middle of a strenuous workout when he died," Holmes says. "He was in rigor so fast that I would have thought he had been dead for several hours. Other people were with him, though, so I knew exactly when he died."

At the other end of the extreme, Holmes examined people who he knew had been dead fifteen hours yet didn't have any rigor. They had been bedridden for so long that their muscles had atrophied to almost nothing.

Holmes knew a little about lividity and rigor mortis from his experiences as a mortician, but the importance of body temperature was new to him. So were the variables.

Bodies cool down after death until they become the temperature of the room they are in or the surrounding environment. In the first hour, body temperature actually can go up a degree or two due to the chemical reaction of dying. After that, though, it goes down one to two degrees every four hours until it reaches the ambient temperature.

Many death investigators, including Holmes, take a decedent's temperature the old-fashioned way, by sticking their hand on the person's forehead and in an armpit. A lot of it is feel.

"If someone's body temperature was close to my hand temperature," he says, "which was less than ninety-eight degrees—it was probably ninety-five or ninety-six degrees because it had been out in the air—then the person probably had been dead an hour because I had to account for a slight increase at first. The exception was if the decedent had a fever. Then I asked why. Oh, she was on ecstasy? Ecstasy increases your body temperature two to three degrees immediately. Methamphetamine can increase a person's temperature five degrees. A person can have a fever of 103 to 105 degrees for days on end if he or she stays on meth."

In some instances a person's body temperature was near the ambient temperature but Holmes knew that the person had been dead only a couple of hours based on witness testimony, lividity, and lack of rigor mortis. This meant the body might have been moved, in which case he started recording actual temperatures—of the body, of the room where the body was found, and also outside.

On *CSI* and other popular TV detective shows, investigators use liver sticks to determine the exact temperature of a dead person. With a liver stick, the investigator pokes a tiny hole in the liver with a scalpel and inserts a thermometer. Some real-life coroners still use liver sticks, but most have gotten away from them because it doesn't make much difference. The liver is the densest organ in the body and takes the longest to cool down—that's the theory.

"You're just as well off taking someone's rectal temperature, though," Holmes says, "because the rectum is protected." He adds with a wry smile, "It's not as good for television viewing, though."

Household temperatures vary depending on the room. Attics are warmer than the rest of the house, while basements are cooler. Most garages aren't insolated so they are warmer on hot days and cooler on cold days than the main house. Anytime Holmes investigated a case, he asked police officers whether windows in the room where the person was found were open or closed when the officers arrived, because that can affect a body's temperature. If the decedent was found on a floor, Holmes noted whether it was a tile floor, which tends to be cool, or a carpeted surface, which tends to be warm. If a body was found in a bathtub, pool, or spa, he took the temperature of the water and bottled a sample for testing purposes.

Determining the time of death as well as the circumstances surrounding it can be meaningful for a family. Oftentimes loved ones need to know for their own benefit that nothing could have been done, that Walter died while his wife was out of town, visiting her mother, not while she was running errands.

"At some level the information helps absolve feelings of guilt and enables people to manage their grief," Holmes says.

AUTOPSIES

The word "autopsy" means "see for yourself." It is the examination of a human body externally and internally following death using surgical techniques, laboratory analysis, and medical records. Ideally, autopsies would be performed following every death because each one furthers our understanding of diseases and contributes to our body of medical knowledge. Autopsies also reveal undiagnosed or misdiagnosed illnesses that may be hereditary and important for family members to be aware of, as well as provide peace of mind to loved ones by eliminating some of the uncertainty surrounding a death. In addition, autopsies can validate whether environmental hazards were a factor in someone's demise, or call into question the competency of medical care that a person received, in both instances opening the door for potential litigation. In practice, however, autopsies tend to be performed only when the cause of death isn't clear, and sometimes not even then. As local governments grapple with budgetary constraints that impact services, funding for death investigations is often restricted, and limitations are set on the number of autopsies that can be conducted in a given year. Whenever this happens, medical science, the needs of families, and the community suffer. Infectious diseases go undetected, rightful compensation is lost, and people literally get away with murder.

Typically, the autopsy room in a mortuary is small, about the size of a modest living room. It's not sterile because the risk of disease exists only for the living people in the room. At one time the only special clothing pathologists wore was gloves, an apron, and a mask if the smell was bad. Today, personal protection equipment—a Tyvek jumpsuit with eye guards—is common, especially if the decedent is known to have a contagious disease.

The floors are linoleum or tile, and there are one or more stainless steel tables with locking wheels. The tables are angled slightly with the head on the left and the feet on the right. There is a lip all the way around the table, and at the bottom is a drain hole that sits over an open sump. A tub that is lined with a plastic bag is placed between the calves of the deceased. When the pathologist has finished removing, examining, and weighing an organ, he or she places it in the bag. At the end of the autopsy, a mortician takes the bag, which contains the person's heart, lungs, stomach, liver, and brain, and adds embalming powder. The powder absorbs any leftover liquids, controls any odors, and preserves organs. Then the whole bag is put back inside the chest cavity. The chest is stitched up and so is the head, although there's nothing in it since the brain has been removed; it's just the skull. After that the body is washed with a hose—not before, because the pathologist doesn't want to wash off anything that might be evidentiary—dried, placed in a clean body bag, and put in a cooler until instructions are received from next of kin regarding disposition.

In the early days the pathologist had a Dictaphone, and as soon as the autopsy was finished he or she recorded the findings. Later, pathologists began using voice-activated tapes, dictating the results as they went along. This was easier for doctors, although it created problems for transcribers since the clanking of surgical tools against stainless steel tables can make it difficult to hear. Moreover, sounds tend to echo in an autopsy room. Today, digital recorders are common.

The average autopsy takes one to two hours, with homicides typically lasting three to four hours. Microscope slides are made and analyzed a day or two later, adding another hour or more to the process. When the toxicology report comes back with the results of blood, urine, and gastric juices testing, time is spent scrutinizing this, too.

Autopsy results often provide another element in determining the time of death. Food is digested at a fairly predictable rate, usually breaking down in about twenty minutes. If the autopsy is done shortly after death, a pathologist often can tell exactly what foods a person ate last. As with lividity and rigor mortis, there are variables, however. Food doesn't break down as fast if the person was dehydrated, super-active, or had some sort of chemical imbalance.

The timing of the autopsy can have an effect, too, because digestion continues after death for as long as food enzymes are working in the stomach and small intestine—generally four to eight hours. Almost coincidentally, but not predictably, decomposition starts then, so food begins to decompose at the same time that the interior lining of the stomach begins to decompose. This is why bodies are refrigerated prior to autopsy, to stop the digestive system and retard decomposition.

Oftentimes, especially in cases that go to trial, a defense attorney or prosecuting attorney asks the coroner how long the person had been dead before his or her body was found. This is common on TV shows. There are so many variables, though, that Holmes learned not to rely on any of them until he knew everything he could about somebody, which might take several weeks depending on how many people he needed to talk to, how quickly he was able to contact them, and when the autopsy and toxicology reports would be back. After that he would give the broadest range he could, within reason. If it looked like the person had been dead two days, for example, he gave a range of one to three days. This way if someone came forward later and said that he talked with the decedent the day before he was found,

Holmes didn't look foolish by having said that the person had been dead exactly two days.

"Lividity, rigor, body temperature, and digestion help determine time of death," Holmes says, "but it's not a science. That's one of the first things I learned. Depending on the circumstances, there may be pressure from multiple entities to be as precise as possible, as quickly as possible. It's folly to do that, though. Better to be slow, deliberate, and get as much information as you can first, then provide a reasonable estimate, not an exact one."

LOOKING FOR BOOGEYMEN

Another thing Holmes learned—although it took time—was to trust his instincts. When he was being trained, first at the police academy and then on the job, he was told to take nothing for granted.

"Question everything people tell you," his trainers said, "family members, friends, doctors, nurses—everyone. Don't be too trusting."

Most of the instructors at the academy were police officers, and Holmes's supervisor, Keith Craig, was a retired cop as well. Since their focus was on wrongdoing, they expected people to lie to them and were suspicious of anything they were told. The same level of skepticism didn't play out well in the coroner's office, though. It was important for coroners' investigators to question, but not to assume that everything they heard was less than the truth. That kind of attitude distances coroners from families and is why the relationship between coroners' offices and families tends to be better in counties where the operation of the coroner is separate from law enforcement.

Because of the way he was trained, Holmes started out suspecting people of equivocating or withholding information. "I found myself looking for boogeymen where none were to be found," he says.

An example of this was the death of a twenty-seven-year-old woman named Brie. "She was beautiful," Holmes says. "Brown hair, green eyes—every man's idea of a knockout."

She also was the consummate party girl, going so hard and so long that few people could keep up with her. Whether it was alcohol, drugs, or sex, she embraced it eagerly and hungrily. Her lifestyle caught up with her, however, after a wild night in a motel room.

Brie invited two men her age who barely knew her to the room. Then she unloaded a duffel bag full of sex toys, condoms, lubrication, hard rock CDs, a portable player, and an assortment of drugs.

The three of them went at it, starting with marijuana and beer, then moving on to hard liquor and heroin. Brie showed them how to inject themselves, and she drank lots of Gatorade so that she would urinate often and flush the drugs through her system. Eventually the two men had to turn down her demands for more sex because they were exhausted. They fell asleep in the room, only to wake up the next morning and find her lying dead next to them. She was still holding a cigarette that had burned down to the filter, there were empty liquor bottles and used condoms in a trash can, and on a nightstand next to the bed were drug paraphernalia and heroin.

Police officers questioned the two men one time, and decided that they didn't have enough information to charge them with a crime that would stick. Holmes wanted to continue investigating, however. He spent nearly three full days interviewing both of them because he thought they were partially responsible for Brie's death.

"They claimed that she rented the room, provided the drugs and booze, and masterminded or scripted the marathon sex between all three of them," Holmes says. "It sounded too concocted, though, a story better suited to the pages of *Penthouse* magazine than a coroner's report."

He adds, "They were alone in the room for a long enough period of time to have built their story," which enhanced his suspicions.

During his investigation, Holmes talked with other people who knew Brie. They confirmed that she was a needle user and on a crash course for an early demise. He also talked to acquaintances of the two men and was told that they weren't sophisticated enough to have scored the drugs and come up with a plan to use Brie, then kill her. Except for minor marijuana use, both were clean.

Just to cover all the bases, Holmes went to the hotel and checked the heater in the room. It wasn't likely, but he wanted to rule out any chance that there had been a carbon monoxide leak. The heater functioned perfectly.

By now a different picture of the event had taken shape in his mind. It was helped by the fact that both men were visibly shaken when Holmes talked to them, and their stories never wavered. One man was in tears through most of Holmes's first two interviews with him.

Among other items found in Brie's duffel bag were Alcoholics Anonymous books and a journal. Another investigator in the coroner's office contacted Brie's AA sponsor, who said that the two of them talked almost every day, and Brie had been sober more than seventy days. The sponsor hadn't heard from her in the past four days, however.

Holmes says, "I could have saved myself a lot of time if I had been more open-minded at the outset. Not that I resented the time I put into the case, but if I had been less suspicious in the beginning, I could have reached the same conclusion faster."

It wasn't clear whether Brie's death was an accident or suicide, so Holmes ruled that the manner of death was undetermined. In the end, he was confident that it wasn't a homicide, though.

"I believe she overdosed by cumulative effect," he says, "but not intentionally. She built a high early in their night and tried to keep it with beer, hard liquor, and heroin. I think she lost track of the quantity, and died after they all passed out."

CHAPTER 06

THE OVERDOSE THAT WASN'T

When Carol Filipelli died under mysterious circumstances, and Ken Holmes investigated her death, he discovered facets of her life that were eye-opening. It was the stuff of bestselling novels and popular movies—in fact, a well-known writer heard pieces of it from a doctor who treated Carol, and wanted Holmes to discuss it. Holmes refused. In his mind, the public didn't need to know the story. Even Carol's parents and brother didn't need to know more than the basics of what happened to the twenty-six-year-old onetime model, Holmes believed. What good could come from describing secrets that Carol kept hidden from everyone? It is only with the passage of nearly forty years and his retirement as the coroner of Marin County that Holmes discusses the case now.

On Tuesday, January 24, 1978, police officers were called to a two-story luxury apartment in Sausalito by a neighbor who requested a welfare check on the person who resided there. Carol Filipelli hadn't answered when the neighbor knocked on her door and phoned her. That wasn't unusual since Carol traveled frequently, but what concerned the neighbor was that Carol's dog had been outside, loose, for several days. Carol never let the dog out on its own.

Sausalito is one of the most affluent communities in Marin. It was that way in 1978, and it's that way today. Multimillion-dollar homes are perched on hillsides with panoramic views of San Francisco Bay. The waterfront resembles a chic seaside village with fancy boutiques, expensive restaurants, and high-end art galleries. The Sausalito Yacht Club is home to impressive sailing and racing vessels. Located just north of San Francisco, at one end of the most famous bridge in the world, the Golden Gate Bridge, Sausalito also serves as the gateway to California's fabled wine country, redwoods, and northern coast.

Carol Filipelli's apartment had the same breathtaking views as the most expensive homes in Sausalito. The furniture was tasteful and expensive. A late-model Mercedes was parked in the garage.

At 2:40 P.M. that Tuesday, police arrived to find Carol's front door locked. They went around the side and gained access through an unlocked sliding glass door in the rear of the apartment. Carol's body was upstairs, in the master bedroom. Dressed in a maroon robe and black socks, she was lying at an odd angle on the floor, as if she had fallen from her king-sized bed. The receiver of her phone was off the hook, and an alcoholic drink was on a nightstand nearby. The closet doors in the bedroom were closed, and the sliding glass door leading to an outside balcony was locked.

Bill Thomas was the coroner's investigator who was on duty at the time. He checked in with the responding officers, then examined Carol's body. There was no evidence of trauma and no unusual markings. Lividity, the process by which blood settles after it ceases to circulate, was pronounced and fixed. Rigor mortis—the stiffening of muscles—had passed, and her body was room temperature. These signs indicated that Carol had been dead at least twenty-four hours, and probably longer. Upon moving her body, Thomas noted a clear fluid coming out of her mouth. He took nasal, vaginal, and vitreous humor swabs (the latter is the fluid behind the cornea), which is standard practice in cases like this. He also preserved the drink on the nightstand.

Searching the apartment, Thomas found miscellaneous papers and checks, assorted jewelry, designer clothes in the master bedroom closet, and $889 in cash. It was in the master bathroom that he discovered the apparent cause of Carol Filipelli's death. The wastebasket had five empty pill bottles. All were for prescriptions in Carol's name that had been filled recently. One was for 500-milligram capsules of Doriden, a sedative for insomnia. The prescription, thirty-six pills, was only four days old, yet the bottle was empty. Two other empty bottles had contained Valium. The fourth bottle once held Quaalude, an antidepressant, while the last bottle was for Minocin, an antibiotic used to treat bacterial infections, including those caused by sexually transmitted diseases. Three different physicians had prescribed the medications, and the bottles, collectively, had contained 260 pills at one time.

Thomas knew from experience that unless additional information surfaced during the autopsy or in conversations with Carol's family and acquaintances, it was unlikely that the reason for her death could be determined. The cause—a drug overdose—seemed obvious, but the manner—whether it was accidental or intentional—wasn't clear. Without compelling evidence such as a suicide note, there was no way for the coroner to rule one way or the other.

After Thomas completed his examination, Carol's body was delivered to a funeral home in Mill Valley where the autopsy would be performed. Carol's dog, as well as a caged bird, were turned over to the Marin County Humane Society.

The autopsy confirmed Thomas's initial assessment. There was no indication of trauma—no bruises, lacerations, or punctures. There was nothing unusual about Carol's heart, lungs, liver, kidneys, brain, bile, or body cavities, either. Samples of Carol's blood, urine, and gastric fluids were sent to a lab in Oakland. The results wouldn't be known for several weeks, although that wasn't a concern. Given the empty pill bottles in the bathroom, no one doubted what the toxicology report would show.

In the meantime, Thomas had phone numbers for Carol's parents in Brooklyn and her brother, John, in Florida. He thought it best to notify John first and have him tell his parents. They might receive the news better if it came from their son rather than a stranger. Thomas called police in Florida and asked them to inform John that his sister had died.

When police knocked on his door, John told them that they had made a mistake. He said his parents lived in New York, but he didn't have a sister named Carol or any relatives in California.

An officer relayed this information to Thomas, who was puzzled. Among the personal items that he'd found and held on to for her file was Carol Filipelli's address book. John's address and phone number were there, exactly as Thomas had noted them. Moreover, written in parentheses next to John's name was the word "Brother."

Thomas asked police to go back to John's residence and have him phone Thomas. The officer told Thomas afterward that John was reluctant and had to be badgered to make the call. Eventually, he admitted to Thomas that he had a sister named Carol who lived in California. His excuse for not admitting it earlier was that he thought the cop "was a bill collector or something." He said that he and his sister weren't in touch with each other.

When Thomas told him about his sister's death, John merely said, "Thanks. I'll tell my parents." He didn't ask any questions.

The next day, Carol Filipelli's father phoned the coroner's office. Thomas wasn't on duty, and Ken Holmes took the call. Without preamble, the father cried, "What's happened to my baby?"

Holmes told him that the investigation hadn't been completed yet, but it looked like Carol overdosed. Her father was stunned and at a complete loss to explain how or why that happened. At one point he told Holmes, as if offering a kind of testimonial, "She's a hardworking girl. We talk to her once a week on the phone."

Later in the investigation, Holmes collected copies of Carol's phone bills for the six months prior to her death. Her father was right; every Sunday, like clockwork, she called home.

After the autopsy, Carol's remains were released to her parents. They said they were going to bring her home to be buried, but instead they had her cremated in California and her ashes sent home. That proved to be unfortunate because when the toxicology report came back several weeks later, it held a big surprise: there was no trace of drugs in her system. Carol hadn't overdosed. Because her body already had been cremated, however, it wasn't possible to reexamine it.

THE INVESTIGATION

A short time later, a San Francisco attorney walked into the Marin County Coroner's Office and said he wanted to speak with someone who was familiar with the Carol Filipelli case. When asked why he was interested in it, the attorney said he was representing a client in the dissolution of her marriage, and the case had some bearing on it.

According to the attorney, his client, named Martha, and Carol Filipelli were in the same profession. Both were high-priced prostitutes. Martha was fearful of her husband, who knew Carol, and refused to be alone with him at the present time, the attorney said. Then the attorney asked a curious question: During the autopsy, had Carol's skin been examined closely to see whether any kind of "esoterical substance" had been rubbed on it? Bill Thomas told him that the autopsy had been thorough and nothing unusual had been found.

During the conversation, the attorney noticed Carol's driver's license in Thomas's case file and asked to see her photo. When Thomas showed it to him, the attorney was dumbfounded. He said that the two women, his client and Carol Filipelli, shared a strong physical resemblance. Both had brown hair, brown eyes, and light skin, and were beautiful.

Thomas asked the attorney about the occupation of Martha's husband. The attorney said that he was a marine biologist with a PhD.

After the attorney's visit, Thomas phoned Martha's husband, whose name was Eddie. Thomas's impression of him was that he was a meek, milquetoast kind of guy. Eddie admitted that he knew Carol Filipelli and had even been to her apartment. He said that Carol was security conscious and it was unlike her to leave any door unlocked. Also, she didn't let her dog out unattended. In addition, she was secretive, to the point of removing mailing labels that were affixed to magazines she subscribed to. Recently, he noticed that she had an issue of *Newsweek* opened to an editorial titled "A Good Death."

It was clear to Thomas that Eddie was more than just a casual friend of the deceased. While Eddie didn't seem particularly moved by Carol's death, he knew things about her that belied a passing interest. Thomas looked to see if there were any gifts from Eddie in Carol's apartment. There weren't, nor did Thomas find a passport for Carol despite the fact that Eddie said she had traveled to Mexico recently, as well as to Hawaii. When Thomas asked Eddie about Carol's secret life—the same secret life as Eddie's wife—Eddie denied any knowledge of it. He said that Carol must have had a dual personality, and if he had ever married her then found out about it he would have killed himself. It was an odd comment, and Thomas noted it in his investigative report. Then he moved on to other cases. Inasmuch as no one was likely to know anything more, he couldn't justify looking into it further.

Ken Holmes wasn't willing to let the case go, however. It would be a recurring theme in his work. Carol's apartment with its fabulous view rented for more money than Holmes's monthly salary at the time, yet Carol's occupation, according to her neighbor, was hairdresser. Even if she was, in fact, a high-priced call girl, how could she afford such luxury? There had to be more to it, Holmes thought.

Holmes went to Carol's apartment, which was still secured and untouched. Near the hearth, he felt a bulge under one foot. Using a pen to peel back the carpet, he found two passports, three thousand dollars in cash, a checkbook, and a driver's license. The passports and driver's license had Carol Filipelli's photo, but the names of different women.

Now Holmes's curiosity was piqued, and he began searching the whole apartment carefully. A number of shoe boxes were perched high on a shelf in the closet in the master bedroom. One shoe box contained copies of an ad that Carol had placed in the personals section of the *Wall Street Journal* and other publications. The ad was a teaser, and Holmes handed a copy to me.

"Former bunny, five-five, 125 pounds, dark hair and eyes, would like to meet generous gentleman over 40. I will light your cigarettes and take off your shoes if you treat me sweetly. Write to Michelle."

The shoe box also contained dozens of responses to the ad, from men all over the country. Holmes showed me these, too. On some of them Carol affixed brief comments. "He's a private pilot." "He owns his own company." "He has three kids." The information was relevant, it seemed, in helping her decide which men were the best candidates to pursue.

A second shoe box contained copies of a letter that she sent to men who responded, as well as a photograph of her. The letter was handwritten but xeroxed with space for Carol to add the person's name in the salutation, as well as a signature at the end. She didn't presign it, because she used different names in the ad—Michelle, Maureen, Jade, Rose.

The letter said, "Thank you for answering my ad. A little something about myself. I'm 26, five-foot-five, light-skinned, brown hair and eyes, 125 pounds, and I do enjoy being feminine. I'm looking for a soft and warm friendship with no complications or misunderstandings. Since I have received several answers, I cannot reply to each letter individually by giving my telephone number because privacy and discretion are of utmost importance to me. Therefore it would be more convenient if you would give me your number and a particular date and time you'd like me to phone you with politeness and discretion assured. I'm hoping to meet you soon."

The photograph, of which there were several dozen copies, was in color and taken with a Polaroid camera. It showed Carol in enticing lingerie, kneeling on the same bed in her bedroom in Sausalito and holding a wineglass with red liquid. She was wearing a big, floppy-brimmed hat that hid most of her face, and her head was tilted down, further shielding her.

A third shoe box had individually written follow-up letters that she sent to the best prospects. Usually it was a wealthy businessman who was married and traveled frequently. He told her when he was going to be in a particular city and where she should meet him.

Holmes says, "The deal, I learned, was that Carol would join the man at a conference and do everything he wanted her to do. She would escort him to meals and functions, being more than arm candy because she was well read and conversant, and also provide sexual services while there."

Inside a manila envelope that had been taped shut, Holmes found other photos, which he showed to me. These were much different, and appeared to be for personal viewing. There were no copies, just single prints, all in black-and-white. They were eight-by-ten in size, of professional quality, and taken when Carol was nineteen, according to the date on the back. In all but one photo she was nude and on a beach, either frolicking in the surf or lying outstretched in the sand. Her full body was on display, unabashed and free. The lone exception was a close-up of just her face with the collar of a blouse visible. In it she looked pensive, unguarded, and, if possible, even more alluring.

"The black-and-white photos had the photographer's name stamped on the back," Holmes says, "so I tracked him down. He said he hadn't seen Carol in years; nevertheless, he was brokenhearted when I told him why I was calling. He said that Carol hired him to take photos of her after she moved to San Francisco. A short time later, the two of them became lovers."

Once Holmes learned that Carol wasn't who she pretended to be, he pursued the case with even greater vigor. In addition to her apartment in Sausalito, he learned that she maintained two other apartments in San Francisco under the same phony names that she used in the ads. She had bank accounts in those other names, too, as well as credit cards.

The more he uncovered, the more absorbed Holmes became. His next stop was San Francisco, where he found, through word of mouth, three other former lovers of Carol Filipelli. While the photographer kept a low profile, these men had social standing and owned businesses. Also unlike the photographer, they were married. Holmes assured each of them that any information they provided wouldn't be part of his report. His inquiries were intended solely to help fill in the blanks regarding how and why Carol died.

From one of the men Holmes learned that Carol's latest boyfriend frequently hung out at a bar on Lombard Street in San Francisco. Taking his wife with him as cover, Holmes chatted up the bartender, thinking he might know the boyfriend. He didn't seem to, but that didn't stop Holmes and his wife from going back to the bar seven nights in a row with the hope of running into Carol's boyfriend.

"Later," Holmes says, "I found out that the boyfriend was a fringe player in Hollywood. He did frequent the bar, but only when he happened to be in town."

Eventually, Holmes tracked down Carol Filipelli's Hollywood lover. His name was Romano, and when he came to Holmes's office he was accompanied by his attorney. Romano said that he first met Carol when he was visiting the Bay Area and she was walking her dog on Stinson Beach, in Marin County. They began a conversation that evolved rather quickly into an intimate relationship. He said she told him what she did, which didn't bother him. She also told him that oftentimes after a rendezvous with a client she went to the beach and swam in the ocean, as an act of cleansing.

It was Romano who told Holmes about Eddie, Martha's marine biologist husband. Eddie was Carol's sugar daddy, Romano said. He was independently wealthy and paid for Carol's apartment in Sausalito. He provided the Mercedes, too, and gave her $1,500 per month in spending money. When she told him that she wanted to visit her parents in New York and also do a little shopping, Eddie gave her $3,500. He didn't know that she actually was visiting someone else.

Romano told Holmes several other pieces of information that were helpful. The first was that Carol used Quaalude and Valium heavily, and sometimes talked about suicide when she was drugged but, to the best of his knowledge, had never attempted to kill herself. If nothing else, Romano said, she loved her dog too much to leave it uncared for.

The second piece of information was that Carol had frequent doctor's appointments. That was how she was able to keep getting refills on her medications. Romano said that one of her physicians was something of a lothario who was happy to trade drugs for sex.

"I talked to two of the doctors," Holmes says, "but didn't ask whether either one had had a personal relationship with Carol. It never crossed my mind. I did ask if Carol had ever expressed any suicidal tendencies, and both doctors said no. The first doctor said that Carol was afraid her boyfriend might kill himself, which caused her to have difficulty sleeping. That was why he prescribed a sedative for her. He didn't know that she was getting prescriptions filled by other physicians as well, he said. The second physician, a gynecologist, said Carol came in so frequently to be tested for a venereal disease that he wondered whether she was prostituting herself. Each time she told him that she was taking a trip and the thought of it made her nervous, which was why she needed medication, to calm her down. On one occasion she claimed that she had lost her prescription."

Another thing Romano told Holmes was that Carol's going rate—which wasn't in any of the ads—was three thousand dollars for a weekend. It didn't include airfare, meals, or other expenses, which the client paid for as well.

The most important thing Romano told Holmes was that Carol and Eddie had had a big fight several days before she died. This was after Eddie found out about her and Romano. Eddie thought he was the only man in Carol's life, or at least the only one who mattered. Certainly he had paid handsomely for the privilege.

Holmes listened to everything Romano said with a sense of wariness. Romano was circumspect, measuring his words in order to avoid saying anything that might be incriminating. The fact that his lawyer accompanied him added to Holmes's distrust.

"In my experience, only people with something to hide bring their attorneys with them to the coroner's office," Holmes says.

At the end of their conversation, Romano told Holmes that he had changed his name after he was charged with dealing marijuana and jumped probation, that Romano wasn't his real name. Holmes wasn't surprised.

Nevertheless, like each of Carol Filipelli's other lovers whom Holmes interviewed, Romano seemed genuinely upset by the news that she had died. Talking about her many months later, his voice still caught at times. That led Holmes to think that Romano probably was telling the truth. It didn't make things any clearer, however. On the contrary, the more Holmes learned from Romano, the more confusing the case became.

During the course of his investigation, Holmes had three face-to-face meetings with Eddie. While soft-spoken, slight in build, and of average appearance, Eddie was smart and exhibited a steely resolve.

"In the first meeting," Holmes says, "Eddie played the grieving boyfriend, never letting on that he knew about Carol's other boyfriends or about how she earned money beyond what he gave her. The second meeting was at Eddie's house, an impressive residence in Tiburon. [Tiburon is next to Sausalito and even more upscale.] Eddie let me in, but was cagey and didn't admit anything. When I returned several weeks later, Eddie met me at the door and said, 'I prefer that you don't come in.' I tried to ask him several questions while standing in the doorway, but Eddie demurred, saying politely but firmly that he was done talking."

Holmes is silent for a moment, replaying the conversations with Eddie in his mind. They happened long ago, but the memory of them is still fresh.

"So you don't know whether he killed her?" I say.

"Oh, I think I figured it out," Holmes says. "It took a while, and I can't prove it, but I know. During the latter part of my investigation I learned that Eddie's specialty as a marine biologist was poisonous fish—pufferfish, stonefish, lionfish, boxfish. They store or excrete toxins that, in sufficient quantities, can be lethal to humans if swallowed or absorbed through the skin."

The toxicology tests that were done on Carol's body didn't reveal any trace of barbiturates, morphine, Doriden, Librium, Quaalude, methamphetamines, or other common drugs. They also didn't show any evidence of lead, mercury, strychnine, or arsenic. Tests weren't conducted for more exotic and unusual substances, however, because no one knew that that was a possibility. Similarly, the drink on her nightstand, which subsequently was discarded, wasn't tested for tetrodotoxin or other fish poisons. Once her body was cremated, the case was closed. It has been that way ever since.

"And you never talked to Eddie again?"

He shakes his head. "I had no reason to. The only thing I did was check periodically to see whether he was still alive."

"And?"

"He died several years ago from natural causes." Holmes adds with a touch of bitterness because his certainty can't be confirmed, "If he was responsible for Carol's death, he took the knowledge to his grave."

CHAPTER 07

INVESTIGATING HOMICIDES

For coroners, murder investigations are time-consuming. Police are involved throughout, autopsies are longer, and unless a suspect pleads guilty, courtroom testimony follows, orchestrated by a district attorney.

In many instances the cause of death is fairly obvious, but there are cases where things aren't what they seem. The Ladd case is one example. Gloria Ladd was a forty-eight-year-old former teacher and unemployed realtor whose husband, a NASA test pilot, had drowned in Florida sixteen years earlier. Her two sons, John and James, ages nineteen and eighteen, lived with her in a modest one-story, wood-framed house in San Rafael. Holmes was called to the house on a warm night in August 1975.

At the time, John was on summer break after finishing his freshman year at the University of California, Davis. He was on the school's cross-country and track teams and was a premed student. James, meanwhile, had graduated from high school and was set to attend UC Davis in the fall.

Earlier that evening an elder had come by the house to pick up James for a church outing. On the door was a note: "We're all sick. Jim is unable to go. Thanks for coming by."

When the elder called the house later and spoke with Gloria Ladd, her incoherence alarmed him and he contacted the police. The scene that officers walked in on when they arrived was the same scene that greeted Holmes. The front door was ajar, and Mrs. Ladd sat quietly in the dining room, smoking a cigarette. Meanwhile, John Ladd was in his bedroom, lying on the floor. He was dressed in boxer shorts, his head was on a pillow, and his body was partially covered by a blanket. Holmes noted that he was cold to the touch, in full rigor with marked lividity in the dependent portion of the body (that is, on the side facing the floor). There were no external signs of trauma—no abrasions, lacerations, or gunshot wounds.

James Ladd was lying on his bed in another room. He, too, was dressed in boxer shorts, as well as a white T-shirt. Like his brother, he was cold to the touch, in full rigor with marked lividity, indicating that both young men had been dead roughly twelve hours.

On a desk in the kitchen were two brief handwritten wills. They were signed by each brother, dated the day before, and said the same thing: "In the event of my death, I leave all of my material possessions and my money to my brother. If not surviving, to my mother, Gloria Ladd. If not surviving, to be equally divided among my aunts and uncles."

Near the wills, on the kitchen table, were bankbooks for the two brothers, indicating that each had inherited thirty thousand dollars recently from a grandmother. On another table was what appeared to be a partially completed, unsigned note in Gloria Ladd's handwriting indicating a possible suicide attempt.

Because portions of the police report and investigation wouldn't be released to the media, Holmes suppressed corresponding information in his own report. Later, he added it as a confidential addendum to the file. In this supplemental report he noted Gloria Ladd's confession to Bart Stinson.

Holmes had been on the job only four months, but already he knew Stinson because he was the police officer who questioned Marlene Olive and Chuck Riley about the deaths of Marlene's parents, James and Naomi Olive. Over the years, Stinson had gained a reputation as "Marin's toughest crime fighter"—this was the title of a newspaper article about him when he retired—in part because he didn't look or sound anything like it. On the contrary, he had a confiding nature, and his soft southern accent lulled people in. This was the case with Gloria Ladd. Her motive for the murders seemed to be financial gain, but it took only a few minutes for Stinson to learn that she killed her sons because she thought it was the only way she could save them. She was certain that the world was coming to an end soon, and killing them would preserve their souls.

"The wills confused many people," Holmes says, "because they thought she did it for the money. I sat and listened to her talk with Bart for half an hour, though, and she absolutely was convinced that she had done the right thing. Money had nothing to do with it."

As she recounted to Stinson, Gloria Ladd told her sons that she had been exposed to hepatitis, and her doctor suggested that both boys take prescribed medicine as a preventative measure. She crushed thirty phenobarbital tablets in water for each one and saw that they consumed this tonic before they went to bed (phenobarbital is a barbiturate that is used as a sedative and also to treat certain types of seizures). Both boys were small—James was five foot five and weighed 135 pounds while John, the older of the two, was five foot nine and weighed 150 pounds—and she thought each dosage would be fatal. Instead, she found her sons alive the following morning.

At that time she gave each of them three delamine pills (delamine is an antihistamine). These had no apparent effect. That night, just before bed, she gave each son fifteen more phenobarbital tablets in water. During the night, both boys were groggy, got out of bed, and stumbled around. Once again, though, they didn't die. The next morning she placed a plastic bag over the head of one boy, then the other, suffocating them. She couldn't get John back into bed before doing this so she left him on the floor. The same morning she took the family dog to the Marin County Humane Society.

Holmes learned that at one time Gloria Ladd had been a mental patient at Napa State Hospital. Her brother told Holmes that five years earlier she had attempted suicide and was treated at both Marin General Hospital and a community mental health clinic. In the aftermath of John's and James's deaths, these agencies were criticized for not taking the boys away from their mother at that time. Child welfare workers don't like to break up families, though, and she hadn't abused or neglected her sons.

"I'm sure they were so obedient and trusting," the church elder told Holmes, "that they took the pills without question."

When Holmes talked with Gloria Ladd's physician, he was told that a month earlier she had asked for a prescription of one hundred phenobarbital tablets. The physician refused and instead prescribed thirty delamine pills. When she asked again for phenobarbital a short time later, he prescribed another twelve delamine capsules. It was unclear where she secured the phenobarbital.

"She was a quiet lady, and her sons were good kids," Holmes says, "not into drugs or causing trouble. She was sure that the world was ending and this was what she had to do."

THE STEPHENSES

It's virtually impossible for a double homicide to have any kind of happy ending. After Bill and Tasia Stephens were murdered, however, there was one bright spot.

A friend of Bill Stephens went to their house after Stephens hadn't shown up for work in two days or answered his phone. Through a locked sliding-glass door, the friend saw the couple lying next to each other, unmoving and covered in blood, on the bed in their master bedroom. He called the police, who confirmed that the Stephenses were dead from multiple gunshot wounds. Police then called Holmes and also Child Protective Services because next to the Stephenses' bed was a crib with a nine-month-old infant in it, alive and unhurt.

Mr. Stephens, age forty-five, was dressed in boxer-style shorts and a T-shirt. He had been shot three times—twice in the head and once in the chest. There was no evidence of powder staining, indicating that the weapon was more than a couple of feet away when it was fired.

Mrs. Stephens, forty-three, was wearing black pants and a white blouse. She had been shot twice in the head, and there was no gunshot residue on her body, either. Like her husband, she was cold to the touch, in full rigor, with moderate lividity in the dependent areas, indicating that death probably had occurred the previous day.

As usual, Holmes took oral, nasal, rectal, and vitreous fluid swabs from both bodies, as well as fingernail scrapings, fingerprints, and samples of Bill's and Tasia's head hair and pubic hair. Some of this information was used to confirm the decedents' identities. In addition, vaginal swabs were done when the possibility existed that a woman had been sexually assaulted and the perpetrator's semen might be present. Rectal swabs were taken as well, to eliminate the possibility of drug stashing (that is, people hiding drugs in a body cavity to avoid being charged with possession). The latter didn't seem likely in the Stephenses' case; however, as many swabs as possible were collected in all cases like this because it was the only opportunity that the coroner's office would have.

"We did everything we could do because we knew that we'd never have that body again," Holmes says.

There was another reason for the swabs, which was to be able to say in court that something wasn't there. Holmes learned that the absence of something can be as important as its presence.

"If the defense asked whether we found any cocaine in a person's nose, for example," Holmes says, "and we said we didn't check, then it called into question everything we did. 'Why didn't you check?' the defense might say. 'It could have exonerated my client.'"

After he left the Stephenses' house, Holmes sought out some of their friends to get information on next of kin. Mr. Stephens had a twenty-one-year-old daughter from a previous marriage who lived in

Texas, while Mrs. Stephens had siblings who lived in Massachusetts, as well as parents who lived in Greece. Holmes notified everyone he could reach regarding the Stephenses' deaths, telling them that a full-scale police investigation was under way.

In homicide cases, the first suspects are family members. That didn't apply to the Stephenses since their families were out of state. Both Mr. and Mrs. Stephens owned small businesses, chains of video stores and hair salons respectively, and the next tier of suspects included potentially disgruntled employees. That proved not to be the case as well, until police questioned the Stephenses' housekeeper, Yolanda Segura. She was twenty-five, from Guatemala. The Stephenses had fired her recently for being lazy, but that wasn't what she told her boyfriend, Zohelin Diaz, also twenty-five and from Guatemala. She said that she had quit because Bill Stephens kept making passes at her and had tried to rape her.

"It was a ridiculous lie," Holmes says. "The Stephenses were happily married, with a new baby boy. Moreover, the housekeeper weighed over three hundred pounds. She wasn't someone most men would hit on." He shrugs. "The police said it was a matter of Latino jealousy. I wouldn't want to characterize anyone's motives in a case like this, but it was hard to argue against it."

Segura and Diaz were arrested south of San Francisco, at a motel in Daly City, after a clerk at the motel recognized photos of them that were shown on TV. Segura was convicted of manslaughter for her role in the Stephenses' murders and sentenced to six years in prison. Diaz was sentenced to life in prison and subsequently killed himself while incarcerated.

The one positive was that the infant boy was reclaimed by the teenage mother who had given him up for adoption. During her pregnancy, seventeen-year-old Tracy Medeiros stayed at a home for teenage mothers in Northern California. There she met the Stephenses, who desperately wanted to adopt a baby. Medeiros, in turn, wanted her son to enjoy a better life than she could provide, so she agreed to let them have him. The Stephenses were present for the birth, and all three adults collectively chose the baby's name—Travis. A year later, when Medeiros was notified that Travis's adoptive parents had been murdered, her son's safe, secure future suddenly vanished.

"I thought, I love him," Medeiros decided. "I want him to be with me."

She was living with her mother in Massachusetts and working at a state hospital for the mentally ill. She successfully applied to regain custody and arranged child care so that she could continue to work.

"It was a senseless tragedy," Holmes says, "but at least there was a good outcome for the baby. That was something."

WORST OF ALL

When I read the file on Tammy Vincent, my initial reaction was that the case was too heinous to include in this book. Indeed, when I mentioned it to Holmes, he said, "In terms of what the victim went through, this was the most gruesome homicide I ever dealt with. The Trailside Killer was evil, and his victims experienced awful deaths, but I don't think any of them experienced the trials and tribulations that Tammy did."

Ultimately, I decided that it was too important to omit. When the unidentified body of seventeen-year-old Tammy Vincent was found on a beach in Tiburon in September 1979, Holmes was still in the early portion of his career as a death investigator. When she finally was identified, it was 2007 and he was in his third term as coroner of Marin County.

"In the end we knew the story," he says, "but in the beginning, of course, we did not."

In the end, what Holmes and others learned was that Tammy had been brought to California from Washington State, where she had been working in a brothel. Her employers not only intended to kill her but wanted to send a message to others of what would happen if they were crossed. In all likelihood, two men were involved, although this isn't known for certain. What is known is that her assailants showed her no mercy.

The area where Tammy was taken looks much different today than it did in 1979. Today it's a lush green meadow known as Blackie's Pasture. It features the life-sized sculpture of a swaybacked horse named Blackie who stood there, day after day in the same spot, for more than two decades. In 1979, however, it was a sandy beach with several dunes and a row of trees that blocked most of the beach from the roadway. A gravel pathway ran through the dunes from the street and connected near the water to a paved pathway that ran along the bay.

Long after dark, Tammy's assailants led her down the gravel pathway to the middle of the beach, then knocked her to the ground. Holmes was the investigator who responded to the scene, and he found her blood on the pathway, so he knew where she fell. In addition, there were pieces of gravel embedded in one of her cheeks, indicating that she landed face-first.

Much more blood was found ten feet away, in grayish-white sand, surrounded by all sorts of footprints, none distinct enough to provide any clues. Tammy either ran or staggered to this spot, where she was stabbed forty-three times. In newspaper accounts the weapon was described as an ice pick, but it actually was an awl with a red handle and a spike. Holmes knew this, as did the police, because it was left at the scene. Obviously, whoever killed her didn't care that it was found.

Also left at the scene were two cans of acetone, one empty and one open. A receipt for the awl and acetone was nearby and indicated that the items had been purchased the night before from a Woolworth's store in San Francisco. Police tracked down the salesclerk, who remembered the buyer. He was described as a white man wearing a white leisure suit. With him was a teenage girl, about five foot six and 125 pounds, with light brown hair that was tightly curled—an apt description of Tammy Vincent. The man bought acetone—a colorless, flammable liquid found in nail polish remover and paint thinner—enamel paint, and an awl, the clerk said.

Tammy's stabs wounds, while numerous, weren't deep, and she managed to get up and stumble several feet. That was when her assailants doused her with acetone and set her on fire with a cigarette lighter. A witness reported seeing a bonfire on the beach shortly after 3 A.M., then a van that sped away.

The fire burned off most of Tammy's clothing on one side of her body, all the hair on her head, and one side of her face. She was still alive, however, and even ran ten yards before collapsing. At that point she was shot once in the head, execution-style.

A jogger discovered her body at daybreak. Fortunately, the jogger came from the opposite direction and didn't contaminate the scene. The awl was lying in the sand with fresh blood on its tip, and the solvent containers were near it, along with the lighter. Police tested each item for fingerprints, but only found two partials on one paint can that weren't sufficient for identification.

What was left of Tammy's clothing was parts of a black blouse, yellow halter top, and tan jeans. Also found were her shoes—high-heeled and Italian made.

The three people who were there the morning Tammy's body was found—Holmes and two detectives from the Tiburon Police Department, John Kim and Rich Dunn—had visceral reactions upon seeing her body. It was that horrific.

Kim and Dunn worked night and day on the case. For Kim, it would lead to his own death. He was young but somewhat overweight, and one night while reviewing the evidence again he had a heart attack and died.

Over the next two months, police checked hundreds of leads, but none of them panned out. When Tammy Vincent's body was buried, her identity was still unknown.

In many counties, an indigent person is cremated, meeting the state constitutional requirement that if someone dies and no one can be held responsible for dealing with his or her remains, then the county where the body is found has to provide a minimal disposition. This wasn't the practice in Marin County, however.

"We always felt that if you cremate them, there's no going back," Holmes says. "For a little more expense, if you work with the right cemeteries, you can inter somebody so that if you need to exhume the body one day because of new evidence that has come to light, you can."

In Tammy's case, and others, the coroner's office paid the cemetery a nominal fee for a simple wooden casket and burial. The decedent's body was put in a plastic-zippered body bag and placed in the casket, which was then laid in a four-sided concrete grave liner with a concrete lid. There wasn't a bottom because the county couldn't afford interment in a concrete vault, which meant that water could seep into the body bag from below and break down bones, making it more difficult to get a good DNA sample. The person's probable identity needed to be established first, however, before a DNA test could confirm it.

Instead of a headstone, there was a bronze medallion, set in the ground, with a number on it. The cemetery had a map showing where every grave was, and in the section of the cemetery reserved for county burials there was a record of each one, indicating that John Doe #6-85 was buried in grave #19, for example.

At the time that Tammy Vincent's body was found, Holmes took numerous swabs and also pubic hair samples (since all of the hair on her head had been burned away, he couldn't take samples there). He sent everything he had to the Department of Justice lab to be analyzed, but because this was before DNA testing was well established, relatively little was learned. When the samples were returned to him, Holmes filed them.

Twenty-two years later, in 2001, the Marin County Sheriff's Office, at the request of the Tiburon police chief, reopened the case. With all of the advances that had been made in DNA analysis during the previous two decades, there was new hope that Tammy's body and the bodies of other John and Jane Does could be identified. Holmes provided Tammy's pubic hair samples to the sheriff's office, which in turn submitted them to the Department of Justice lab for new testing. Ironically, the breakthrough in Tammy's case, when it came, was the direct result of a series of murders in another state that had nothing to do with her murder.

"That never happened before or since," Holmes says, "but it happened with her."

In 2003, researchers at the University of North Texas were commissioned to build a large database of DNA samples from suspected victims of a serial killer in Washington State. The killer, named Gary Ridgway, picked up young women—primarily prostitutes—near Sea-Tac Airport, a major transportation hub for drug and sex trafficking. After he killed them, Ridgway left their bodies near the Green River, which runs south of Seattle. So many young women and girls were reported missing in the 1980s and 1990s that police investigators decided a database was needed to identify them all. In the course of building it, researchers input every missing-person report they could find, including that of seventeen-year-old Tammy Vincent.

Tammy was a headstrong girl from Okanogan County, Washington—about 140 miles northeast of Seattle. She ran away from home multiple times, often disappearing for weeks at a stretch. In 1980, her mother filed a missing-persons report that included oral swabs from herself and her other daughter. It contained a significant mistake, however. Tammy's mother didn't know the date when her daughter went missing, and estimated that it was sometime earlier that year. In fact, Tammy already had been dead six months by the time the report was submitted.

It was standard operating procedure that whenever the Marin County Coroner's Office had a body it couldn't identify, the investigator issued a found-unidentified report. This is the opposite of a missing-persons report in that it notes that a body has been found without identification. Public and private investigators who are looking for a missing person go through these reports, of which there are thousands, to see if there is a match.

Holmes doesn't know how his found-unidentified report from Marin County ended up in the database that was created for Washington State, but it did. Because of the discrepancy in dates, however, his report wasn't matched with the report filed by Tammy's mother. After the database was developed, it automatically generated matches every Monday morning. Since Tammy was listed as dead half a year before she was listed as missing, her DNA wasn't compared with her mother's and sister's DNA.

"It was another part of Tammy's unfortunate life," Holmes says.

In 2007, he received an unexpected phone call. University of North Texas researchers told him that they had found a match for Jane Doe #4-79 from Marin County. A report was run from the database in which dates were ignored, and that's when Tammy Vincent's name came up.

Researchers thought initially that Tammy might be another victim of the Green River Killer, aka Gary Ridgway. She was from the same general area, and involved in prostitution, although the fact that she died in Marin was perplexing. In November 2001, Ridgway had been caught, and as part of a negotiated deal he pled guilty to forty-eight counts of murder, including forty-two of the forty-nine Green River victims. He showed police where the bodies were buried in exchange for the death penalty being waived. He never admitted to Tammy Vincent's murder, however, and in retrospect almost certainly had nothing to do with it. Nevertheless, he was the reason why she was able to be identified, because of the database that was created to identify his victims. Since then, the database has been expanded and is part of the University of North Texas's national Center for Human Identification (UNTCHI).

Once Holmes learned of the match, he notified Tammy's mother and sister. They were overwhelmed by the news that after nearly thirty years Tammy's remains had been identified. He asked them what they wanted him to do, and Tammy's mother said she wanted the remains exhumed and cremated, and Tammy's ashes returned to her. This was done.

As for Tammy's killer, the most likely suspects were members of the Gypsy Jokers, a motorcycle gang that reportedly controlled prostitution, drugs, and guns in the Seattle-Tacoma area, although their network was much broader. Tammy was working in a scam house run by the Jokers. Seattle cops told Holmes how the houses worked.

"Men traveling on business were lured by young women to come to a residence for sex, not with them but with another woman," Holmes says. "At the front door the first woman left and the john talked with someone else. They discussed prices, he paid, then he was sent down a hallway to the door of a room where he was supposed to get laid, only the door led outside where a big bouncer was waiting and told the guy to get lost. If the guy protested, the bouncer said threateningly, 'What are you going to do about it?' The answer was nothing because no one wanted to mess with the Jokers. They're the only motorcycle gang that Hells Angels are afraid of—at least, that's what I've been told."

Police raided a residence where Tammy was staying, rounded up her and others, and offered her immunity if she testified against five men who were accused of forcing women and girls into prostitution. Tammy was young and afraid. She agreed but never showed up for the trial. According to one report, she was last seen getting into a silver Lincoln Continental that was owned by one of the suspects in the case. It was speculated later that she was driven to California and put to work at the Palace Theater in the North Beach section of San Francisco, although this wasn't proved.

The defendants in Seattle were convicted of promoting prostitution and sentenced to prison terms ranging from five to eight years. No other charges pertaining to Tammy Vincent were filed against them.

In 2007, after Tammy's identity had been established, Marin

County Sheriff Robert Doyle expressed optimism that her murderer would be found. It was only a matter of time.

"I'm confident we'll ultimately be able to make some arrests and bring those responsible to justice," he told the media.

Ken Holmes wasn't so certain, and he turned out to be right. To date, no one has been charged with Tammy's murder and there have been no further developments. From the point of view of the coroner's office, the case is closed. Tammy's remains were identified, exhumed, and returned to her family, and the cause and manner of her death were determined.

From the point of view of law enforcement, it's still open, her killer or killers still free or incarcerated for other crimes but not for her murder. The case grows colder every day.

CHAPTER 08

THE TRAILSIDE KILLER

When Edna Kane's body was found on Mount Tamalpais in Marin County in the summer of 1979, naked except for socks, it was clearly a homicide. The forty-four-year-old married bank executive had been raped, stabbed repeatedly in the chest, and shot in the head while she was kneeling, execution-style, perhaps pleading for her life. Most of her clothes, along with her glasses and a black waist pouch containing her wallet, were missing. Searchers discovered Edna's body the following day after she failed to return home from a hike. Her husband and friends had gone looking for her, concerned that she had fallen and was in some inaccessible place. When they couldn't find her, they called the police. No one could explain why she had been attacked. It seemed most likely to be a crime of opportunity—a woman on her own in a remote area—although that was even more puzzling. Most murderer-rapists operate in cities, where they blend in with the crowd, can find isolated victims easily, and are able to disappear without being seen. What was a murderer-rapist doing on the mountain? No one had an answer, nor were any weapons found.

The following spring, there was a second murder on Mount Tam. Twenty-three-year-old Barbara Schwartz, known as "the bread lady" because she sold homemade breads and cakes to local restaurants, had been hiking with her dog, a black Lab, when she was attacked and stabbed twelve times in the chest while kneeling in the dirt. Bill Thomas had been the coroner's investigator in Edna's death, and Ken Holmes was the investigator for Barbara's. This time there was a witness, a female hiker who had seen the attack through the trees. She ran for help while Barbara's dog barked, and police responded as quickly as possible. They weren't quick enough, though, as the assailant managed to escape.

As with Edna's murder, the police couldn't find a weapon, but now they had a general description of the suspect. Unfortunately, it proved to be erroneous in almost every way, hindering rather than helping the investigation. While authorities focused on finding a thin, athletic-looking man in his twenties with a hawk nose and dark hair that possibly was pulled back in a ponytail, they ignored the fact that other hikers said they had seen an older man in the area who was alone, balding, had glasses, and was wearing a raincoat even though it hadn't been raining.

Wanting to see the scene again, which was still cordoned off by police tape, Holmes returned later that day, after dark, and found a pair of glasses off the trail where the murder had taken place. They were obscured by leaves and twigs, and he saw them only because the lenses were reflected in the beam of his flashlight. During daylight everyone had missed them. A fine splatter of blood was on the outside of the lenses, and the Department of Justice laboratory subsequently confirmed that the blood was Barbara Schwartz's. When the glasses were shown to an optometrist, he said that it was an unusual prescription. One eye was markedly different from the other, and the wearer had to be nearly blind without the correction. It seemed like an important clue, but the police didn't pursue it aggressively. They were still focused on the witness's description, and she hadn't mentioned glasses.

Several days later, some teens found a ten-inch boning knife three hundred yards from the crime scene. The knife had dried blood on it and turned out to have been purchased at a chain grocery store, although police couldn't determine the specific store. In the course of reporting the story, a female TV reporter inexplicably handled the knife and obliterated any fingerprints that might have been on it. Other than being the probable murder weapon, the knife now had little value.

MORE MURDERS

The third murder on Mount Tam occurred seven months after the second and, for me, was personal. Anne Alderson, twenty-six, was my sister's best friend and had vacationed with my family when she was younger. She was smart, pretty, independent, and loved animals and the outdoors. After graduating from UC Davis with a master's degree in animal husbandry, en route to becoming a veterinarian, she joined the Peace Corps and spent two years in Bogotá, Colombia, studying animal genetics. She had just returned to her parents' home in Marin County the week before, and in all likelihood didn't know that there had been two murders on Mount Tam. A caretaker at the park said later that he saw her sitting alone in the five-thousand-seat amphitheater watching the sunset. He was tempted to warn her but decided that she might not want to be disturbed. He also said that earlier in the day he had seen a lone man, about fifty years of age, in the area, but he didn't match the killer's description on posters that were being circulated.

Like Edna Kane, Anne was shot in the head with a single bullet from a .38-caliber pistol, and probably was in a kneeling position at the time. She was fully clothed, but apparently had been allowed to get dressed after being raped. Her body was a quarter mile from the outdoor theater, on Telephone Line Trail. Holmes was glad that he wasn't on duty when her body was found. He knew Anne's parents, as did I. Both were physicians—Bob Alderson was our family's doctor—whom Holmes sometimes asked to sign off on death certificates.

Over the next year, there would be four more murders on Mount

Tam, as well as two murders and an attempted murder in the Santa Cruz Mountains south of San Francisco, all committed by the same person. In addition, the day after Anne Alderson's body was discovered, police responded to the scene of a double homicide at a residence near the foot of Mount Tam. The victims—seventy-four-year-old Helen McDermand and her forty-year-old son Edwin—had been shot by someone who left an angry handwritten note that made the killer seem like a good suspect for the trailside slayings, too.

Police had come to the house in response to a neighbor's request for a wellness check. The neighbor hadn't seen the occupants in more than a day, yet lights were on in the home.

Off the garage, beneath the house, was a single room with a mattress on the floor. The door was locked and police had to force entry. Attached to the inner door handle was a note.

"Dear Shitheels: By the time you read this you will be <u>way</u> too late. The next time you see me it will be on the news or on a slab. Either way I will still look the same, ugly." It was signed, "Mr. Hate."

The room was dirty and had an acrid smell. There were spent .38-caliber casings, live rounds of .22-caliber ammunition, and ankle holsters for a handgun and a knife.

When Holmes arrived, he saw that Edwin had been shot multiple times and his mother once. Edwin's body was in a hallway to the left of the living room, and Mrs. McDermand's body was lying on a bed, covered by a blanket. The house was cluttered and disheveled, but there were no obvious signs of a struggle. The only things out of place were the spent casings from the killer's weapon that were scattered across the floor.

Holmes told the police that the McDermands had been dead three or four days. That meant the murderer could be far away by now, but at least there was an obvious suspect. Mark McDermand, thirty-five, lived with his mother and brother, in the basement room. He had been working as a short-order cook at Denny's and was wanted on a no-bail warrant for embezzling money from a local 7-Eleven store.

McDermand didn't have anyplace to go, as it turned out, and remained in the area, in part to be able to follow news coverage of his crimes. He took to writing letters to local newspapers and the Marin County Sheriff's Office in which he claimed responsibility for his mother's and brother's deaths. A handwriting expert said that the person who wrote the letters was the same person who wrote the note that was tacked to the basement door.

McDermand said in the letters that he "was as dangerous as a coral snake in a sleeping bag" and never would be caught alive. Nevertheless, the six-foot-four, 190-pound killer surrendered to police eleven days later without incident in front of an International House of Pancakes restaurant in neighboring Solano County. He was sitting on the hood of his car with his hands clasped in his lap—a pose that had been arranged in advance by police in a phone call with him. He had a loaded .38-caliber revolver on his right hip, and inside his car, a yellow Chevy without license plates that police had been searching for, were a .22-caliber pistol, twelve-gauge shotgun, and ammunition. There was also a metal box filled with hypodermic syringes and vials of insulin. McDermand was a diabetic.

He said he wrote the letters not for publicity but to correct erroneous information about his case, including speculation that he was responsible for the Mount Tam slayings. Those were committed by somebody else, he said. His motive for killing his mother and brother was that his mother was an invalid who wouldn't live much longer and his brother had schizophrenia and he didn't know what would happen to him after their mother died. Inasmuch as McDermand confessed freely and didn't match the description police had of the Tam suspect, the police tended to believe him. A jury found him guilty of two counts of first-degree murder, and he was sentenced to death.

Any further thoughts that he might be the Trailside Killer, as the murderer on Mount Tamalpais was being called, were dispelled when none of McDermand's weapons matched the bullets used on Edna Kane and Anne Alderson. Moreover, even after McDermand was jailed, the murders continued. Mount Tam became a place for everyone—and especially single women—to avoid.

ACCIDENTAL DISCOVERY

On November 29, 1980, while searching for two women who didn't know each other and were reported missing after getting separated from friends on hikes in two different parks, police chanced upon the decomposing remains of two other people. Both had been shot in the head and then stashed in a small hideaway off one of Mount Tam's trails. Once again Ken Holmes was called to the scene, only this time there were different challenges.

"The toughest part of a decomposed body," Holmes says, "is determining how long the person has been dead. The more time you're dealing with, the harder it becomes. The victim's gender can be determined fairly easily. The collarbone, jawbone, and area behind the ear are more prominent in men than women. Women who have birthed children can be identified by changes in the pelvic area."

The victim's age can be determined by analyzing the cellular structure of the center of bones. Throughout a person's life, bones "remodel"—that is, they make new, microscopic tubes called osteons, which contain blood vessels. The older a person is, the smaller his or her osteons are. Additionally, the number of osteon fragments is greater as new osteons form and disrupt older ones. Younger adults have fewer and larger osteons.

As for determining the cause of death, this depends on the condition of the body. Knifings and strangulations are the hardest, gunshots the easiest. In some stabbing cases a bone is nicked, while in cases where someone is strangled there may be damage to the neck bones. With gunshots, sometimes the bullet is inside the body.

In this instance, the coroner's office was spared a lot of work because the two victims were able to be identified from dental charts in their missing-persons reports. One was nineteen-year-old Richard

Stowers. He was on the verge of graduating from radioman's school at a Coast Guard training center near Petaluma, and was considered AWOL after failing to show up for a class. The other victim was his fiancée, eighteen-year-old Cynthia Moreland, vice president of her senior class at Rancho Cotate High School. She had been one of two honors students selected to speak at commencement ceremonies and was a finalist for the school's homecoming queen. She also had been selected as a varsity song leader her senior year, but dropped out in order to work a part-time job at the training center's commissary. That was where she and Richard met. He was scheduled to begin working soon at the Coast Guard Communication Station in Point Reyes when he disappeared. Both had been missing for six weeks.

Police might not have come across the remains of Richard Stowers and Cynthia Moreland if they hadn't already been looking for the two women who were missing more recently. One woman, twenty-two-year-old Diane O'Connell, had been hiking with friends on Mount Tam when she slipped away, unnoticed. Meanwhile, twenty-three-year-old Shauna May was supposed to meet friends in nearby Point Reyes National Seashore the previous day, but never showed up. Their bodies were found on the same Sky Camp Trail on Mount Tam, in a heavily wooded area, within minutes after searchers discovered the skeletons of Richard and Cynthia. Both Diane and Shauna were nude, lying side by side, and, as their autopsies subsequently revealed, had been raped. Their clothing and backpacks were next to them, and there were no signs of a struggle. Diane had been shot once in the head and Shauna twice. Police speculated that the killer intercepted one of the women in her hike and the other woman happened to come along right afterward. Police also speculated that the recent killings were intended to draw attention to the area so that the earlier deaths, which occurred within a few days of Anne Alderson's murder and only fifteen feet away, could be found. Holmes didn't believe this, because if Diane's and Shauna's bodies had been discovered first, the search probably would have ended there.

After learning that a man and a woman had been killed, and two women one right after the other, police began to rethink the notion that the murders were committed by a single person. The fact that at least one victim—Shauna May—supposedly had been hiking in Point Reyes, not Mount Tam, and was killed, along with Diane O'Connell, six weeks after the second set of deaths raised the horrifying possibility that there were two predators roaming the area. A ballistics test confirmed that the same gun used in Anne Alderson's murder also was used to shoot Diane and Shauna, however, which reaffirmed the one-killer theory. It was a small measure of comfort, at best.

THE END

The discovery of four bodies in one day—two by happenstance—raised the possibility that there were more dead bodies on the mountain that hadn't been found yet. An aerial search team was called in. Using infrared cameras that detected contrasts in temperature, the team photographed the mountain with special sensitized film that was capable of shooting through foliage and soil. Even dead deer registered on the film. To everyone's relief, no other unexpected remains were detected.

Hikers in both parks were warned not to hike alone, although being with another person hadn't helped Richard Stowers and Cynthia Moreland. It also wouldn't prove to help two people who were hiking in a state park near Santa Cruz, roughly eighty miles south of San Francisco, five months later.

On March 29, 1981, Ellen Hansen and Stephen Haertle were accosted by a man brandishing a gun. The man told Ellen that he was going to rape her. Haertle begged him to let them go instead. When Ellen refused to cooperate, the killer shot her twice in the head and once in the shoulder. All three shots were at point-blank range. Then he turned the gun on Haertle and shot him in the neck before fleeing.

Haertle survived and was able to crawl for help. In describing the killer, he said the man had crooked yellow teeth, was about fifty, under six feet, roughly 170 pounds, wore glasses, and was balding.

Once this description was released, other hikers in the area told police that they had seen a man resembling the gunman get in or out of a red, late-model, foreign-made car. The car, his age, and the fact that he was alone attracted their attention.

A month later, a San Jose man reported that his girlfriend, Heather Scaggs, twenty, was missing. He said that she was last seen en route to buy a car from a man named David Carpenter. He worked in the same print shop she did and, apparently, had told her specifically to come alone to pick up the car. When police questioned Carpenter, they noticed immediately his strong resemblance to the man Stephen Haertle had described. A small red Fiat with a bent tailpipe was in his driveway.

Carpenter, fifty-one, lived with his elderly parents in San Francisco. He was a habitual sex offender but hadn't shown up in a records check that police conducted of released inmates because of a technicality. When Haertle identified Carpenter in a lineup as the man who killed Ellen Hansen and almost killed him, officers made the arrest. In Carpenter's car were books of Bay Area hiking trails and trail maps.

Ten days later, the remains of Heather Scaggs were found by hikers in Big Basin Redwood State Park in Santa Cruz County. She had been executed with the same .38-caliber gun that was used to shoot Ellen Hansen and Stephen Haertle. She had been raped as well, and the killer had tried to hide her body under a pile of brush. Her identity was confirmed through dental records.

In investigating Carpenter, police linked him to another death. The partial remains of a seventeen-year-old high school student named Anna Menjivar were found June 4, 1980, in Castle Rock State Park in the Santa Cruz Mountains. Her murder had seemed like an isolated killing until police learned that she was a friend of David Carpenter and often let him drive her home from work.

Once authorities in Marin heard about the Santa Cruz killings, they zeroed in on David Carpenter as the prime suspect for the Mount Tam murders. Ballistic tests from the two slayings in Santa Cruz tied Carpenter to five of the Marin County homicides, and he was charged with the deaths of Anne Alderson, Diane O'Connell, Shauna May, Cynthia Moreland, and Richard Stowers.

To Holmes's frustration and dismay, Barbara Schwartz wasn't named as one of the Marin victims. He believed that the glasses he found with Barbara's blood on them were Carpenter's. Despite the unusual prescription, however, and the fact that Barbara and Carpenter reportedly had the same eye doctor, which may have been how he targeted her, police decided that there wasn't enough evidence to charge Carpenter with her murder, or Edna Kane's, either. The view of law enforcement and the district attorney's office was that it didn't matter whether Carpenter was convicted of additional murders. He would receive the death penalty regardless, so there wasn't a compelling reason to spend time collecting or presenting evidence on other homicides he committed.

In two separate trials, both held in Southern California because of the publicity that the cases attracted, Carpenter was charged with first-degree murder and rape. In 1984 he was convicted of murdering Ellen Hansen and Heather Scaggs in Santa Cruz, plus the attempted murder of Steve Haertle. In 1988 he was convicted of murdering Anne Alderson, Diane O'Connell, Shauna May, Cynthia Moreland, and Richard Stowers in Marin County. Throughout both trials Carpenter maintained his innocence.

At the conclusion of the first trial, which took place in Los Angeles, Carpenter was sentenced to die in San Quentin's gas chamber. Judge Dion Morrow told the court, "The defendant's entire life has been a continuous expression of violence and force almost beyond exception. I must conclude with the prosecution that if ever there was a case appropriate for the death penalty, this is it."

The second trial, in San Diego, resulted in a similar verdict. Since then Carpenter has submitted multiple appeals, all denied.

From time to time, Holmes has toyed with the idea of trying to talk to Carpenter to see if he might tell him anything different from what he told police when they arrested him, or the judges and juries when he was being tried, or the appeals board when he has sought a new trial. As one of the people who were intimately involved in the case and have been haunted by it, Holmes continues to seek answers that he knows, realistically, he'll never find. Carpenter has never admitted guilt so it's unlikely that he would agree to talk to Holmes or tell him something that he hasn't told anyone else.

Still, it's tempting to think that a man might confess with the end of his life approaching. And it is approaching. Born in 1930, Carpenter is now in his mid-eighties. At last report, he was the oldest inmate at San Quentin.

CHAPTER 09

INSIDE SAN QUENTIN

San Quentin Prison owes its existence, in large part, to the California Gold Rush. Many fortune seekers were rough and unsavory as well as greedy, and their frequent fights were a problem for communities in northern portions of the state. County jails couldn't hold them all, and the need for a state prison became increasingly clear.

In 1852, a large wooden prison ship named the *Waban* anchored in San Francisco Bay. During the day, inmates were ferried from the ship to Point San Quentin, an impressive promontory in Marin County that was named after a Miwok Indian chief. The state of California had purchased twenty acres of land there several years earlier, and the convicts were put to work building a prison. Within a few months the first cell block was completed and San Quentin opened.

Today San Quentin is twenty times its original size and one of the largest penitentiaries in the United States. One thousand correctional officers, four hundred medical and mental health staff, and several hundred administrators preside over nearly five thousand inmates while contending with facilities that have deteriorated considerably and are out of date. In fact, a court-ordered report in 2005 determined that San Quentin was "old, antiquated, dirty, poorly staffed, poorly maintained with inadequate medical space and equipment, and overcrowded," and little has changed since the report came out.

The prison consists primarily of four medium-security cell blocks, which are known by their cardinal coordinates: North, South, East, and West. In addition, there is a smaller medium-security block called the North Segregation unit ("North Seg"), as well as a medium-security dormitory facility called H unit and a maximum-security cell block called the Adjustment Center.

Inmates at the Adjustment Center have the tightest security and the fewest privileges. It's where every new inmate is placed initially and where the worst inmates remain indefinitely. By worst one might think that this refers to those individuals who have committed the worst crimes, the serial killers and murderer-rapists. In fact, though, being assigned to the Adjustment Center—as in attitude adjustment—is based on an inmate's behavior while incarcerated. Inmates who can't be managed elsewhere are placed there, as well as inmates who are being punished for an offense or an assault. One psychologist at the prison told me, "It's for the baddest of the bad and the sickest of the sick." Correctional officers—referred to as COs, not guards—don't have the ability to let themselves out. They are locked in with California's most dangerous criminals and can exit at the end of their shift only after several gates, manned by other COs behind bulletproof glass, are opened for them.

COs must be alert at all times. The slightest distraction can result in death—and not just for a CO. An inmate who doesn't take advantage of an opportunity to assault a CO can be punished by other inmates. COs in the Adjustment Center wear face shields and stab-proof vests, and inmates who have a penchant for kicking prison staff are shackled in leg restraints when they are being moved outside their cell for one hour per day of exercise in a solitary yard or for a solitary shower every other day.

California's only gas chamber is at San Quentin, and all of the state's male death row inmates are housed at the prison. While the term "death row" conjures images of a specific area that is devoted to those who are awaiting execution, death row is a classification rather than a location. Death row inmates are housed in three separate sections—the Adjustment Center, North Seg, and East Block.

North Seg was the original death row. It's six stories high and has sixty-eight cells. The elevator goes to only two floors—one and six. The most compliant inmates are housed there now, and are let out of their cells for five hours a day. In contrast to the Adjustment Center, they can walk the tier freely and exercise together in a recreation yard, making North Seg highly desired.

Death row inmates are classified as grade A or B. Grade A inmates tend to follow the rules, while grade B inmates don't. East Block ("E Block") has only grade A inmates, and the majority of condemned men—more than five hundred—are here. Just because they're classified grade A doesn't mean that they are in any way docile, however. Most of them have nothing to lose—and maybe something to gain—by hurting someone. Demonstrating toughness through violence is the way that inmates achieve respect among peers. It's also the way that they survive in prison. Inherent is the message to fellow inmates: Don't mess with me.

E Block is five stories high, and each cell is four and a half feet wide, ten and a half feet long, and seven and a half feet high. At forty-eight square feet, it's just big enough for a twin bed and a toilet. Like their counterparts in the Adjustment Center, correctional officers in E Block wear face guards and stab-proof vests. They're not worried too much about being shot, because it's difficult for inmates to get access to a gun, but weapons that cut, puncture, strangle, or bludgeon can be fashioned out of almost anything.

One of the few areas of the prison open to the public is a small museum that includes a weapons room. On display are daggers, knives, chains, and garrotes fashioned from things like bolts and rulers. Heavy-gauge wire, filed to a point on the concrete floor of a cell and stuck in a whisk broom, makes a lethal weapon, and there are examples in the museum. Paper clips, copper wire from a TV antenna, and heavy-duty staples that have been pried from cardboard boxes can be made into darts, then slingshot with elastic bands that have been removed from socks or underwear. Alternatively, they can be launched from a makeshift blowgun in which tightly wound newspaper has been hardened with dried oatmeal. Word of an attack is shared with other inmates by attaching notes to dental floss and shooting them across cell block floors. It's called "fishing."

Inmates are subject to frequent searches, and officers check inmate cells regularly for weapons. That leaves body cavities as the primary place where knives and razor blades are hidden.

"Sticking a sharp object up your ass seems crazy," Holmes says, "but inmates generally don't care. It's more important to them that they have a weapon they can pull out in the moment to attack somebody or defend themselves than that their insides get cut up from storing it."

During his time in the coroner's office, Holmes accumulated his own collection of weapons that were found on San Quentin inmates during autopsies. One man used a candle to melt both ends of a toothbrush. At the end with bristles he inserted a pin, while at the other end he inserted a razor blade. After the plastic hardened, he had a dual weapon. He could poke someone in the eye with the pin to blind him, then cut his throat. The weapon was found in the inmate's rectum after he died.

INITIAL VISIT

The first time Holmes was called to the prison was at night, when all of the inmates were in their cells. Many of the inmates don't sleep, though, so it's noisy. The fact that the prison is made of concrete and metal makes it worse because every sound reverberates off the walls.

"If you're on one tier, and anybody coughs or farts or sneezes on any other tier, above or below you, it echoes all over the place," Holmes says. "It's also cold, because it's concrete, and a lot of the windows are broken out, so the wind rushes in off the bay. Even in summer, it's cold."

A correctional officer walked with Holmes on the ground floor of one of the cell blocks. The tiers above them formed an overhang of eight to ten feet on each side, and the CO, who was on the inside, closest to inmate cells, told Holmes to stay on his shoulder and not drift out near the end of the overhang.

"Why is that?" Holmes asked.

The CO was matter-of-fact. "Because you'll be hit with piss and shit."

He then explained that inmates use mirrors to detect the shadows of people passing below. Anytime they see a shadow, they hurl a container of stored, fermented urine or feces, trying to hit whoever is down there. With correctional officers, inmates aim for the face, knowing that if nothing else they are splattering the officer's protective shield. It's called "gassing."

Holmes had never been inside a prison before and didn't know what to expect. Several times when he went to San Quentin and walked the tiers, he heard a splat behind him. He always managed to avoid being hit with thrown excrement, but it was unnerving. So were the catcalls.

"You're walking on the tiers, past inmate cells, and you're fresh meat," he says. "Inmates are saying, 'Hey, baby, let me bend you over,' or, 'You want to suck on this?' all the time. They can say anything they want because there's nothing anybody can do about it. They're already in jail. They may lose one of their privileges, but they don't care."

One of his first cases at San Quentin concerned a twenty-six-year-old inmate named Concelio Carrasco. He had been stabbed multiple times earlier in the day in one of the prison's exercise yards and taken by gurney to Neumiller Hospital, within the prison, where he was admitted without a pulse. Prison doctors were able to revive him, but his wounds proved to be fatal. At 12:35 A.M. he was pronounced dead and the coroner's office was called.

When Holmes examined Carrasco's body, he noted six knife wounds. He measured the length and circumference of each wound, as he had been trained to do, and recorded them on a chart. He also noted various tattoos. One, on Carrasco's left arm, consisted of the letters *EME*.

In the course of his investigation, Holmes learned that two weeks before he was killed, Carrasco had requested an appointment with prison medical staff to have the "EME" tattoo removed. The information was relevant because among San Quentin's many gang members are individuals affiliated with the Mexican Mafia, sometimes known as La Eme (Spanish for *M*). In this case, having the tattoo removed might have saved Carrasco's life by making him less of a target to members of other gangs in San Quentin, including La Nuestra Familia, the chief rival of the Mexican Mafia. Then again, it might have contributed to his death if other incarcerated members of the Mexican Mafia heard about his request. That was for prison investigators to pursue, however. Holmes's work ended after he confirmed a ruling of murder and issued the death certificate.

LEARNING HIS WAY AROUND

In the beginning, a correctional officer escorted Holmes from the first gate through an open courtyard into whichever cell block the decedent was in. Entering a cell block meant passing through an air walk and then a series of closed chambers, each chamber secured by locking steel gates and thick iron doors that were manned by other officers. There were at least two doors between anywhere and outside, and usually three or more. No door could be opened until the door behind it had closed with a loud bang. Each CO who manned a door looked through a peep hole to make sure that the person wanting in was authorized before the door was opened.

After a few years, Holmes had been at San Quentin often enough that most COs recognized him. When he got to the open yard between cell blocks, the CO escorting him stopped, pointed across the way to a chain-link fence with a gate that wasn't locked, and told him to go through the gate to the next cell block, where another CO would meet him. All of the inmates were locked up so no one was in the yard. Still, it was eerie, especially in the middle of the night when the shouts of angry, sleepless, and deeply disturbed men filled the air. Holmes would walk thirty feet into the yard, look around him, and start to think, what if? What if some guy did get out? Holmes would be a sitting duck.

"I was always armed when I arrived at the prison," he says, "but a person doesn't go into San Quentin with a weapon so I would check my gun at the front gate. I was never in danger, but I was never certain of that, either."

Florenzo Ramirez's death was typical of many others. The twenty-seven-year-old was stabbed in the prison's South Dining Hall with the right side of a pair of scissors. He was crying for help and trying to climb the security fence between Section 1 and Section 2 in the dining hall while another inmate, Daniel "Termite" Roberts, made repeated thrusts into his back. A third inmate stood close by with a smirk on his face, according to a correctional officer who was the first guard on the scene.

Roberts fled the dining hall as Ramirez was taken by gurney to Neumiller Hospital at the prison. He was then transferred to Marin General Hospital, where physicians pronounced him dead on arrival. Holmes examined him there, supine on a morgue table. Ramirez had multiple puncture wounds and lacerations across his shoulders, arms, and back. His muscular body also featured numerous tattoos. Holmes took seventeen photos of the wounds and tattoos, then Ramirez's body was removed to a local mortuary for autopsy. The medical cause of death was no surprise—traumatic injuries, including stab wounds. The manner wasn't a surprise, either—homicide.

Another time, early in Holmes's career, two inmates got into a fight with knives and one was killed. Holmes was called out to investigate and, as usual, brought his camera as well as his other equipment. The prison didn't have its own investigative unit at the time, and the officer in charge of the case asked Holmes if he would mind taking a few pictures of the assailant.

Wanting to be helpful, Holmes said okay, adding, "Does he have injuries?"

"Nothing serious," the officer said, "but both of them were wearing boxer shorts and his knees are all scraped up. I need pictures of them for my report."

The inmate was cuffed and flanked by two correctional officers. He stood while Holmes knelt in front of him and snapped photographs of his knees. All the while, Holmes had a foreboding feeling.

So many things can go wrong right now, he thought. He has just killed a guy, and here I am, on my knees at his knees, taking pictures and wondering what's going through his mind. He can raise one leg and hit me square in the forehead, or hit the camera and drive it right into my eye, just because he wants to. Thank God these two mountainous COs are here.

Inmates know the score—they can be executed only once. No matter what they do, the only recourse for officers is to write them up. This gives inmates considerable leverage, and they use it to full advantage. In this instance, the inmate had no interest in Holmes. Instead, he addressed the officers.

"Motherfucker deserved it. Won't be shooting off his mouth no more."

When Holmes got to his feet, he breathed a sigh of relief. He also knew that if a similar request was made of him again, he would think twice before he agreed to it.

GANG WARFARE

Gangs tend to operate in depressed areas, so one wouldn't expect them to be present in Marin. Yet the Marin County Civil Grand Jury noted in a 2011 report that numerous gangs, starting with the Norteños, Sureños, and Mexican Mafia, and moving on to smaller gangs such as the Young Hawgz, KUMI-415, Aryan Brotherhood, Crips, Bloods, and Zetas, exist in the county. The title of the report, "Gangs of Marin: A Tale of Two Counties," referred to the disparity between wealthy Marin, where "affluent citizens walk safe streets with lives largely insulated from the majority of criminal influences found in neighboring counties," and gangland Marin, where homicides, fights, and graffiti are more commonplace. According to the report, Marin's geographic isolation, overall affluence, and natural beauty serve to discourage gangs from taking hold. There are only three main routes into and out of the county—two by bridge and one by highway—and police can close these off quickly to prevent someone who commits a crime from escaping. The high cost of living has been a buffer because many gang members can't afford to live in the county. As for aesthetics, Marin County residents tend to be intolerant of the vehicles that often are favored by gang members: flashy cars and banged-up clunkers.

Offsetting these factors are others, though, that serve to foster gangs. The most notable one is the heavy use of drugs in the county. Much of the dealing, particularly of illegal drugs like heroin, cocaine, and methamphetamine, is done by gang members.

A second factor is that gang activity is high in surrounding counties, and there is spillover into Marin. "The same people who estimated Marin gang members in the hundreds," said the grand jury report, "estimated up to 1,000 in Richmond [Contra Costa County] and somewhere around 4,000 in Santa Rosa [Sonoma County]. That does not begin to account for other proximate gang regions like Vallejo, Napa, and Oakland." Each of those communities is only a half-hour drive from Marin County.

Last but not least is the fact that many gang members end up incarcerated at San Quentin. Kingpins can continue to run the gang from their cells, and those in "middle management," who are free and on the street, want to stay close enough to the kingpins to take and act on orders.

During Holmes's career, gang-related murders occurred outside San Quentin infrequently, if only because they weren't recognized as such unless both the decedent and assailant were multiple offenders who were known to local law enforcement. Witnesses rarely talked, so the primary way that gang membership was determined was by the person's tattoos, which constituted another part of Holmes's education. There was "X3" for the Sureños and "MS-13" for Mara Salvatrucha-13. A sombrero denoted membership in the Norteños while a shamrock symbolized the Aryan Brotherhood. There also were more universal tattoos such as "ANT," short for "Ain't No Talking," meaning no squealing to police, and a square composed of four dots with a dot in the middle—the four dots symbolizing prison walls and the inner dot representing the inmate.

The placement of tattoos had meaning as well. A gang-related tattoo on the neck, head, or face, for instance, indicated that the person was an upper-echelon member of the gang. The tattoo of a tear below one eye signified that the person had killed for the gang. The tattoo of a wristwatch without hands meant that the person was "doing time"—that is, serving a long prison sentence.

Gang-related tattoos and their placement have to be sanctioned, according to the grand jury report. Any tat that isn't authorized yet purports to symbolize "work" done for the gang might be removed with a blowtorch or flayed off the person's skin, the report said. Holmes never heard an instance where that happened, but it was a threat espoused by gang members in order to inhibit other members from inking false claims and also dissuade non–gang members from getting tattoos that made it appear as if they had the power of the gang behind them.

In recent years the number of homicides within San Quentin has decreased dramatically, for two reasons. Neither one has anything to do with improved security, better inmate control, upgraded facilities, or effective rehabilitation efforts. Instead, when Pelican Bay State Prison opened in 1989 in Crescent City, three hundred miles north of

Marin, many of San Quentin's worst gang members were transferred there. That reduced some of the inbred animosity that inmates at San Quentin had for one another, with the result that assaults declined. They weren't eliminated by any means, but they became less frequent.

The other reason for the drop in homicides was that drugs at San Quentin, always available, became even more prevalent. One might think that this would upset prison officials, but they had been aware of it for years and recognized that inmates who self-medicated were less volatile and easier for staff to handle. Stopping incoming drugs was virtually impossible, and officials knew that turning a partially blind eye was one way to keep the lid on a festering cauldron of pent-up anger.

"Over the years, I had many conversations with some of the guys in San Quentin's Investigations Service Unit," Holmes says. "We talked about all of the drugs that are there—those that are smuggled in from outside and the ones that inmates manufacture out of anything they can lay their hands on. ISU knows which guys are selling and which guys are using, and they're thankful because if it wasn't for the seller, who's getting cigarettes or sexual favors or whatever, those guys would be absolute animals. It might seem like they're that way now—and some of them are—but it would be so much worse. The assault rate would climb for everyone—inmates, COs, prison administrators, and medical staff. It's wrong to condone all of the drug dealing that goes on in the prison, but without it San Quentin would be on fire all the time."

Early in his career, Holmes examined dead inmates in their cells if that was where they were found. He searched the cell, always with a correctional officer so that there was a witness. They tipped the mattress, looking for cuts that indicated something was hidden, and flattened the pillow to determine whether anything was inside. Other than that, there wasn't much to check. Later, ISU did that and informed Holmes of anything that was found.

Executions were an exception. The coroner wasn't involved because there was no reason for an autopsy, much less an investigation. Prison doctors knew the exact time an inmate died, as well as the cause of death—electrocution or cyanide. For manner, Holmes wrote "judicial homicide" on the death certificate because the death was court ordered.

During Holmes's career, thirteen men were executed at San Quentin. Holmes never observed an execution, not because he was squeamish about it but because he didn't feel like he needed to. He had been inside the execution chamber and knew how the mechanisms worked because he was part of an oversight committee that was formed when capital punishment was reinstated in California in 1978. (Executions in the state ended in 1972 due to a decision by the California Supreme Court and were reinstated in 1978.)

Because San Quentin is antiquated, there has been talk from time to time of lifting the requirement that all male death row inmates be housed there (women on death row are housed at the Central California Women's Facility, in Chowchilla). Also, with capital punishment on hold, there is less of a reason to place condemned inmates in the only prison that has an execution chamber. Offsetting this is San Quentin's proximity to federal and state courts in San Francisco, as well as to metropolitan airports that enable attorneys to have relatively easy access to inmates in preparing challenges to convictions and sentences. In addition, supportive services to death row inmates and their families are established in the area.

Whether the policy will change in the future is unknown. One thing that won't change, though, is a prevailing sentiment that surprises people outside the system: many death row inmates are in favor of capital punishment. The reason isn't intuitive, but makes sense after it's explained. Condemned inmates receive special privileges, such as private cells and personal treatment, including the ability to request meetings with their attorney regarding their defense, meetings in which the state is required to pay the attorney's airfare and hotel costs. If capital punishment is overturned, then death row inmates will lose these privileges. More important, they no longer will be separated from the rest of the prison population. Even with many gang members transferred to Pelican Bay, those who remain at San Quentin tend to dominate. They are young, tough, and fearless, whereas most death row inmates are in their forties, fifties, or older. They may have been young when they were first incarcerated, but after spending decades on death row they have aged and are no match for young gang members. In 2012 and 2016, the last times a bill was on the California ballot to repeal capital punishment, psychologists at San Quentin worked extra shifts on election night in anticipation of a rash of suicide attempts if the bill passed. When it didn't, they were able to go home.

CHAPTER 10

AN UNNECESSARY DEATH

In 1986, a brouhaha developed in Marin over whether coroner's investigators should receive the same safety retirement benefits as police officers and firefighters. Because of the inherent dangers posed by their jobs, cops and firefighters received higher pensions than other county employees. Also, if they developed any serious health problems while they were working, such as heart disease or stomach cancer, it automatically was assumed that the problems were job related and fully covered. As the coroner, Dr. Jindrich argued that his investigators should be treated similarly. Like cops, they carried a gun. Like firefighters, they had to deal with the stress of being woken up in the middle of the night out of a deep sleep, jumping out of bed, and racing to a scene. In addition, every time an investigator went to San Quentin, his life was in danger because inmates often walked unshackled in open areas.

Even though there were only three investigators, county administrators didn't want to incur any added expenses, and Jindrich's request was denied. Moreover, he was told that if it was dangerous for investigators to go to San Quentin, they shouldn't go there. As a result, from that time forward all deaths at the prison were examined in an outside hospital or mortuary.

That was where Sammie Marshall's body was taken in June 1997 after he was forcibly removed from his cell by five correctional officers—three big men who went into the cell to get him, and two female COs who observed from outside. Holmes was the assistant coroner at the time, and one of his investigators, Don Cornish, was the one who observed Sammie's body at the mortuary. Cornish noted minor abrasions on Sammie's face, hands, and one knee, plus torn fingernails. In addition, clear liquid was exuding from Sammie's nose.

Holmes reviewed Cornish's written report as well as written reports that were filed by prison personnel afterward. According to the watch commander, when the three male correctional officers came to Sammie's cell, he barricaded himself inside and tied the door shut. The officers used OC spray (commonly known as pepper spray) to subdue him before they dragged him out. Shortly thereafter, Sammie had some sort of seizure and died. That didn't make sense to Holmes, and he asked prison officials for permission to interview selected staff.

It was a delicate situation, and Holmes knew that he had to be careful and not accuse anyone of wrongdoing. It was his responsibility to determine whether prison protocols were followed, however, and whether Sammie's death could have been avoided. To do that he needed to understand how a man with no obvious health problems died while being extricated from his cell.

Sammie Marshall was fifty-one years old, African-American, and big. He had been incarcerated at San Quentin nearly ten years, after being convicted of killing a prostitute in Los Angeles. Three psychiatrists had testified that he wasn't mentally competent, but the judge in the case overruled them. Prison psychologists subsequently diagnosed Sammie as "actively psychotic" and his condition as "chronic."

Holmes says, "Sammie was somewhat overweight, but still formidable. He only had a grade school education and was easily confused, sometimes paranoid. When prison officials told him that they were moving him to another cell, he didn't understand. He had been in the same cell a long time and didn't want to leave it. No one bothered to tell him why he was being moved."

Over the course of four days, Holmes was able to talk to all but one of the key participants at the prison and piece together the story. The one exception was a correctional officer who, Holmes was told, had been injured recently and no longer was at San Quentin.

Holmes explained at the beginning of each interview that his purpose was to gain more insight into the circumstances surrounding Sammie's death. The written reports described the actions of everyone, he said, but didn't include any spoken words, feelings, or impressions of the event as it unfolded. Also, the autopsy and toxicology reports didn't explain why Sammie died, and Holmes was attempting to substantiate or rule out the possibility that Sammie had a condition known as "excited delirium," in which a person becomes agitated, incoherent, hyperaggressive, and displays extraordinary strength— characteristics that were hinted at in the reports.

Three of the correctional officers were forthcoming and expressed genuine interest in assisting Holmes with his inquiry. One male CO was reluctant to answer Holmes's questions, saying that he would need to refer to his written report before commenting. All said that they were surprised by Sammie's death, which seemed sudden to them. Each had participated in cell extractions before, and said that this wasn't the first cell extraction involving Sammie.

By this time Holmes had enough firsthand experience to know how prison officials operated. "The way a prison system handles someone who isn't obeying orders," he says, "is to overpower him, and Sammie knew that. As the COs slid his cell door open—it doesn't open very wide—they shot pepper spray from a few inches away into Sammie's face. It irritates a person's eyes, causing pain, tears, and temporary blindness. Each burst was two seconds, they said, as per regulations, with an appropriate interval in between. All of them were spraying Sammie at once, however, multiple times, and probably for more than two seconds."

Sammie's eyes were blistering and his throat no doubt felt like it was on fire. He held his mattress in front of him to stop the spraying, but the COs pulled the mattress down and continued to squirt him. He tried to push them out of the cell—three huge men, each one younger and stronger than Sammie—and for several seconds was succeeding. Collectively the COs were mightier, however, and they got Sammie down on his stomach. Two men pinned him to the ground, with one man placing his knee in the middle of Sammie's back.

"Sammie had more than four hundred pounds on his torso," Holmes says, "compressing his diaphragm. It was the worst possible situation for an older, overweight man to be on his belly with all that weight on him after being sprayed and sprayed and sprayed."

Sammie kept saying, "I can't breathe! I can't breathe!" but the COs ignored him, thinking that it was a ploy to get them to let up.

Still with a knee in his back, and his shoulders, arms, and legs held down, Sammie was handcuffed, then leg restraints were applied. As Holmes wrote in his supplemental report, "At about this point Marshall began to exhibit signs of seizure or convulsion, although it was not a violent reaction, mostly described as uncontrolled shaking. There was no vomiting, gagging, or flailing."

Sammie was facedown on the cement floor, "trussed like a pig," Holmes says. One of the female COs advised turning him on his side and this was done, then a litter was wedged into the cell and Sammie was loaded onto it. According to all the COs, Sammie was coherent and communicating with them as he was being carried to the infirmary. Holmes found this highly questionable, however. In talking with other prison staff he was told that Sammie seldom communicated with anyone, and if he did it was widely described as mumbling. Several people said that they had never heard Sammie speak.

As soon as Sammie arrived at the infirmary, a paper mask was placed over his mouth and nose. His mouth was bloody, and he was known to have spit at prison personnel before. It was unclear to Holmes what everyone in the infirmary did after that, even though each person filed a formal report on their involvement. There were six to eight people tending to Sammie, including three correctional officers (because Sammie was a death row inmate), a nurse, and a physician. Holmes talked with the medical staff, who said that Sammie's blood pressure was taken twice, but that appeared to be all that was done. His breathing was described as shallow but not labored. Twenty minutes after he entered the infirmary, Sammie was hooked up to an EKG monitor. It showed a flatline heart rate; Sammie had no pulse.

Holmes found nothing in Sammie's medical history to indicate a known heart disease, and Sammie had not been on any heart medication while at San Quentin. Holmes determined that the prison physician had access to blood pressure, pulse, and respiration information when Sammie first arrived, well before pronouncing him dead. The doctor didn't initiate CPR at any time, and Holmes wondered whether Sammie's seizure was misinterpreted as cardiac arrest.

Holmes noted that Sammie didn't appear to have been choked, accidentally or otherwise, to the point of losing consciousness and causing anoxia, a condition in which brain cells begin to die because they lack oxygen. The autopsy showed no abnormalities other than the expected congestion of the mucosal linings of the larynx.

The one correctional officer whom Holmes wasn't able to talk to because he no longer was at the prison was the videographer. Seeing a videotape of Sammie being removed from his cell would have been helpful in assessing what took place and the sequence of events. Holmes was told that the camera "malfunctioned," however, so there wasn't a tape.

Two and a half months after Sammie's death, Holmes received the results of a tryptase test that was done on Sammie. Tryptase is a substance found in the blood, and an elevated level indicates anaphylaxis—an allergic reaction that can cause a sudden and dramatic drop in blood pressure, sometimes with fatal consequences. Individuals have reported eating shellfish and seafood throughout their lives and then, on one particular occasion, they developed an anaphylactic reaction from it and almost died. Sammie's tryptase level was elevated well beyond the normal range, leading Holmes to conclude that Sammie had an allergic reaction to the OC spray, since no other substance was involved in the cell extraction or in the infirmary.

During a subsequent and formal coroner's inquest, Holmes brought to light all of the factors that made Sammie's death a potential homicide—the excessive pepper spraying, the compression of Sammie's diaphragm due to all the weight on him, Sammie's pleas that he couldn't breathe, the fact that Sammie had no known heart problems, and the lack of proper medical care. Holmes was convinced that Sammie's death wasn't accidental or due to natural causes, and it obviously wasn't a suicide. Neither the police nor the district attorney was willing to file charges, however. Prison officials, in their own investigation, concluded that Sammie died from exertion because he was overweight and his heart gave out. The correctional officers and medical staff were absolved. Holmes ended up saying that the manner of death was undetermined. He felt bad about that, and regrets it to this day.

"The COs were complicit and the system was complicit," he says. "I'm not an advocate for inmates or anybody who does something bad, but I'm an advocate for doing something the right way, and they did it wrong. Sammie Marshall didn't need to die, and he didn't deserve to die, certainly not under the circumstances of moving him from cell to cell."

A lesson Holmes learned early on echoed in his brain. "When the guy with the badge says stand up, if you don't stand up you're a bad guy. If the guy with the badge says sit down and you don't sit down, he feels like he's being challenged and it escalates from that point. It shouldn't be that way. What they should have done was have a counselor come and talk to Sammie, tell him, 'Sammie, it's going to be *better* if you move.' They all knew him, he had been in the system a long time. They knew he wasn't educated. He wasn't an idiot by definition, but he wasn't far from it."

Sammie had a brother who lived in the South. When Holmes notified him of Sammie's death, the brother couldn't understand it.

"Sammie's not a violent person," he said. It was true.

"Sammie was a big guy," Holmes says, "and had been convicted of murder, but other than a few psychotic episodes he wasn't a threat to anyone."

Four months before Sammie died, the California Supreme Court unanimously reversed his death sentence. It was only the second time in five years that the court found grounds to reverse a death sentence on direct appeal (eighty-four death sentences were affirmed during the same period). The basis for the reversal was that Sammie's attorney, a Long Beach lawyer named Ron Slick, never told the jury that another man had been witnessed leaving the murder scene just before the victim's body was discovered. Slick also never told the jury that the semen found in the victim's vagina didn't match Sammie's DNA. In fact, Slick rested his case without presenting a single witness.

After Sammie's sentence was reversed, he was never informed of it. Letters from his lawyers were returned unopened. Meanwhile, day after day Sammie continued to sit in his cell, rocking back and forth on his steel bed, certain that prison staff were poisoning his food and that his lawyer was conspiring with them. He wasn't that far wrong.

CHAPTER 11

INVESTIGATING SUICIDES

In the United States, 40,000 people die by suicide every year. By comparison, there are 18,000 homicides in the country annually. The average person doesn't know it since it's rarely the subject of news stories, but more than twice as many Americans die by suicide as are murdered. Coroners know it, though. They deal with suicides every day. Some take place in homes, garages, and hotels, while others occur outdoors, in parks and recreational areas.

The Golden Gate National Recreation Area (GGNRA) consists of 80,000 acres of protected open space, much of it formerly used by the U.S. Army. Unlike other parks, it's not continuous; rather, it comprises multiple areas that stretch south, from Marin County through portions of San Francisco and into the northern part of San Mateo County. Included are fifty-nine miles of bay and ocean shoreline, a number of decommissioned army bases, and destinations as diverse as Alcatraz Island and Fort Mason. The bulk of the GGNRA is in Marin County, with the Marin Headlands, Muir Woods, Stinson Beach, Muir Beach, and Tomales Bay among the most prominent locations. More than fifteen million people visit the GGNRA annually. Not surprisingly, it has been the site of numerous suicides, too.

A seventeen-year-old girl was lying on the floor of a van that was parked in the Marin Headlands. Her feet were hanging out a rear cargo door, a gun was on her stomach, and there was an entry wound in her right temple and an exit wound on the other side. Her body was warm, she was fully dressed, and there was slight rigor and lividity. Holmes found several sealed envelopes in a jacket pocket, displayed prominently. The notes were dated the same day that her body was found and were addressed to family members and friends. One note said that she stole the gun from an aunt's boyfriend. When Holmes talked to him, he said that he kept the gun in plain view in his bedroom. Another note said, "There was nothing you could have said that would have changed my mind. I wasn't trying to get back at anyone, and it wasn't anyone's fault. . . . I wasn't as strong as I thought. . . . Forgive me."

Mount Tamalpais State Park consists of three hillside lakes and miles of hiking and biking trails, many offering panoramic vistas. When a thirty-seven-year-old woman disappeared after leaving a suicide note for her boyfriend, he called the police in a panic. While sheriff's deputies searched the area, the boyfriend and two of his friends began looking for her on the 2,700-foot-high mountain. Her body was found sixty feet down an embankment that wasn't accessible by foot. A police helicopter was used to retrieve her remains. She could have been the victim of an accidental fall, but during the investigation Holmes learned that she had a history of depression, was being treated by a local psychologist, and had attempted to jump from the Golden Gate Bridge the previous year but was stopped. The note she left her boyfriend, which he shared with Holmes, indicated her intent.

"I'm so sorry to all my family and loved ones," she said in the note. "Life seems so scary because I feel incapable of doing just the simple daily tasks that most people do to function in life. . . . I wish I could make myself stay alive for you. But I'm drowning, inside, by a lack of self confidence, extreme sense of inability, laziness, and general dissatisfaction of how I've conducted myself in this life. . . . I just can't struggle any longer."

Another suicide was of a fifty-one-year-old writer named Calvin Kentfield, who jumped from a cliff at Point Reyes National Seashore. The night before, his backpack was found abandoned at the top of the cliff, and his white 1960 Volkswagen bus, unlocked and with the key in the ignition, was located blocking a fire gate.

Since it was dark, park rangers contacted the U.S. Coast Guard's air assistance service to help locate him. The helicopter search was unsuccessful, however, so people returned early the next morning. At 9 A.M., Kentfield's body was sighted on the beach, 280 feet below the cliff. A rescue party with a Stokes litter—a long, shallow stretcher with sides—went down a steep trail to the beach, retrieved the body, which was nude, and brought it up to the road, where Holmes was waiting. He observed numerous abrasions, befitting a fall from a cliff, and was given a typed suicide note that was on the front seat of the van. The note, signed by Kentfield, said he was tired of living and was going to kill himself. Also inside the van was an unpublished manuscript, plus a book contract with an East Coast publisher.

Kentfield had written several novels, as well as a recently published memoir. According to the toxicology report, his blood alcohol content was .19—no surprise to Holmes since by now he knew that many suicidal people drink excessively beforehand to dull their senses and overcome self-preservation instincts.

BROTHER AND SISTER

Whenever someone dies by suicide, loved ones of the deceased ask, Why? Why did he or she do it? There's no one answer because suicidal behavior is complex. A variety of social, psychological, and physiological factors are cited. According to the National Institute of Mental Health, 90 percent of the people who die by suicide have a diagnosable mental illness; however, the majority of people with mental disorders don't kill themselves. Similarly, events such as the end of a relationship, death of a loved one, financial problems, legal issues, or declining health can lead to a suicide attempt, but most people who face these or other personal crises don't resort to suicide.

Holmes knew that psychological pain and extreme feelings of helplessness and hopelessness were important pieces of the puzzle. They produced the desire for death, of a release from one's physical, emotional, and mental anguish. Anytime Holmes talked with family members, friends, or physicians who treated a suicide victim, he asked them about the decedent's frame of mind.

The other important factor was developing the capacity to kill yourself. This wasn't something that Holmes knew when he started, but he came to understand it the longer he was on the job. Through practice and repeated exposure, individuals can become habituated to death. Some suicides, particularly by younger people, seem impulsive, but most victims develop a fearlessness about dying. This results from previous suicide attempts, from frequent witnessing of deaths—one reason why soldiers and police officers have high rates of suicide—and from suicides by family members and friends. It's aided by having access to lethal means, which becomes the centerpiece of a plan.

One of Holmes's first cases concerned the suicide of a twenty-year-old man named Skip. He had tried to kill himself by overdosing on Seconal, a barbiturate most commonly prescribed for insomnia, after his girlfriend had killed herself several weeks earlier overdosing that way. Skip survived the attempt and was hospitalized on a psychiatric hold for seventy-two hours, during which time he refused to see a doctor. As soon as he was released, Skip vowed to continue making attempts until he died.

Skip had two sisters. Bonnie was three years older and a striking beauty with brown hair and brown eyes. Patty, the oldest, was a reserve in the San Anselmo Police Department. Skip knew that Patty kept a service revolver somewhere in her house; also, she was away much of the day because she worked at a local veterinary office. Patty's husband, Art, was out of the house often, too.

While Patty and Art were gone, Skip went to their house. He knew where they kept a key and let himself in. Rummaging around, he found Patty's gun on a shelf in her bedroom closet. He took a chair from another room into the bedroom, sat down with his back to the closet, and shot himself in the head.

Holmes responded to the call, which was how he got to know Patty, Art, and Bonnie. All three were beside themselves with grief. After that, Art and Holmes developed a friendship. They had coffee together several times, and generally stayed in touch.

Art was the one who found Bonnie's body. It was several months later, and he didn't call his wife. Instead, he called Holmes. When the call came through, Holmes knew something was wrong. Art was so choked up that he could barely say Holmes's name, but Holmes recognized his voice. He thought maybe it was Art's wife, but Art said no, it was Patty's sister. She had shot herself with the same gun, in the same chair, facing the same direction, as her brother Skip.

Ever since Skip killed himself, Bonnie had suffered from fits of depression. Three months earlier she had attempted suicide by overdosing on phenobarbital, after which she was hospitalized for seven days. Lately she had been seeing a psychiatrist. Like Skip, she used the hidden key to enter Patty and Art's house while they were out.

"I'm not going to tell Patty until you get here," Art told Holmes.

When Holmes arrived at the house, Patty was still at work. The house was within walking distance of the veterinary office, and Art decided that it would be best if the two of them went there rather than told Patty when she came home. Art realized that if Patty saw Holmes, though, she would know that something was wrong, so he told her boss to tell her to come out in back of the office, away from her coworkers. There, with Holmes standing at his side, Art told her that Bonnie had shot herself.

Patty's lips quivered and she looked on the verge of fainting. Without anyone saying it, she knew that that wasn't the whole story, as terrible as it was. She didn't have to ask her husband or Holmes to know that there was more to it, that Bonnie had killed herself with

Patty's gun, in Patty's bedroom, just as Skip had done. She could see it on their faces.

Following Bonnie's death, Patty got rid of the gun and quit the police force. She and Art kept in contact with Holmes for a while but gradually lost touch. As much as he tried to provide comfort and support, Holmes was a reminder of the twin tragedies of their past. It was easier for them not to see him.

PAINKILLERS AND HARD DRUGS

When Holmes started working in the coroner's office, he had a good understanding of medicine and firearms, which proved invaluable in doing death investigations. One subject he knew next to nothing about, however—and had to get up to speed on fast—was drugs, both legal and illegal. There was only one way to do it, and that was by constant studying.

"Whenever I encountered a new drug or brand-name variation, I would go to the books," he says. "The *Physicians' Desk Reference* was an amazing resource, before the Internet. Now I can look up almost any chemical compound on my phone, but in the early days that wasn't an option."

Just looking up information wasn't enough, however. He needed to be able to retain it, which proved to be harder.

"When it came to drugs, memorization was difficult for me. I found myself looking up the same compounds on many occasions. After a while I was able to remember the basics, but still I found myself continually referring to books on drugs and prescription medications."

In upper-class areas like Marin County, painkiller addiction is rampant. According to the California Department of Justice, doctors in Marin and other Bay Area counties wrote out 2.2 million prescriptions for opiate painkillers—OxyContin, Vicodin, Percocet, and the like—in 2013. That is nearly one prescription for every three people who live in the region. Hard drugs often follow. According to the federal Substance

Abuse and Mental Health Services Administration, nearly 80 percent of people who use heroin have a history of abusing prescription painkillers.

Holmes used to keep a large glass jar on his desk. It was filled with three of every pill that he and other investigators in the office found at the site of drug overdoses.

"These are the kinds of things that you have in your medicine cabinet," Holmes told parents. "Every pill in this jar came from a bottle that we retrieved after someone died overdosing on them."

It wasn't just their own medicine cabinets, Holmes said, that parents had to be concerned about. It was the medicine cabinets of strangers, too.

"Adults are smart," Holmes says, "but when it comes to drugs, kids are smarter. During real estate open homes, they go into bathrooms and look in medicine cabinets. They also go to garage sales, estate sales, and moving sales, asking whichever adult is there, 'Do you mind if I use your bathroom?'"

As for hard drugs, Holmes kept samples in his office of white, brown, and black tar heroin, plus cocaine and methamphetamine. "This is what heroin looks like," he told parents. "If you see this on your teenage daughter's dresser, you know that she's using drugs. Stop telling yourself that she's safe. She's not; she's using drugs."

What Holmes tried to impress on kids when he talked with them about drugs was that users didn't always know what they were buying. The consequences of that ignorance could be deadly.

"I may go to you for my weekly fix," he told them, "and I trust what you're selling me because you're my friend or the friend of a friend or have been my regular supplier, but then one day you're not there, you're in jail or whatever. I go to somebody on the street because I'm sick and really need help, and they could sell me anything—it might be shoe polish, or maybe it's baking soda. I prepare it the same way I prepare the stuff I'm used to, inject it into my arm, and could be dead before I even pull out the needle." It was a sobering message.

When a fourteen-year-old girl named Diana deliberately overdosed, Holmes found her parents, particularly her father, surprisingly blasé about it. Her body was discovered by her best friend, named Emma, lying on the water bed in her bedroom, under a comforter. A suicide note was next to the bed, along with a plastic bag containing codeine and other prescription painkillers.

She had told her parents that she wasn't feeling well and wasn't going to school. Her father said he would check back later to see if she was feeling better. Instead, after work he called Emma and asked her to look in on Diana, then he went to a gym to exercise.

At Emma's request, Holmes talked with her alone, out of earshot of Emma's parents. Emma said she had known Diana since first grade, and while Diana didn't seek out friends, she was well liked. At the same time, she was pessimistic and mentioned suicide periodically.

"Did Diana say how she would kill herself?" Holmes asked.

"Pills," Emma said. "Always pills. A year ago she experimented with tying things around her neck to see how long it took for her to become unconscious, but she told me pills were how she planned to do it. She experimented with overdosing two or three times, taking pills—mainly Valium, I think—and then falling asleep."

"Did you know that she was stockpiling medications?"

Emma bowed her head and said softly, "Yeah. Two weeks ago she showed me the bag."

Holmes considered this. "What else did Diana tell you?"

"She told me she'd written several suicide notes and hidden them in her room."

"Did you see any of them?"

Her voice was faint. "No."

"Did you tell anyone about Diana's suicidal thoughts or previous attempts?"

"I told my mother."

"What did she do?"

"She told Diana's parents."

Emma said that Diana had been nearly blind since birth, and because her eyesight was so bad she never knew what she looked like since she couldn't see her image in a mirror very well. Then, with her fourth corneal transplant six months earlier, she could see herself clearly for the first time and didn't like what she saw.

After talking with Emma, Holmes talked with Emma's mother. "Emma said you told Diana's parents you thought Diana might try to kill herself soon," he said.

Emma's mother nodded. "I did. I said that in addition to her other problems, I thought Diana was fearful of going into high school next year and said they might want to get counseling for her. I was surprised they didn't do it."

"Do you know why they didn't?"

"I guess they decided she didn't need it or that it wouldn't help."

Next, Holmes talked with a sixteen-year-old boy named Justin. One of Diana's suicide notes was addressed to him and said, in part, "I loved you and still do very much. I'm so so so sorry!"

"How long had you known Diana, and how did you meet?" Holmes asked. Being two years older, Justin was in high school while Diana was in middle school.

Justin said, "We met five months ago, through Emma."

"How would you describe your relationship with Diana?"

"We were friends," Justin said. "Not boyfriend-girlfriend, but good friends."

"Did she ever mention suicide to you?"

Justin hesitated before answering. "Yeah, a couple of times. She said her parents didn't love her, they only pretended to. The last couple of days she seemed better, though, not depressed."

"Did she tell you about experimenting with suicide?"

"No, just that she thought about suicide sometimes."

"Did she tell you that she had written notes a month earlier, or that she had stockpiled pills?"

Justin shook his head.

"Did you know about her medical problems?" Holmes said.

"Yeah," Justin said. "She told me that for her recent eye surgery she had been in the hospital four or five days and her father never visited her, never called her, never sent a card or flowers. That reinforced her feelings that her parents didn't love her."

Holmes talked with Diana's father three times. The first time was a day after Diana died. He said she was "upbeat," did well in school, and had no problems. The second time, Holmes questioned him about Diana's medical history, which included jaw reconstruction surgery and the corneal transplants. Diana's father downplayed them, saying that she recovered and that her vision after the fourth transplant improved considerably. He was more concerned about who was going to pay for his front door, which had been kicked in during the 911 response.

"Who do I call to seek reimbursement and also investigate who did the kicking and why?" he said. In addition, he wanted to know if anyone was going to investigate Justin and why "a guy so much older was hanging around young girls."

In their third conversation, Diana's father said that Diana, Emma, and Justin "may have had a suicide pact of some sort because there is something fishy about the whole thing."

"Why do you say that?" Holmes said.

The father said, "It's just a feeling, based on the other suicide notes we found in Diana's bedroom, dated a month earlier, and knowing that she stockpiled pills."

"Did you ever seek counseling for Diana?"

"No. Why would we?"

"It sounds like she had a lot of issues to deal with, being nearly blind since birth, having a deformed jaw, going through multiple surgeries, taking a lot of medications. All that would affect a young girl's sense of self-esteem, I would think."

"She always had everything she wanted," Diana's father said, "and really had no problems."

Holmes was getting a good idea of what Diana's life probably had been like. "I'm sorry for your loss," he said. There was nothing else he could say.

CHAPTER 12

THE BRIDGE

The Golden Gate Bridge is one of the most beautiful man-made structures in the world. Spanning the mouth of San Francisco Bay, and joining the city and county of San Francisco with Marin County, it's an architectural and engineering triumph. For all of its grandeur, however, its magnificent setting, elegant design, and storied construction, the Golden Gate Bridge has a dark side. From the day it opened in 1937 until now, it has been the world's top suicide site.

There are several reasons why the bridge is so deadly. One reason is that it was the first bridge in the world to span a major harbor, so it had to be tall enough to accommodate large ships passing underneath. The roadbed is 220 feet above the water, making jumping from it equivalent to jumping from a twenty-five-story building.

Another reason is that access is easy. There are walkways on each side of the bridge—on the west side for bicyclists and on the east side for pedestrians—that run the bridge's length and are open year-round. In addition, there are parking lots at both ends, and buses to the bridge operate frequently.

A third reason is that some people believe jumping from the bridge spares family members the agony of finding their body. A person's remains are either swept out to sea, never to be seen again, or retrieved by the Coast Guard. Either way, there is no gruesome cleanup for loved ones.

Then there is the lure of the bridge. Suicide sites, by virtue of their repute, tend to attract depressed people to them, and no site exerts a stronger pull than the Golden Gate Bridge. Each new death adds to its siren's call.

These reasons wouldn't be important if the bridge had a suicide deterrent, but to date it doesn't. In fact, the Golden Gate Bridge is the only major international landmark without one. The existing railing is only four feet high—short enough for almost anyone to jump or climb over it. Original plans included a higher railing specifically to prevent suicides, but in a last-minute design decision the railing was lowered to enhance the view.

Ken Holmes wasn't always in favor of a suicide deterrent on the bridge. He didn't oppose one, but he didn't think it was a high priority. Until 1990, the Marin County Coroner's Office handled one or two cases a year where the body of a Golden Gate Bridge jumper either washed up in the county or the person jumped on the Marin side close enough to shore that he or she struck land rather than water. Holmes knew that the coroner's office in San Francisco handled a few more cases because Coast Guard Station Golden Gate, which retrieved the bodies of jumpers, was based in the city and delivered them there, but he didn't know how many more. No one really did. Unlike Marin, the San Francisco Coroner's Office didn't track Golden Gate Bridge suicides as a separate category of deaths. Instead, cases were lumped in with jumps from other structures, such as hotels. In 1990, however, Station Golden Gate relocated to Marin County and Marin assumed responsibility for investigating most of the suicides from the bridge. That was when Holmes realized the problem was much bigger than he had thought. Instead of one or two cases a year, Marin began handling thirty to forty cases annually.

In one case, a thirty-two-year-old San Jose man murdered his wife, grabbed their three-year-old daughter, and drove to the Golden Gate Bridge. Two Bridge Patrol officers noticed him acting strange and stopped their car mid-span to talk to him. Seeing them, the man stood with his back to the railing, lifted his daughter over his head, and threw her off the bridge. Before the officers could get close to him, he followed her over the railing.

Father and daughter were recovered in the water by the Coast Guard within fifteen minutes, only five feet from each other. CPR was started immediately on both of them by Coast Guard personnel, then continued by paramedics when the boat docked. The father died shortly thereafter. Holmes observed him still lying on a Stokes litter, covered with a blanket. He noted "extensive subcutaneous emphysema over the entire upper half of the body, most notably to the mouth, face, neck, and upper chest, resulting in marked distension of all facial features." Subcutaneous emphysema is a condition in which air gets into tissues under the skin, causing the skin to bulge and producing an unusual crackling sound when the skin is touched. Typically, it results from a collapsed lung due to a rib fracture, or to fractured facial bones, a ruptured bronchial tube, or a ruptured esophagus. Coast Guard members told Holmes that the man wasn't distended when they recovered him from the water, but his distension grew as they continued CPR.

The daughter, named Kellie, was still alive, and emergency room doctors at Marin General Hospital worked on her frantically for ninety minutes. It was a losing battle, however.

When Holmes examined her, she was supine on a backboard in the emergency room. An immobilization collar was still around her neck, and there was an endotracheal tube in her mouth, a catheter below, and IV lines in one wrist and ankle. Holmes could see subcutaneous bruises and multiple fractures. He didn't take fingerprints because she was too young for matching prints to be in a database.

Kellie's death was the third documented instance of a child who was thrown over the short railing of the Golden Gate Bridge by a suicidal parent, who jumped afterward. Holmes could only hope that she was the last.

DUANE GARRETT

One of the suicides was a prominent Bay Area lawyer, radio personality, and Democratic Party fund-raiser named Duane Garrett. His jump wasn't witnessed, but two girls spotted his body floating in the water underneath the bridge. There was nothing on his person to indicate who he was, however, and no one recognized him, so his identity wasn't known immediately.

When someone is found underneath the bridge who doesn't have identification, the Bridge Patrol and California Highway Patrol begin searching bridge parking lots. They note all of the cars that are there, then return thirty minutes later because turnover is rapid. If after two hours a car hasn't moved, that's probably the jumper's car. Once officers know which car it is, they usually are able to get inside it. Oftentimes the doors aren't locked and the keys are in the ignition because the person is past the point of caring. Police might find the individual's wallet or purse, which may be left behind and have ID. They also may find a suicide note on the front seat.

In this instance the California Highway Patrol found an abandoned dark blue 1993 Lexus. The vehicle was registered to Garrett, the driver's-side door was unlocked, and papers inside confirmed that the heavyset man with straight brown hair and a short beard who had jumped the day before from the bridge was, indeed, Duane. He was forty-eight.

His name didn't mean anything to police on the scene or to Gary Erickson, the investigator who was on duty when the call came in. It didn't mean anything to Holmes, either, who was now the assistant coroner and Erickson's supervisor. Holmes rarely listened to the radio, and never to talk shows.

Erickson went with an officer from the Tiburon Police Department to the Garrett home to do the death notification. When he told Mrs. Garrett, she was shocked. She said she had no idea her husband was worried or depressed. Erickson expressed condolences and said that he would come back the following day with her husband's personal effects.

When he returned, he was met outside the front door by two men in dark suits. Both of them were stone-faced, wore dark glasses, and had earpieces.

"What do you want?" one man said. His tone of voice wasn't welcoming.

Erickson showed them his identification and said he was there to give Mrs. Garrett her husband's effects. Both men eyed him carefully, then one man opened the front door to get Mrs. Garrett. When he did, Erickson could see a group of people inside, two of whom he recognized immediately—Vice President Al Gore and his then wife, Tipper. That explained the presence of the Secret Service agents.

Unbeknownst to Erickson or Holmes, Duane Garrett was a close personal friend of the Gores. He had managed political campaigns for Al Gore as well as other Democratic candidates. As soon as the Gores heard about Garrett's death, they had flown out from Washington, D.C., to be with the family.

Garrett was well known in political circles, and the coroner's office fielded so many inquiries regarding Duane's death that Holmes issued a press release. It was a way to control some of the rumors that were circulating, one of which was that Duane killed himself because of mounting financial troubles and allegations of impropriety. He owned a sports memorabilia business that had been heavily leveraged when the market for baseball cards collapsed, and was accused of selling fake memorabilia. In a letter to his attorney and personal friend, Duane said that he had been misled and didn't profit personally from the wrongdoing. Still, his reputation was impugned, and for someone in his position, reputation was everything. The public didn't need to know the details, though, Holmes decided. Besides, there was no reference in the letter to suicide.

KILLED ON THE WAY DOWN

Three months after Duane Garrett's suicide, Holmes was involved in the investigation of another jump from the Golden Gate Bridge. This one didn't attract media attention, which was a good thing considering that the coroner's investigator who responded failed to notice a critical piece of information.

Denise Atchison, age forty-two, was a card dealer at a gaming business. At 3 A.M. she stopped her car on the bridge and went to the pedestrian walkway. This was before the walkway was closed after dark. The fog was heavy, only a few cars were on the bridge at that hour, and no pedestrians were around. A female motorist driving home from work saw Denise climb over the rail. What the motorist didn't know, and neither did the police officers who responded or the coroner's investigator who was called out, was that Denise was dead before she hit the water.

A Coast Guard crew found her body—no small feat, especially in the dark and given the conditions.

"I have nothing but admiration for the crew members who retrieve the remains of Golden Gate Bridge jumpers," Holmes says. "They go out in all kinds of weather, in choppy seas, day or night, oftentimes battling strong currents, and get to the spot within minutes after being called. They're just amazing."

The coroner's investigator on duty, Ray Nichols, met the Coast Guard boat at the dock and took several photographs of Denise's body. Then he followed the mortuary van to the funeral home, where he undressed her, fingerprinted her because she didn't have identification, took some mug-shot-like photos, measured her height, and estimated her weight because he didn't have access to a scale. Nichols also recorded the labels on all of Denise's clothing, noting the manufacturer's name and clothing size because sometimes that was the only information the coroner's office had to work with when trying to determine a person's identity. After that Nichols wrote a brief report, which accompanied the body so that Dr. Jindrich, the coroner, had that information when he did the autopsy. A fuller report would be prepared later, for the files. Then Nichols drove home to bed.

Seven hours later, at eleven o'clock in the morning, Holmes was at his desk when he got a call from Jindrich. "Who handled this case?" Jindrich said. Jindrich rarely lost his temper, but this time there was anger in his voice.

"Nichols," Holmes said. "Why?"

Jindrich had hired Nichols to replace Holmes when Holmes was promoted to assistant coroner. Nichols was a former mortician who had been working in the sheriff's office and wanted to transfer. On paper he seemed like a good fit. He was comfortable dealing with death, and he had been through the police academy so he could hit the ground running. From the outset, though, he had presented problems, the main one being that he was neither observant nor curious. He was good working with families, but that was all. A big man—six foot four and 250 pounds—he had strong opinions and ended up alienating his coworkers.

"Did he say anything about the gunshot wound?" Jindrich said.

Holmes's jaw dropped. "What!"

"She has a gunshot wound in her head," Jindrich said.

As soon as he got off the phone, Holmes called Nichols, waking him up. "Are you trying to keep the gunshot a secret?" he said.

There was a pause, then Nichols said, "What do you mean?"

"Doc just called. Your bridge jumper from last night has a gunshot wound in the head."

Nichols was incredulous. "That can't be."

"Well, it is," Holmes said.

One of the things that investigators did in cases where the decedent's identity wasn't known was wash off any blood or dirt that was on the person's face and comb his or her hair back so that a clear picture could be taken. In this instance, Denise's face didn't have any blood on it, mainly because she died immediately and her blood stopped circulating, but also because bay waters washed away what little there was. In addition, she had a lot of hair, so that even when it was combed back the wound was covered. Still, Nichols should have seen it.

The question now was whether someone shot her and threw her over the short railing. In every questionable death, the coroner's office proceeded as if it was a homicide.

The motorist who called it into the toll plaza said, "I saw her climb over the rail and let go." She didn't mention seeing anyone else.

Holmes went to the Golden Gate Bridge District, got the motorist's name and contact information, and went to talk with her. The woman told him that there wasn't anyone else around. She saw Denise only because Denise was wearing a white shirt under a dark jacket. The flash of white caught the motorist's eye. Also, Denise was a big, heavyset woman, and it wasn't easy for her to get over the side.

A fingerprint match confirmed Denise's identity and the fact that she lived in San Francisco. Holmes arranged for someone to go to Denise's residence. A female roommate was frantic because Denise hadn't come home, but had left a note. The note said that Denise was going to jump from the bridge and planned to shoot herself on the way down because she didn't want to feel the impact of hitting the water. Denise had a long history of depression and previously had told her roommate that if she decided to kill herself, this was how she would do it: she would shoot herself as soon as she jumped. The roommate said that in the past few months Denise had purchased a 9-millimeter semiautomatic handgun from a private party. The gun was never found—no one attempted to look for it—but that didn't matter. It was enough to know that it was a suicide.

"Thank God for the note," Holmes says. "Without it, Denise's roommate could have been a prime suspect, even though the motorist didn't see anyone else. Maybe the roommate was on the other side of the rail, out of view, inciting her to jump. You never know. We were lucky that she wrote it down rather than just told somebody."

BRIDGE OPERATING PROCEDURES

When the Golden Gate Bridge Patrol or California Highway Patrol sees or is notified that someone has jumped, an officer goes to the location on the bridge as determined by the light pole number. The bridge has 128 light poles, and each one has a number painted on it. Even-numbered poles are on the west side, illuminating the bike lane and facing the Pacific Ocean, and odd-numbered poles are on the east side, lighting the pedestrian walkway and facing San Francisco. The poles are spaced evenly from the parking lot at Vista Point in Marin County to just before the toll plaza into San Francisco.

If the jump is witnessed—75 percent are—an officer drops a nineteen-inch-long marine location marker into the water. Known as "smoke floats," the markers are supplied by the Coast Guard and are stored on the bridge for easy access (they're not reusable). They emit both smoke and a flare for up to thirty minutes. In addition, they are weighted and indicate which way the tide is moving, enabling the Coast Guard to develop search patterns. On the bridge, officers follow the marker with binoculars and maintain radio communication with the Coast Guard.

When the body of a Golden Gate Bridge jumper is recovered, Coast Guard crews bring it to shore at Fort Baker in Marin County. The coroner's investigator meets first with the California Highway Patrol officer who is handling the case, and the officer relates any information he or she has, such as whether the jump was witnessed, whether a purse or wallet with identification was found, and whether the jumper left a suicide note. Then the investigator goes to work.

In most instances, the decedent has "pattern injuries"—deep bruises, broken bones, and damaged internal organs—that are consistent with a fall from a great height. About 5 percent of jumpers also have water in their lungs, indicating that they survived the fall and subsequently drowned. In these cases the person's last seconds are filled with excruciating pain and terror.

"Some people think that jumping off the bridge is a light, airy way to end your life," Holmes says. "I'd like to dispel that myth. When you jump off the bridge, you hit the water hard. It's not pretty."

During the four-second fall, jumpers' bodies travel at a speed of seventy-five miles per hour. The impact is equivalent to a pedestrian who is struck by a car driving that fast. The outer body stops abruptly, but internal organs are still moving. They hemorrhage or are lacerated by broken bones, which is one reason why only a small number of people survive the fall.

The biggest challenge in some cases is determining the jumper's identity. Even if people have a wallet in their pocket when they jump, their clothes can be shredded on impact and any belongings lost.

In one case, a man's foot in a white cotton sock and a black canvas Rockport shoe, size seven and a half, washed up on Stinson Beach, eleven miles away. That was all; nothing else.

Holmes turned to local media for assistance. He placed an article in multiple newspapers asking for help in connecting the foot to a person. An inventive headline proved to be the key.

"If you just say 'Coroner's office is trying to identify an unidentified person,'" Holmes says, "few people will notice it. If you say 'Foot found in a shoe in the bay,' though, they'll read it."

Several days later, a woman who had seen the article called Holmes. She was a nurse at a hospital in San Francisco and said that one of her coworkers, a forty-nine-year-old man named Julian, had disappeared two months earlier. He was depressed because he had been diagnosed with AIDS, she said, and had transitioned from being a nurse to a patient. She added that he always wore black Rockport shoes with white socks.

Julian's apartment had been cleaned out by his brother, but police were able to find a razor and a toothbrush. They also found suicide notes and a diary hinting at a possible jump from the Golden Gate

Bridge. DNA samples from the toothbrush and razor matched the bone marrow samples taken from the foot. According to his brother, the shoe size was a match, too.

BRIDGE RAIL FOUNDATION

On October 26, 2003, a twenty-six-year-old student at the University of California, Santa Cruz, jumped from the Golden Gate Bridge. Kathy Hull drove her white Honda Accord an hour and a half to San Francisco, crossed the Golden Gate Bridge at twilight, and parked at Vista Point on the Marin side. From there she began walking across the bridge. Midway, near light pole seventy-one, she laid down her purse and cell phone, climbed over the railing, and jumped.

Several suicide notes were in her car. One said, in part, "Spirit is the glue that holds mind and body together, but mine is broken. It was held together for a very long time, and now it has crumbled. I don't seem to care anymore. I can't keep the pieces together."

A bridge worker found the phone, looked at Kathy's contact list, and pressed her home number. Dave Hull answered.

"Did you lose your cell phone on the Golden Gate Bridge?" the man asked.

"No," Hull said, confused.

"Did your daughter lose her phone? Her purse was found on the bridge."

Hull and his wife, Jean, sat in stunned silence. Later that night, they were contacted by the police. Kathy's car had been found at Vista Point, and her body had been retrieved by the Coast Guard after someone on the bridge had seen and reported it.

Dave Hull's world stopped, and he didn't want it to go on. "It was as if I could be closer to her if nothing changed," he says. "It was Joan Didion's magical thinking; just a few hours separated me from Kathy alive. That's not much. Isn't there something I could do that would change that?"

Hull's own thoughts turned to suicide, but he had another child, a son, at home who needed him. Still, Hull remembers how close he came. "Suicide is contagious," he says. "It puts everyone else at risk."

In time, Hull resumed elements of his life. He wrote poetry about Kathy. He returned to his job as the principal librarian at the San Francisco Maritime National Historic Park. He disposed of Kathy's possessions, including her car. Each step was painful.

Hull also began talking about the need for a suicide barrier on the Golden Gate Bridge. With two other people—Patrick Hines, whose son Kevin was one of the few people to survive a jump from the bridge, and Paul Muller, whose business partner lost a relative to the bridge—Hull founded a nonprofit, all-volunteer organization called the Bridge Rail Foundation. It had one mission: to end suicides from the Golden Gate Bridge.

The organization didn't have any funding, but it did have a core of passionate volunteers, many of whom were grieving the jump of a loved one. Holmes was an early recruit. He didn't have any kin who jumped, but two good friends did, including a police detective whom he had worked with on many cases.

For a long time, Holmes was opposed to media stories about Golden Gate Bridge suicides—particularly stories that included a chronological count. He thought they incited more people to jump. If the number wasn't publicized, he believed, suicidal people wouldn't be encouraged to go to the bridge. Over a fifteen-year blackout period, however, when local mental health professionals lobbied the media not to report bridge jumps in order to avoid a contagion effect, the number of bridge jumps didn't go down. On the contrary, it increased.

Once he realized that limiting media coverage wasn't helping to save lives, that all it was doing was hiding the problem, Holmes decided to try a different tack. If silence wasn't working, then maybe it was time to be vocal about it.

In 2007, Holmes issued a report with the Bridge Rail Foundation that stated the total number of recorded suicides to that point. It was nearly 1,500, even though hundreds of other suicides were excluded because they couldn't be confirmed—a body was never found or it was found far enough away that the death couldn't be attributed with certainty to the bridge. The number received a lot of press because during the blackout period no one knew that suicides were continuing or that there had been so many.

Holmes's report summarized demographic data on Golden Gate Bridge suicides over the previous ten years. The majority of bridge jumpers were white, male, under forty (making them younger than most suicide victims in the country), and lived locally. Despite the myth that the bridge attracted jumpers from all over the world, 85 percent of the victims lived in the Bay Area, and 95 percent lived in California. Fewer than 5 percent came from out of state or another country.

The release date of the report coincided with the seventieth anniversary of the bridge's opening and also its first suicide, by a forty-seven-year-old World War I veteran named Harold Wobber. He walked partway out on the span, turned to a passerby, and said, "This is as far as I go," and leaped over the side. Shortly thereafter, three other men jumped, and the parade of deaths was under way.

In 2008, Holmes issued a second report. This one covered the previous fifteen years and, among other things, listed the occupations of jumpers. No names were mentioned, but by listing the occupations the report allowed readers to see the societal impact of bridge suicides. Included were doctors, nurses, engineers, artists, caregivers, homemakers—people from all walks of life. The most common occupation was student. The second most common was teacher.

Both reports put new pressure on officials at the Golden Gate Bridge District to end these deaths from the structure that they managed. For his work in bringing the problem to the public's attention, Holmes was honored by the American Association of Suicidology at the organization's next annual conference, which happened to be held in San Francisco.

In October 2008, the Bridge District board voted to add a marine-grade stainless steel net under the bridge to prevent suicides. It was a historic step—the first time that the board approved a suicide deterrent for the bridge—but only a start. At the same time that board members approved the net, they voted not to allocate any bridge monies to pay for it. As a result, the deaths continued.

Ironically, a net was strung the length of the Golden Gate Bridge at the time it was being built to protect construction workers. The net cost $120,000 in 1937 ($2 million in today's currency) and saved the lives of nineteen men who, at various times, fell into it accidentally. Four months before the bridge was completed, a section of scaffolding broke away and tore through the net, killing ten workers. Another $120,000 was spent to have a new net installed. Once the bridge opened, the net was removed.

Holmes and other Bridge Rail Foundation volunteers (myself included) began working on a variety of fronts with Bridge District staff to identify and leverage funds. It all came together in 2014 when the board reversed its six-year-old decision and voted unanimously to allow bridge revenues to be used to match funds for the project that were committed by three other sources—the Metropolitan Transportation Commission, the California Department of Transportation, and the state's Mental Health Services Act—for the net.

"We did it!" shouted Sue Story after the final vote was cast. She was a Bridge Rail Foundation volunteer whose twenty-eight-year-old son jumped from the bridge in 2010.

Family members in attendance who had lost loved ones to the bridge stood and applauded the board, prompting board members to stand and applaud family members in return. Everyone acknowledged that it was the willingness of family members to be public with their grief that had turned the tide and resulted in the decision.

It was one of the most satisfying moments in Holmes's life. He knew that the families who had been victimized by the lack of action on the part of the Golden Gate Bridge District had made a huge sacrifice. For more than seventy-five years, since the bridge opened in 1937, there had been an endless procession of unnecessary deaths. Once the net was up, these tragedies wouldn't be known to future generations who would be spared. When the net was in place, families and friends wouldn't realize that their loved one who was troubled remained alive because the world's top suicide magnet no longer exerted a deadly pull. They wouldn't know—except in a general way—of the losses that others had suffered, largely in anonymity, or even that their loved one would have been at risk because jumping from the bridge was so easy. There wouldn't be any thought given to the fact that the bridge was now safe from suicide, much less any thanks to the people who had been responsible for making it happen. That was okay. It was enough to know that everyone would be able to enjoy a magnificent structure because the tragedies associated with it had ended.

CHAPTER 13

THE GERMAN TOURIST

It's rare for an intact body to remain unidentified. Oftentimes someone reports the person as missing, maybe not immediately, but at some point paperwork is filed. Fingerprints can be checked in national databases for a match. In a worst case, labels in clothing and jewelry can be tracked to determine where and when various items were made.

None of that existed in this instance. The man, six foot four, in his twenties, with long, flowing brownish-blond hair swept back, was found in 1986 on Marin land at the foot of the Golden Gate Bridge. Based on his injuries, it was apparent that he had jumped. He had no identification, and his face was so damaged that it wasn't possible to put his picture in the paper. As it turned out, that wouldn't have helped, but Ken Holmes didn't know it at the time. A police artist created a concept portrait based on a small portion of the man's face that wasn't damaged, and it proved to be fairly accurate. Even so, Holmes learned later that the only people who might have been able to recognize him were several East Bay masseuses who, if they had seen the rendering, couldn't have provided much information anyway. They didn't know the man's real name or anything about him.

There were no witnesses to the man's jump, and no one reported him missing. Holmes took fingerprints, but they didn't produce any hits when he entered them into a national database. The man was well dressed in an expensive sport coat, nice slacks, and a white dress shirt, but the labels had been removed from each item. If not, Holmes would have known at the outset to start his search abroad. The only thing he found on the man's body was the business card of a Bay Area limousine company.

Holmes waited a week, thinking someone—a family member, girlfriend, or roommate—would come forward, but no one did. After that he put an article in local papers, without a photo, saying that a young man had jumped from the Marin side of the bridge and landed in the rocks. No leads came from it.

With nothing else to go on, he called the limo company and talked with the owner. He told him why he was calling, and the owner said he didn't remember anyone matching the description.

"How many drivers do you have?" Holmes asked.

"It's just me and my brother," the man said.

"Have many cars do you have?"

"Two."

Holmes asked to talk with the brother, and was told that he wasn't there. "Would you ask him if he dropped off anybody at the Golden Gate Bridge recently?"

The man said he would, but after two days Holmes hadn't heard back so he called the limo company again. This time the brother, named Dennis, was in. Dennis told Holmes that several days earlier he did drive someone to the bridge.

"Can you describe him?"

"He was foreign; I think German. He was real tall and had lots of blond hair."

Holmes's mystery man. "Did you get his name?"

"No," Dennis said. "Why would I?"

"You're right," Holmes said. "You wouldn't have a reason to."

Holmes told Dennis that the man had jumped from the bridge. Dennis was upset to hear it.

"He was really nice to me," Dennis said. "And seemed so happy."

Holmes gave him a few seconds to digest the information, then said, "How did he pay you?"

"With cash," Dennis said. "Always with cash."

"You mean you drove him more than once?"

"I picked him up several times," Dennis said. "He had been using a different limo company before, but something led him to us. I drove him for three days, and he always asked for me so my brother never saw him."

"Where did you pick him up?"

"At the Concord Hilton."

The Hilton was forty miles east of Marin, in Contra Costa County. If the man had been staying there, the hotel would have a record of him.

"Where did you go?"

"We went to dinner a lot," Dennis said.

Holmes couldn't contain his surprise. "You went to dinner?"

"He would take me to dinner. He wanted to eat, and he always would buy me dinner."

"Did you go to nice places?"

"Only nice places. He also had me drive him to a massage parlor in Berkeley. He paid for me to have a massage, too."

"What!" Holmes exclaimed.

"Honest to God, I got massages along with him each of those three days."

"Just a massage?"

Dennis was silent for a moment, then said, "His included sex."

Holmes didn't ask what Dennis's massage included; it wasn't relevant. He did ask Dennis for the name of the massage parlor. Dennis said he thought it was Interlude.

The last day, the man paid for an hour at the same massage parlor, Dennis said. After that, he and Dennis ate dinner in San Francisco, with the man again paying for both meals. At 9:30 P.M. Dennis dropped him off at the bridge. The man said he was meeting a friend, and the friend had a car.

When Holmes called the Concord Hilton, he was told that a man matching the description of the deceased had registered five days earlier under the name Nils Exeter Edison. Hotel staff couldn't confirm that that was his real name because he hadn't presented any identification and had paid in cash.

"It wasn't the hotel's practice to accept cash," Holmes says, "but he was cute and had a German accent, so they let him."

Holmes asked when Nils Edison checked out.

"He didn't. His luggage is still here."

Thinking that it might contain the man's ID, Holmes asked the clerk if he could pick it up. The clerk wanted to know why.

"Because I'm investigating his death and need to be able to identify him and contact his next of kin," Holmes said.

The clerk was reluctant to release the luggage, but agreed to go through it and let Holmes know if there was anything of value to the coroner's office. There wasn't—no paperwork, passport, airline tickets, airline tag on the handle—nothing, not even a toothbrush. The two soft bags just had clothing, none of it with labels.

"We'll probably dump it in a few weeks," the clerk said. "Do you want to come get it?"

"Not if there's nothing to identify him," Holmes said. "Did you refer him to any limo companies?"

"Yes. Two. I think a limo came every day and picked him up."

Holmes got the name of the other company and contacted it. The story was the same. The young man was picked up at the Hilton on two successive days and driven to nice restaurants and other places. The second day the driver took him to look at a high-rise apartment that was for rent in the East Bay city of Emeryville. On the way there they stopped at Interlude and the man paid for massages for himself and the driver. After that the two of them went to several bars, had drinks, returned to the massage parlor, and subsequently had dinner. The man bankrolled everything, always paying with cash. Both days they went to the massage parlor, the man saw "Debbie," the driver said.

"Did he say anything about himself?"

"He said he was from Sweden and worked as a sound mixer for a rock band named Yellow Submarine. His parents were divorced, and he had been to the United States before."

At one point the man had the driver take him across the Golden Gate Bridge. He asked questions about the bridge's height, the speed of the current underneath, and how the bridge was patrolled.

Holmes called the massage parlor and asked to speak with Debbie. "When she came on the phone, she sounded like she was ten years old," Holmes says. "Just a kid." Holmes told her who he was and why he was calling. When he described the man, she started to cry. She turned away from the phone and said something to one of the other girls, who let out a gasp and started to cry, too.

Holmes asked Debbie if he could talk with her in person the following day. She said okay but called him back several minutes later to say that her boss said Holmes had to pay Debbie for her time.

"Fine," Holmes said. "How much is it?"

"It's a minimum of thirty-five dollars per hour," Debbie said.

Holmes told Dr. Jindrich that he needed his approval to spend thirty-five dollars at a massage parlor so that he could talk with Debbie. Jindrich thought it was the funniest thing he had ever heard. "What do you think the auditor is going to do with that?" he said, laughing hard.

"I don't know," Holmes said. "I guess we'll find out."

Every unusual or nonbudgeted item needed approval from the accounting department. When Holmes presented his request, the woman looked at him with a mixture of disbelief and amusement.

"I've never had anybody have the guts to ask me for money for a massage parlor," she said.

"Honestly," Holmes said, "I'm only going to talk."

"That's between you and them," she replied.

Holmes went to the parlor the next day and talked with Debbie. She said she was nineteen, but he wasn't sure she was even eighteen and of legal age, although for his purposes that wasn't important. He assured her on the phone, and her boss when he got there, that he didn't care what they did at the parlor. Even though it clearly was a brothel, he wasn't there to bust anyone; he just needed to identify the man who jumped from the bridge.

"We went into one of the massage rooms," Holmes says, "and Debbie—if that really was her name—started crying. The whole time we talked she reached constantly for Kleenex. She said she couldn't believe the man killed himself, he was so nice. She said he took care of the limo drivers, paying for happy endings—meaning sex—if they wanted it, and was friendly and generous with everyone."

The last time he was at the parlor, Debbie said, the man saw a woman named "Gina." He told her that he was leaving afterward to catch a plane, and that this would be the last time he would see any of them.

Holmes thanked Debbie for the information. Before he left, he talked briefly with the madam and thanked her for letting him talk with one of her girls during work hours. The madam said that the man not only tipped her, even though she had nothing to do with it other than being the house mother, but took her girls to a neighborhood ice cream parlor where he treated them to sundaes and brought back a cone for her, too.

All of it was interesting but it didn't lead anywhere. Holmes was no closer to identifying his unknown jumper, John Doe #6-86, aka Nils Edison.

Holmes did learn from the limo driver who took the man to the apartment in Emeryville that the realtor who showed it to him was a woman named Ilana. Holmes tracked her down, and she started sobbing as soon as he told her why he was calling. She was twice the man's age, yet they had had several nights of passionate lovemaking and the man had left some clothes in her apartment, which was above Max's Opera House in San Francisco. She looked forward eagerly to his return, and was distraught to learn that he had killed himself instead.

Ilana told Holmes that at one point while she and the man were in her apartment, the man flushed papers down the toilet and plugged it. The only remnants were torn pages from a travel visa, which Ilana recognized because she traveled frequently. She gave them to Holmes, and there was part of a registration number, but not enough to do anything with it.

Running out of options, Holmes talked with the doorman at Max's Opera House. He remembered the man because he tipped him generously, but had no other information.

That left only the Swedish rock group Yellow Submarine. Going through Interpol, the international police organization, Holmes confirmed that the group actually existed, then he was connected with someone in it. The person told him that none of the group's sound engineers was missing, and none fit the description of the decedent.

Holmes was at an end. "I had tracked everything I could," he says, "including at least $3,500 in cash the man spent in just a few days. I had everyone in our office go through all the information I had collected to see if there was anything else I could chase."

This included correspondence and notes from phone conversations that Holmes had with the German consulate, Swedish consulate (because the man told one driver he was from Sweden), and French consulate (because he told another driver that he was born in France), as well as written summaries of every interview Holmes conducted with the limo drivers, Hilton staff, Interlude masseuses, and Ilana, the realtor. There was nothing.

"We had to put it to bed," he says. "We didn't have a choice. There were no other leads to pursue, and everybody else had lost interest. Sometimes you just don't get the person ID'd."

TWENTY YEARS LATER

After two decades, there had been no new developments. Then, one day in 2005, Holmes received an unexpected call. A private investigator in Los Angeles asked him if, by chance, his office had handled the case of a young man who jumped from the Golden Gate Bridge in 1986. Holmes thought immediately of Nils Edison, and his heart began beating faster.

"Yes, we did," Holmes said. "But we were never able to identify him. He didn't have identification, no one reported him missing, and there wasn't a record of him in any database."

"Tall kid?" the PI said. "Big shock of hair, well dressed?"

Holmes couldn't believe it; it almost seemed like a dream. He had to catch his breath before saying, "That's him."

The PI said that he had been hired twenty years earlier by the Fischer family in Germany to find their son, Wolfram. He had disappeared after telling friends that he was going to the United States with a lot of money, which he planned to spend in grand fashion before jumping off the Golden Gate Bridge. For some reason the family had hired an investigator in Los Angeles rather than one in San Francisco, even though it wasn't clear that Wolfram had ever been in Los Angeles. In any event, back in 1986 the PI had contacted the San Francisco Coroner's Office, explained who he was, and asked if anyone matching Wolfram's description had jumped from the bridge recently. He was told no, that everyone who had jumped either had been identified or looked considerably different. The PI told the Fischer family that the coroner didn't have any record of their son, so he must not have jumped.

At that time the Coast Guard was handing over the bodies of Golden Gate Bridge jumpers to the San Francisco coroner. Wolfram had landed on the Marin side, however, so his case was handled in Marin.

"People in the San Francisco Coroner's Office should have told the investigator to check with coroners in other Bay Area counties," Holmes says, "but no one did. Thus the PI didn't know to call me until he happened to read a recent article that said the Marin coroner's office handled most Golden Gate Bridge suicides now. The PI no longer was in touch with the Fischer family, but he thought, what if?"

Holmes was elated by the news, and also upset. "Twenty years of uncertainty and irresolution for the Fischer family, and hundreds of hours of work on my part, could have been saved if only someone in the San Francisco Coroner's Office had told the investigator to call Marin."

The PI got back in touch with the Fischers and informed them that he had found their son. They called Holmes immediately.

"It turned out that Mr. Fischer was an industrial CEO who commuted to work in his personal helicopter," Holmes says. "He didn't fly it; somebody else did. One of the answers to the question, 'How did the young man have so much money?' was because his family had so much money."

Holmes learned that when Wolfram Fischer left Germany in 1986, he took with him more than fifteen thousand dollars in cash. His parents knew it. He had told them that he was coming to the United States to find himself and didn't say anything about wanting to end his life. He had been in touch with friends while he was here, though, and they knew his plan. He had sworn them to secrecy, so they didn't tell his parents. Later, when he didn't come home, his parents got in touch with his friends and they told them what he had said.

The Fischers flew to the Bay Area and met with Holmes and his staff. They had long since given up hope that their son was still alive and were grateful to know what happened to him. Holmes had an arrangement with two cemeteries to bury unidentified bodies in plots without a name but with a marker so that the remains could be exhumed if necessary. This was the case with Wolfram. His body was exhumed, his parents had his remains cremated, and they took his ashes home with them.

"I spent more time on this than on any other case," Holmes says, "except Carol Filipelli and Tammy Vincent. Much of it was my own personal time outside of work. My wife started to get snarly about it, saying, 'Why can't you let it go? You're never going to identify the guy.' The thing is, though, when you just have a skeleton, your chances of identifying the person are slim, but when you have somebody who has been dead only a few hours, it should be easy to identify him. When you can't, it sticks in your craw. In this instance, it took twenty years and some luck, but eventually we did."

He pauses, thinking about it. "One of the most amazing mysteries I ever handled," he tells me, "and with the possible exception of Carol Filipelli, one of the most challenging. But a better outcome."

CHAPTER 14

INVESTIGATING THE UNUSUAL

Most of the time, Ken Holmes and other investigators in the Marin County Coroner's Office were able to make a determination regarding the cause and manner of a person's death. Sometimes, though, too much remained unknown.

A fifty-six-year-old mother of three was found dead in a closed car on a hot day, with a blood alcohol content of .23. She had a history of depression and alcohol abuse, and Holmes learned that she was in an unhappy marriage that included domestic violence. There were no signs of trauma, and no alcohol inside the car. Heat prostration? Alcohol intoxication? Accident? Suicide?

A forty-two-year-old man had a history of somnambulism in which he was able to walk, talk, and even eat while asleep. On the first anniversary of his marriage to his second wife, they were watching TV when he fell asleep in a chair. When the phone rang and she went to answer it, he left the room, came back with a handgun, and shot himself. His wife told Holmes that her husband had been enjoying their anniversary and repeatedly said that he hated the thought of suicide. She believed he was acting out a dream at the time he killed himself and didn't intend to end his life. True?

A thirty-seven-year-old woman was found dead in her trailer after she failed to show up for work. Coworkers told Holmes that she was a dependable employee but recently had seemed exhausted, would become emotional for no apparent reason, and would cry at her desk. She was scheduled to go on vacation the following week and was thought to be flying east to visit her mother. There were no signs of drugs, alcohol, or trauma. The woman was emaciated, however, and had a history of extreme dieting. Holmes found dieting schedules all over her trailer. Was her death accidental or natural, related to an eating disorder? During the course of his investigation, Holmes learned that she was separated from her husband, who currently was out of the area in a rehab program. Friends of the woman described him as "worthless." Was she so depressed that she lost the desire to live, making her death a possible suicide? It was impossible to know.

Coroners—and family members—have to accept the fact that there are times when the story of someone's death is incomplete, and probably will remain that way.

Some deaths, on the other hand, were just head-scratchers, so strange that they defied belief. A thirty-seven-year-old woman was sitting on her front porch watching her neighbor attempt to cut open a sealed fifty-gallon metal drum with an electric grinder when the drum exploded. The lid flew directly at the woman, struck her in the head before she could move, decapitated her, and continued sailing through a window into her house with her head on it as if on a platter. The drum, which had been on its side, was propelled in the opposite direction, where it struck a picket fence and broke several boards.

In another case, a forty-four-year-old roofing contractor was squeezed to death when his body was pinned between the frame and bed of his ancient dump truck. The bed was hydraulic and remained up as long as the motor was running, then returned to the down position when the motor was turned off. The man had been performing routine maintenance with the bed in the up position, but the motor wasn't running when his wife, who was bringing him lunch, found him. A baseball hat and a grease gun were pinned to his body.

In a third case, a thirty-nine-year-old woman was driving on the freeway and was just about ready to go under an overpass when a truck above her overturned. The truck was carrying large boulders, which went crashing down onto the roadway. One boulder landed directly on the woman's Mazda coupe, killing her instantly. Adding to the fluke tragedy was the autopsy report, which indicated that the woman had been twenty-six weeks pregnant.

"You can't make up stuff like this," Holmes says. "You just can't. All you can do is shake your head and say, 'What were they thinking?' or attribute it to fate: wrong place, wrong time. That's all you can do."

ASSISTANT CORONER

In June 1984, Keith Craig, the assistant coroner, told Dr. Jindrich that he was going to retire at the end of the month. A day later, Jindrich called Holmes into his office.

"Keith's going to retire," he said. "I'd like you to be my assistant."

Holmes was surprised and flattered, but thought immediately of his two colleagues, Bill Thomas and Don Cornish. Holmes had been working in the coroner's office nine years by this time, but both Thomas and Cornish had been there four years longer. Moreover, they were the two people who were primarily responsible for training Holmes after he was hired.

"What about Don and Bill?" Holmes said.

Jindrich said, "I don't want them to be my assistant. I want you to be my assistant."

"How is that going to work for them?"

"They don't have to like it," Jindrich said. "I want you to be the assistant, and they can either deal with it or not."

Holmes said, "Can I have a little time to think about it?"

There were advantages and disadvantages to the promotion. The salary was higher and meant that Holmes's retirement benefits would be higher as well. In addition, he would have more authority. Best of all, he would become an eight-to-fiver; he wouldn't work twenty-four-hour shifts anymore, and for the most part, he would have weekends off. On the negative side, he would be on call all the time. The assistant coroner was everybody's backup, and if the investigator on duty was tied up on another case and couldn't respond to a new call, or was sick or on vacation, the assistant filled in. In addition, Holmes enjoyed doing investigations and working with families, and both duties would be curtailed if he became the assistant coroner.

After he talked it over with his wife, Holmes sought out Thomas and Cornish to see how they felt about it. Both men said it was all right with them.

"Are you sure?" Holmes said.

"Yeah," they said. "It's fine."

Holmes told Jindrich that he was interested and asked for more specifics. His only frame of reference was how Craig did the job, and he knew that Jindrich would want more from him.

"Here's what I expect of you as my assistant," Jindrich said. "I do doctor; you do the rest. If we have a personnel problem, I don't want to know about it, I want to know how you handled it. When it's budget time, I approve it, but you do the line-by-line numbers. If the board doesn't like it, I don't want to know it, I only want to know how you worked it out, because I do doctor, and you do the rest."

Implied but not specifically articulated was that Jindrich performed autopsies, signed death certificates, and testified in court when necessary, and Holmes hired and fired employees, supervised the investigators, drafted the budget and presented it to the board of supervisors, dealt with personnel problems and contract issues, handled reporters, responded to requests for community speakers, and took care of anything else that came up.

Holmes accepted the position, and Jindrich was true to his word.

Several times when a lot of things were going on Jindrich jumped in and helped, but mostly he was hands-off.

"It proved to be the best training ground possible for me," Holmes says. "When I became the coroner, I had been doing everything for fourteen years already, except for autopsies. It was no big deal."

A BANK ROBBERY GONE AWRY

Michael Canfield, twenty-six, and Mark Canfield, twenty-three, were brothers from Southern California. Somehow they got it into their heads to rob the Bank of America branch in Valley Ford, a tiny, unincorporated town that lies just across the Marin border in rural Sonoma County. The population of 150 people consisted mainly of farmers and ranchers, and the brothers may have thought that there would be little or no security at the bank, or that Valley Ford was so remote that police wouldn't be able to respond quickly. Holmes still has the dog-eared map that the brothers referred to for directions, and he showed it to me. Marked in blue ink is their planned route to and from the town.

Valley Ford might have looked like it offered easy pickings, but the brothers failed to consider two key facts. The first was that there are only three roads leading into and out of Valley Ford. Each is a country road that doesn't connect with a main artery for miles. The second was that all of the farmers and ranchers in the area did business at this BofA branch. It was the only bank around.

The brothers entered the bank wearing ski masks and collected five thousand dollars in cash and traveler's checks, which they jammed into a pillowcase. After that they fled on a small motorcycle, exchanging it a mile down the road for a thirteen-year-old white Ford sedan they had parked there. As soon as they left, the bank manager made four phone calls. The last one was to the police. The first three calls were to farmers on each of the three roads leading out of Valley Ford.

The brothers headed toward Petaluma on the Bodega Highway,

which, despite its name, is a two-lane road, one lane in each direction. They had only gone a couple of miles when they saw that the road was blocked by a trailer full of hay and a big bulldozer that a farmer had placed there. The brothers spun their car around, went back to Valley Ford, and headed south on Highway 1, another two-lane road. Before they reached the next roadblock, they could see in their rearview mirror units from the Sonoma County Sheriff's Department, Marin County Sheriff's Office, and California Highway Patrol in hot pursuit. Desperate to elude them, the brothers turned onto an unmarked dirt road. They had no idea where it led, but at this point they didn't care. It turned out that the road, which was a mile and a half long, served as the driveway into the Borello Ranch in Marin. When the brothers pulled up to the ranch house, two men came out to greet them, both armed with long guns.

The brothers whirled around to go back out the driveway, only to see half a dozen police cars racing toward them, lights flashing and sirens wailing. The driveway was next to a wide creek with hardly any water in it. It was steep on the other side of the creek, so the brothers jumped out of the car, ran through the creek, and scampered up the other side of the hill, holing up under a canopy of trees. Police officers pulled up in front of the Borello family's homestead and huddled to talk about what they should do. They could see the brothers only intermittently because of the shadows.

Holmes happened to be out on a previous case that was only two miles south of the Borello Ranch at the time this was taking place. A dispatcher with Marin County's Communications Center radioed him and said, "Since you're in the area, go there because they've asked for anybody who's armed to respond to the scene. They think there might be some kind of shoot-out or manhunt."

As Holmes pulled up, one of the cops said, "What are you, a vulture? They're not even dead yet."

Holmes said, "No. No, Comm Center asked me to come."

"Oh," the cop said. "Okay. Good."

For a while everyone stood around, not making a move. From a distance of about two hundred yards, the brothers eyed the police while the police and Holmes watched the brothers, who didn't even have the money they had stolen. It was in the trunk of their abandoned car, along with the motorcycle. Finally, a cop got on a bullhorn and told them to lay down their weapons and come down the hill. The brothers yelled back that they weren't surrendering, that the cops had to come get them. Since the brothers were armed, police officers didn't want to get any closer, so they waited. Meanwhile more cop cars were showing up, plus a police helicopter.

"All of a sudden," Holmes says, "there was a boom."

Soon thereafter Mark Canfield came walking down the hill with his hands up. He had blood all over the back of him and was shaking.

It turned out that the brothers had made a pact. They stood back to back, and each of them was going to shoot himself. After Michael, the older of the two, put a gun in his mouth and pulled the trigger, though, his younger brother felt warm blood and pieces of Michael's brain on the back of his head and couldn't do it. Instead, he surrendered.

Holmes climbed up the hill to where Michael Canfield's body lay. He was dressed in blue jeans and brown boots. A wadded-up pink undershirt lay close to him. At his feet was a twelve-gauge shotgun, and a loaded .22-caliber revolver was nearby. There were two spent casings in the breech of the shotgun, as well as one spent cartridge in the revolver and several unspent cartridges.

"It didn't have to end that way," Holmes says. "They were scared, though, and panicked. Everything that could go wrong did go wrong. They would have been a lot better off picking a bank in any booming metropolis."

THE BROWNLIE BROTHERS

Another set of brothers made news a short time later. The Communications Center called Holmes late one night and told him that there had been a single-car accident in Lagunitas, a small, unincorporated area of Marin County that borders Samuel P. Taylor State Park. One person was dead and another person was seriously injured, the dispatcher said.

When Holmes arrived at the scene, he saw a cream-colored Mercedes, badly damaged, off on the side of the road with twenty-six-year-old Stephen Brownlie dead in the passenger seat. Brownlie had a full beard and was dressed in blue jeans, a blue shirt, lambskin vest, black socks, and brown low-top boots. Among the injuries that Holmes itemized were various abrasions and lacerations, a compound fracture of one leg, and multiple rib fractures. The two cops at the scene told Holmes that the decedent's brother, Gordon Brownlie, age twenty-three, was the driver. He survived the crash and had been taken by ambulance to Marin General Hospital.

Holmes and two cops began to inventory the car. They looked through the glove box and checked under the seats, then Holmes took the keys out of the ignition and popped the trunk. That was when he realized that this wasn't a routine traffic accident. Inside the trunk was an expensive-looking fur coat, but that wasn't the main attraction. There was a large plastic bag filled with money, all wrapped in rubber bands and stacked. It was more money than he had ever seen.

The two cops were still looking inside the car. When they saw the bag in the trunk they were equally wide-eyed. "Now what?" one said.

Holmes said, "We're going to have to count it."

Each of them took about twenty minutes to count the money, which was mostly in small bills, then wrote down the number he came up with. None of the three numbers matched, so they did a recount. This time the three of them got different numbers. It was after 1 A.M. and everyone was beat.

"Look," Holmes said. "We know we're in the ballpark, forty-three thousand dollars and whatever. Let's all initial the bag, then tie it off. I'll take it to the auditor in the morning, and someone there can count it."

The officers agreed, and Holmes hurried back to the coroner's office with the bag. He didn't want to drive around with it, and there was one more place that he needed to go.

The evidence room in the coroner's office was a catchall, serving as a storage room for paper goods as well as for possessions to turn over to next of kin. There was a short hallway with two refrigerators and a freezer that served as the lab. There was also a large, old bank safe and an area with evidence lockers. Each investigator was in charge of evidence for his cases. If a decedent's purse was found, for example, it was noted in the inventory, which was given to the secretary, along with a copy of the case. Then it was logged by the investigator, placed in a bag or plastic container, and put in his locker. The lockers were metal, seven feet tall, with two doors and shelves inside. A logbook attached to the outside noted the date, case number, decedent's name, and evidence collected so that any staff member could see what property was contained within. The key for each locker was kept in a locked key-minder wall box in a back room that was off-limits to anyone but staff. All staff needed access because many times only one person was in the office when a family member came in to claim a decedent's possessions.

Anytime personal possessions were released, the coroner's office got a signed, written receipt. Release was based on the concept of consanguinity, which is a legal doctrine that establishes the living blood relations who are closest to a person. His or her spouse is first. If there is no spouse, then it's children, followed by grandchildren, great-grandchildren, parents, brothers and sisters, nephews and nieces, great-nephews and great-nieces, grandparents, aunts and uncles, first cousins, and so on.

With prescription medications, the investigator took possession, logged them, and kept them for about ninety days. Then they were given to a large firm that burned them at high heat. Street drugs also were burned, unless they were part of a criminal case. Since firearms were the property of the deceased, they were released to the rightful heirs or destroyed if that's what the heirs wanted, except in homicide cases, where the police took possession. A change-of-custody form accompanied the evidence so that every time it changed hands both the person who was relinquishing it and the person who was taking it signed the form. Once the item was released, the form came back to the coroner's office, where it was filed.

In this instance, Holmes locked the money—determined later by the auditor to be $43,700—in the evidence room safe, then drove to Marin General Hospital. He wanted to find out from the surviving brother where his family lived so that he could notify next of kin regarding Stephen Brownlie's death.

When Holmes arrived at the hospital, two young women were there. Both were gorgeous, well dressed, and fully made up, despite the late hour. One was Stephen Brownlie's wife, now widowed. The other was Gordon Brownlie's girlfriend. He was being treated in the emergency room with serious but not life-threatening injuries.

Holmes talked with each woman, telling her what would happen next and asking if there was anything he could do to help. His words barely seemed to register. The wife was too upset to listen, while the girlfriend acted removed and distant.

After that Holmes sat in a chair in the hallway and began writing his report. Among the personal items he found in the car was a small notebook. Thumbing through it at the scene, he had noticed columns of figures next to names and abbreviations: "1 gr.—30.00," "Lumpy—80.00," "1 paper bag—30.00," "½-paper bag—20.00." There were also title papers in the car showing that Stephen Brownlie—the deceased brother—owned a thirty-eight-foot sailboat that was registered in Florida but had a Stinson Beach, Marin County, address. When Holmes searched Stephen Brownlie's pockets, he found a traffic citation that Brownlie had received in Oregon two weeks earlier, driving a Porsche.

While Holmes was writing, Gordon Brownlie's girlfriend came through the emergency room door and headed immediately into a

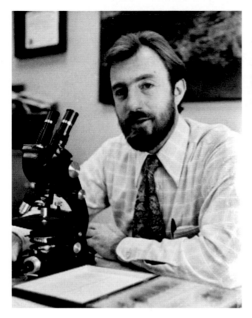

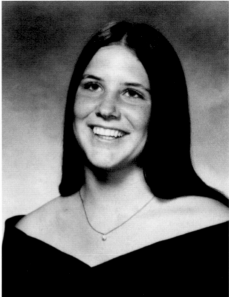

Dr. Ervin Jindrich, Ken Holmes's predecessor and mentor, was thirty-four when he was elected coroner of Marin County in 1974. (Source: *Marin Independent Journal*)

Holmes's first case after he completed training was the murder of nineteen-year-old Terry Listman in 1975. (Source: *Marin Independent Journal*)

Whenever human bones were unearthed, death investigators like Bill Thomas had to determine whether they were fairly recent or dated back several hundred years, to the time when Miwok Indian tribes roamed Marin County. (Source: *Marin Independent Journal*)

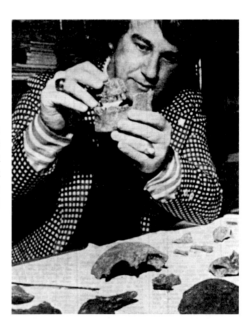

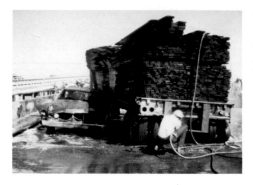

One of the first traffic deaths that Holmes investigated occurred after a car struck a stalled vehicle on the Richmond–San Rafael Bridge, spiraled into a guardrail, was hit by a lumber truck, and burst into flames. (Source: Ken Holmes)

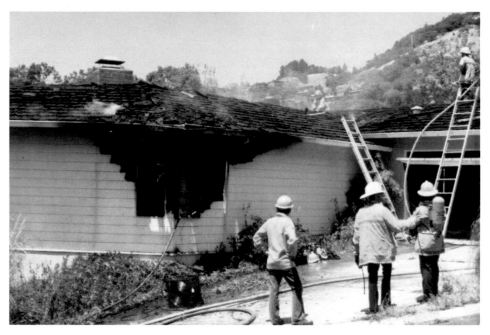

At the scene of a fatal fire, Holmes (center) discussed events with firefighters. (Source: Ken Holmes)

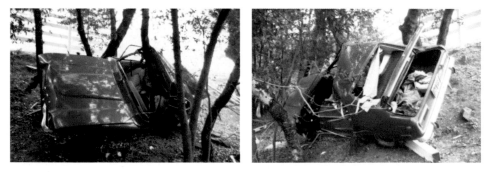

When a professional race car driver's coupe went off the road, down an embankment, and plowed into a tree, killing the driver and his female passenger, the cause was obvious to Holmes, although he didn't note it in his official report. (Source: Ken Holmes)

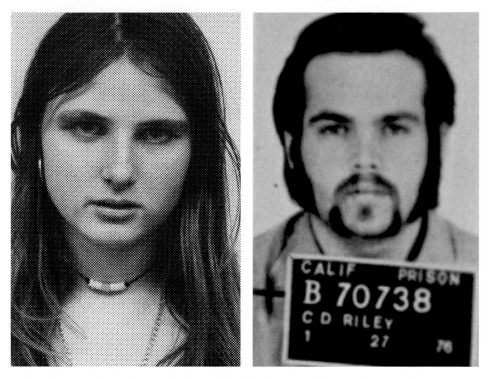

In 1976, in a case that received national attention, Marlene Olive (left), age sixteen, and her nineteen-year-old boyfriend, Chuck Riley (right), murdered her parents and burned their bodies in a barbecue pit in a state park. (Photo of Olive: *Marin Independent Journal*. Photo of Riley: California Department of Corrections and Rehabilitation)

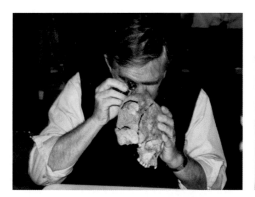

Rodger Heglar, a forensic anthropologist, was on contract with the coroner's office and helped identify human remains, including those of Marlene Olive's parents. (Source: Ken Holmes)

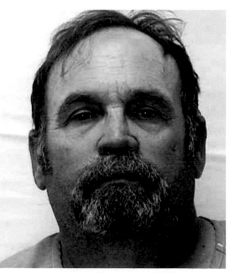

Chuck Riley, pictured in 2013, has been a death row inmate ever since the murders, while Marlene Olive has been free—an injustice, Holmes believes. (Source: California Department of Corrections and Rehabilitation)

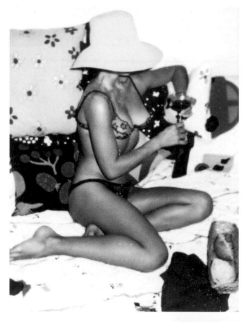

In investigating Carol Filipelli's death, Holmes found copies of this photo of her, which she used to solicit clients. (Source: Ken Holmes)

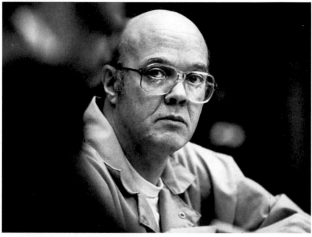

David Carpenter, known as the Trailside Killer, murdered seven people over two years on Mount Tamalpais in Marin County. (Source: California Department of Corrections and Rehabilitation)

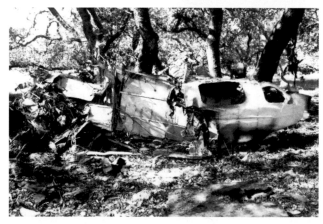

After a twin-engine plane crashed on a mountaintop in Marin, Holmes was called to investigate the pilot's death. (Source: Ken Holmes)

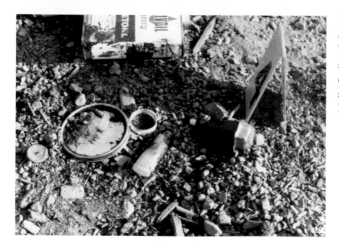

Holmes found these remnants of seventeen-year-old Tammy Vincent's murder at the scene—an awl used to stab her and an empty can of acetone used to set her body on fire. (Source: Ken Holmes)

After forensic anthropologists determined the gender, approximate age, and muscular structure of a dead person based on skeletons that were found, Holmes commissioned artists to sculpt what the decedent might have looked like. (Source: Chris Stewart/*San Francisco Chronicle*/Polaris)

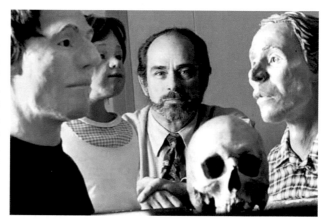

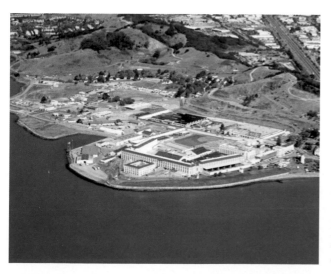

Located on the Marin waterfront, San Quentin Prison houses all of California's male death row inmates, as well as more than four thousand other hardened criminals. (Source: California Department of Corrections and Rehabilitation)

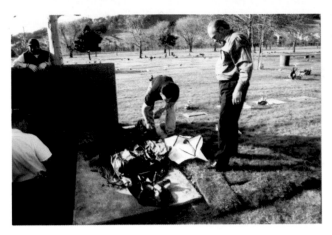

Holmes (right) presided over several exhumations every year. (Source: Ken Holmes)

These medications are typical in quantity and variety of those Holmes found at scenes of a drug overdose. (Source: Ken Holmes)

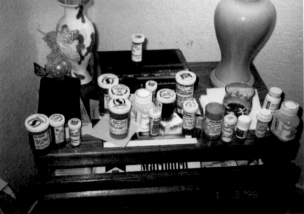
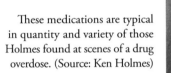

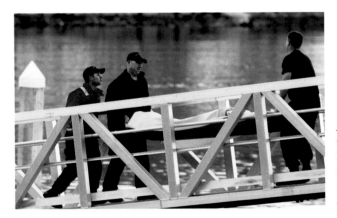

After the Coast Guard retrieves the body of a Golden Gate Bridge jumper, it is delivered to the coroner's office in Marin. (Source: John Storey/*San Francisco Chronicle*/Polaris)

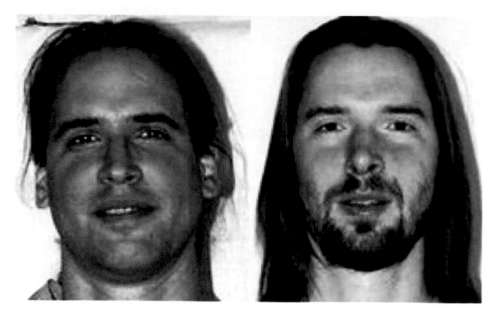

In 2000, Taylor (left) and Justin Helzer (right) proclaimed themselves "Children of Thunder" and murdered five people in a bizarre plot designed to "speed Christ's return to Earth." (Source: California Department of Corrections and Rehabilitation)

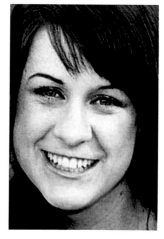

Nearly twenty years after Holmes investigated the murder of porn king Artie Mitchell by his brother, Jim, he investigated the murder of Danielle Keller by Jim Mitchell's son. (Source: *Marin Independent Journal*)

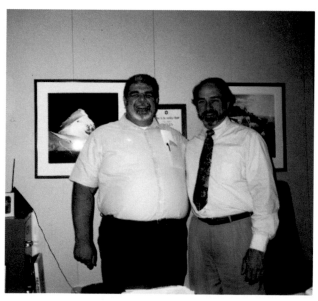

Gary Tindel (left) and Holmes (right) worked together for twelve years, until Holmes retired, the coroner's office was merged with the sheriff's department, and Tindel's position was cut. (Source: Ken Holmes)

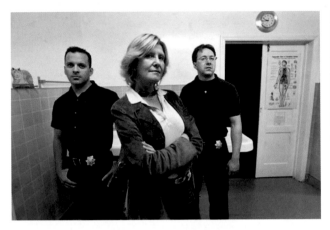

Darrell Harris (left), Pam Carter (center), and Dave Foehner (right) were Holmes's three death investigators. (Source: Christina Koci Hernandez/*San Francisco Chronicle*/Polaris)

Holmes mentored high school and college students in forensics, and one day found this caricature of himself on his desk, drawn by a seventeen-year-old intern who today is a police sketch artist. (Source: Ken Holmes)

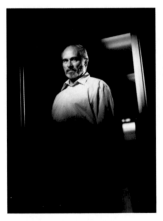

Holmes poses in a doorway in the coroner's office in 2007. (Source: Ken Holmes)

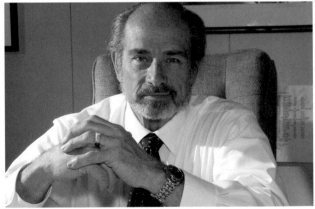

Holmes used this 2010 photo in his campaign after announcing his intention to run for the newly created position of sheriff-coroner. (Source: *Marin Independent Journal*)

pay phone booth. She didn't close the door, and because Holmes happened to be sitting nearby, he could hear everything she said. It was a short message, spoken in a monotone, to somebody's voice mail.

"This is Cheryl. Stephen is dead. I'll call you later."

Then she made another, similar call, and another. In all, she placed more than twenty calls. After a few minutes, Holmes realized what was happening. Using an office phone in a different part of the hospital, he called the San Francisco branch of the federal Drug Enforcement Administration. It was 3 A.M., but someone answered immediately.

"I'm at Marin General Hospital," Holmes said, "after a traffic accident in which one man died and another man is being treated for injuries. I found a lot of money in the trunk of their car, and now this woman is on the phone making calls nonstop, one right after the other, out of a little black book. I think drugs are involved."

Twenty minutes later, someone from DEA was at the hospital, sitting next to him. Holmes shared what he knew, and the man was all ears. Then the man saw the two women, and his eyes lit up.

"We've been looking for these two guys for years," the DEA agent said. "We didn't even know they were back in California. The last we heard, they were in Florida, buying big yachts and taking them out on a sail, then sinking them and collecting the insurance."

He explained the concept of reinsuring whereby a person or company takes out partial or full insurance from another insurer and is covered when an accident occurs. The Brownlie brothers were doing this, and dealing drugs as well. The DEA hadn't been able to find them, however. Now here they were in Marin County.

As the DEA agent and Holmes were talking, the two women walked out the front door, the girlfriend supporting the new widow. The DEA agent let them go; they weren't the ones he was after.

As soon as they left, he went to the pay phone, dialed a number, and said without preamble, "Run this number and call me back." He didn't say this is Agent So-and-So; apparently, he didn't need to. He just recited the number of the pay phone.

Ten minutes later, the pay phone rang and the DEA agent moved quickly to answer it. Without saying a word, he opened a notebook and began writing down what he was being told—all of the phone numbers that the woman named Cheryl had dialed. It was still the middle of the night, and twenty-five years before 9/11, so the government's technological capabilities were nowhere near what they are today; nevertheless, within minutes the agent had the information he needed.

When questioned, Gordon Brownlie said that he knew there was a lot of money in the trunk of the Mercedes, but it belonged to his brother, not him. DEA officials weren't fooled; they knew that both brothers were involved. In a show of chutzpah, Gordon Brownlie later sued to get the money returned to him after it was impounded. If he thought that that might have any effect on his own chances of avoiding prosecution, however, he was mistaken. Federal agents had been waiting years for the opportunity to bust him and his brother.

When the toxicology report came back, it showed that the blood alcohol content of the decedent, Stephen Brownlie, was .28 and there was cocaine in his system. Gordon Brownlie had been heavily intoxicated as well. While he was in the hospital, he was charged in absentia for driving under the influence and for vehicular homicide in the death of his brother. That was just the beginning, though. Government agents had a slew of other offenses lined up.

The Brownlie brothers' traffic accident turned out to have repercussions across the country. Out of it, DEA gained contact information for dozens of drug dealers and made busts in multiple states.

A PROFESSIONAL RACE CAR DRIVER'S DEATH

A week later, Holmes was investigating another accident. This time he was woken up at 4 A.M.

Two California Highway Patrol officers had been called to a winding road in another rural part of Marin because a passing motorist had reported several boards scattered across the road. The boards were from a corral fence that ran parallel to the road. When the officers stopped, they saw that the fence was broken. Beyond the fence was an embankment and a ditch. They swept the area with flashlights and could see, below, that a Capri coupe was wrapped around a tree. The officers climbed down the embankment to the vehicle. Lying next to the car were two bodies. One body was that of the driver. He was on his back, his head pointed toward the rear of the car, while his feet were still inside, wedged beneath the gas and clutch pedals. The other body, of a woman, was partially on top of him. The officers had to lift debris and the shattered remains of the windshield off her before they were able to determine that she was dead, too.

When Holmes arrived, he saw that the tree was embedded in the car and the entire top of the coupe had been peeled back to the rear window on impact. The officers told him that an unidentified person had passed the scene at midnight and hadn't noticed anything, then passed again at 1:30 A.M. and saw wood fencing on the road.

The driver was dressed in a three-piece tan suit with a blue shirt, brown boots and socks, and beige bikini underwear. A sparse amount of blood was on the ground beneath his head, but his left coat sleeve was soaked in blood. His body was cool to the touch, with no rigor mortis and only slight lividity, indicating that death had been recent. Holmes didn't find any identification on him, but upon opening the trunk he found men's clothing with a wallet that had a driver's license. The photo on the license matched the face of the man in the wreckage. Also in the trunk were briefcases that contained toiletries, personal papers, a Texas Instruments calculator, a Colt .38-caliber revolver, and a prescription bottle of Valium.

The woman was dressed in a black velvet top and matching pants. She was wearing pantyhose and a full-length red cloak. Her head was toward the front of the car and her legs were drawn up close to her body. There was blood on her face and on the ground under her head. In her purse was identification.

Later in the day, Holmes was contacted by a fireman whose house was far up from the road where the accident occurred but directly overlooked the area. He said he and his wife had been asleep but shortly after midnight were awakened by a loud crash. It was so loud that he thought someone had come up his driveway and driven through his fence, but when he checked he didn't see anything so he went back to bed, thinking that if the crash occurred in the canyon below someone would have seen or heard it and offered assistance. At 7:30 A.M., as he was on his way to work, he saw a tow truck pulling up a badly damaged coupe from the ravine and realized that it was probably from the accident he had heard. He contacted the coroner's office, and the information helped narrow the time of the accident.

During his investigation, Holmes learned that the man in the car was a thirty-year-old professional race car driver named Daniel. He had come to Marin County to race at Sears Point, a two-and-a-half-mile road course and drag strip in neighboring Sonoma County that is a host to the NASCAR Sprint Cup Series. Daniel had booked a room at the Alvarado Inn (now called the Marin Inn), nine miles away on Highway 101. The hotel was popular with Sears Point drivers because of its proximity to the racetrack. The bar scene there was lively as a result, with numerous young women hanging out, looking to meet the racers. One of them was an attractive twenty-nine-year-old hairdresser named Toni.

She and Daniel hit it off, and she invited him to her house. It was only a few miles away, but the road was curvy and not well lit. He drove and she sat in the passenger seat.

Coroner's reports are public information, often viewed by family members. For that reason investigators tend to omit sensitive details that aren't pertinent to the official summary. These details may have bearing on the case so they are added as a confidential addendum, but they aren't considered something that people outside the coroner's office or law enforcement need to know.

In this instance, Holmes omitted from his report the fact that at the time of the accident, Toni most likely was leaning across the narrow console between the two seats and had her head in Daniel's lap. He wasn't speeding, but his mind no doubt was elsewhere as he approached an unfamiliar ninety-degree turn in the dark. That was why he went too wide and drove through the fence. The police officers and Holmes surmised, based on the vegetation that was damaged, that as the car bolted down the embankment, careening wildly, Daniel fought for control. Then gravity took over and the car descended toward a grove of trees. When it hit one tree head-on, the driver's-side door flew open and the bulk of Daniel's body—all except his feet—spilled out onto the ground. Toni's body followed, landing on top of him.

In his investigative report, Holmes noted Daniel's clothes, but didn't note that at the time of the accident his pants were undone, his zipper was down, and his underwear was pushed aside. It was obvious why his attention had been diverted.

One of the cops joked, "He didn't know whether he was coming or going."

It was the sort of dark humor that first responders often employ. From time to time, Holmes was tempted to join in, but what prevented him was knowing that in nearly every case, the decedent had loved ones, and his next stop after leaving the scene involved notifying them.

AUTOEROTICISM

One of the odder forms of death that Holmes encountered had to do with autoerotic asphyxiation—the practice of becoming sexually stimulated through near suffocation or self-strangulation. Holmes didn't come across it often, fewer than ten times in his career, but when he did it usually was obvious. The decedent, all but one time a male, was naked or dressed in female undergarments, and had pornographic material or sex toys nearby. Typically, he was hanging from a beam or showerhead, and used something that wouldn't leave a mark, such as the sash of a bathrobe. In some cases he was holding his genitalia;

other times there was evidence that he had reached orgasm prior to death. It wasn't a suicide, because he didn't intend to die. He lost consciousness, though, and no one was there to save him.

Twice in his early years, Holmes responded to the scene of an autoerotic death. The phenomenon was so far outside his personal world that he started doing research on it to become better informed. One of the few writers on the subject in this country—autoeroticism is more common in Europe and Scandinavia—was Roy Hazelwood, a former profiler for the FBI. At the time, Hazelwood had written the only books that examined autoerotic deaths from an investigative viewpoint. When Holmes saw that Hazelwood was going to be the featured speaker at an upcoming conference of the California Homicide Investigators Association, in San Francisco, he made a point of attending. Hazelwood talked about the cause, effect, and psychology of autoeroticism, noting that it applied almost exclusively to males. Holmes couldn't help but approach him afterward and tell him that he had handled the autoerotic death of a female. Hazelwood was intrigued and said he would love to see photos from the scene. His obvious but unstated intention was to determine whether it really was an autoerotic case. Since Hazelwood was going to be in San Francisco for a week, Holmes suggested that they have lunch together. Hazelwood accepted and they made arrangements to meet several days later in Sausalito.

The case involved a forty-six-year-old woman, originally from Switzerland, who was found by her boyfriend after he returned home from work. She was nude and hanging by pantyhose that was tied loosely around her neck and attached to the shower faucet. The single-loop looseness of the ligature made it possible for her to step out of it, assuming she was conscious, in contrast to a noose that would have been employed in a suicide attempt. In addition, her hands were in her groin area, and Holmes found evidence that suggested that before she got in the shower she took a bath, then stood in front of a mirror. The mirror was movable and had been placed so that she could see herself in her nylon noose while standing in the shower. He also learned in the course of his investigation that the woman hadn't had sex with her ex-husband during the last six years of their marriage.

Holmes showed Hazelwood the photos he had taken at the scene. Hazelwood barely had to look at them before declaring, "Absolutely. This is autoerotic."

In some instances, individuals who engage in autoeroticism suspend themselves by rope or sash from a beam or door. If he could, Holmes got on a ladder so that he was able to look down on the cross point and see whether there was evidence of chafing, which would provide a clue as to how long the autoerotic behavior had been going on. Was it an early experiment or something that was well practiced?

Another case concerned a thirty-year-old man named Darryl. He was the caretaker of a large recreational vehicle and trailer park who rented an apartment nearby. After he didn't show up to work for two days, the manager of the park went to his apartment and found Darryl hanging in his shower. He was wearing women's black undergarments with a garter belt, corset, and mesh stockings, and had clamped clothespins on certain parts of his body.

After surveying the scene, Holmes asked the manager for Darryl's emergency contact information so that he could notify next of kin. The manager said he didn't have it, but Darryl had a young girlfriend who had been there frequently. Holmes searched Darryl's apartment and found her address, then he took a cop with him and knocked on the girlfriend's door.

Her mother answered. She was blue-eyed, in her forties, and had a Swedish accent. Holmes told her why he was there, that a man had died and the woman's daughter was his girlfriend.

The mother looked at him wide-eyed. "Wow," she said. "What happened to him? He was young and healthy."

Holmes wasn't about to tell her any details. "Well," he hedged, "we're not really sure."

The mother motioned for Holmes and the cop to come in and said that she would get her daughter. The cop told Holmes that there wasn't any further reason for him to stay, so the officer left.

Holmes took a seat in the living room. Several minutes later the mother and daughter emerged from the daughter's bedroom. The daughter was sobbing and the mother had her arm around her.

Darryl's girlfriend almost certainly was underage—sixteen or seventeen, Holmes guessed, although he didn't ask because it didn't matter. What was striking was her appearance. She was so beautiful that she could have been a teenage model. She had long blond hair, flawless skin, and perfect features. That made the circumstances surrounding Darryl's death all the more bizarre.

Holmes asked the girl—she truly seemed like a girl in his mind, not a young woman—if she knew where Darryl's family lived. She said she didn't know; he never talked about them.

"I don't know if he has brothers or sisters or anything," she said.

Holmes nodded. She had used the present tense, as many people do when they refer to someone who has just died, and he did, too. "How long have you been together?"

She paused to think. "Seven or eight months."

"Have you two been sexually active?" It was a question he always felt uncomfortable asking of young people, especially if their parents were present, but it was relevant to the investigation.

She looked at her mom, who nodded. "Yes," the girl said.

At one point the daughter excused herself, saying that she needed to call someone. When she was out of the room, her mother said, "What do you think really happened?"

Holmes hesitated. "I don't know if you understand autoeroticism," he began.

The mother looked at him nonplussed. "Sure."

"Oh," Holmes said. "Well, we're pretty sure this was an autoerotic death. He was found hanging in his shower, wearing ladies' under-clothing. It wasn't a suicide."

"I wouldn't think so," the mother said. "In my country it's quite common. Couples engage in it all the time. Sometimes you're by yourself, and sometimes you're with your partner."

Holmes relaxed a little and thought to himself, Okay, we're cool.

The daughter came back and sat next to her mother on the couch. Holmes was across from them. The mother told her daughter what she and Holmes had been talking about, and said that Darryl hanged himself during an autoerotic episode.

The girl's eyes opened wide. "Really?" she said. She knew exactly what her mother was referring to. "Did he hang himself in the bedroom or somewhere else?"

Holmes was amazed by the openness of the conversation. It was unlike any other that he had had.

"In the shower," he said.

The mother said, "He was wearing women's underwear. Are you missing any undergarments?"

"I don't think so," her daughter said. "I hardly ever take clothes over there and leave them. I don't think I've lost any."

That led Holmes to think that Darryl bought the underwear on his own. It was more his size than hers anyway.

Holmes said, "Did he ever, during your time with him, suggest that the two of you engage in anything like this together?"

She shook her head and said that he was rather conventional when it came to sex, not at all adventurous. As if to prove the point she said, "He never wanted to do it in public."

Holmes just about fell out of his chair. The way she said it made it sound like she had wanted to.

Remembering it today he says, "It was amazing for me to sit there and get that kind of brief education from the mom and daughter. It was like they had already talked about this on their own and were matter-of-fact about it. It served as a reminder that each day in my profession was different and held possibilities of the unexpected."

CHAPTER 15

BONES AND A FROZEN INFANT

Prior to the arrival of English explorer and pirate Francis Drake on the Marin coast in 1589, Marin County was inhabited by Native Americans, primarily Miwok Indian tribes. Long after Drake left and was knighted, the tribes continued to hunt and fish in Marin, and also die there.

Five to ten times per year, on average, Holmes's office evaluated Indian remains. They were buried where they died, not in specified plots, and their bones were unearthed during construction of a new home or business development, or when there was land movement of some kind. Construction stopped until a coroner's investigator determined whether the remains were ancient or more recent. If they were ancient, then it wasn't a concern. No death certificate would be issued. If they were more recent, however, the remains needed to be identified, if possible, and an approximate date of death established, usually by going through missing-persons reports. An attempt had to be made to determine the cause of death as well. Sometimes there were answers, sometimes not.

The bones of a man were found on a hillside west of Bolinas, near an RCA radio tower. An RCA employee had been checking the lines when he came across a bleached skull. Noticing that the jaw of the skull contained dental fillings, the employee contacted the sheriff's office, which in turn called Holmes. He found other bones and also a torn pair of underpants and the bottom portion of a deck shoe. With a shovel and his hands, Holmes sifted through loose dirt and scrub brush and found additional bones, plus three keys, a pair of prescription glasses, some plastic buttons, and small fragments of khaki and woven blue material. Slightly downhill were still more bones, most likely scattered by small animals. He gave the skeletal remains to a forensic anthropologist who concluded that they were of a male in his early twenties, about five foot ten, with heavy musculature. Holmes and others in the office pored through missing-persons reports to try to find a match, but weren't successful. The cause and manner of the man's death remained unknown, as did his identity. He stayed John Doe #2 of that year.

Despite the challenges, the coroner's office was successful much of the time in identifying skeletal remains. Some of it was the result of luck, but mostly it was due to persistence.

"No one should die in anonymity," Holmes says. "Even if that's what a person wants, to just disappear and never be seen or heard from again, I believe his or her loved ones deserve to know what happened."

When it came to human bones, Holmes's most notable case went back forty-four years. One newspaper said that it seemed to be "plucked straight from the plotlines of a late-night TV drama." Holmes, who sometimes watched late-night dramas, agreed.

A groundskeeper at Fernwood Cemetery in Tamalpais Valley had been turning over ground in a remote area that wasn't designated for graves when his tool snagged on what turned out to be a buried wool sweater and a tangle of bones. Digging a little more, the groundskeeper found a broken pair of eyeglasses, two glass lenses, and a 1961 fifty-cent piece. Because no bodies were supposed to be buried there, the coroner's office was called.

"Finding a partial skeleton is one of the biggest challenges a coroner faces," Holmes says, "simply because there isn't much to go on."

In this instance, the skeleton was missing a head and hands. Clearly, someone had removed them thinking that it wouldn't be possible to identify the remaining bones even if they happened to be unearthed at a later date. The position of the bones indicated that the person had been buried in a fetal position, facedown in the shallow grave.

The first step was to determine how long the body had been buried. The only clues were the coin from 1961 and the eyeglasses. The frames of the glasses had the words "American Optical" etched on the arms. Darrell Harris, the investigator on the case, contacted a historian with the company, which was in Massachusetts, who said that that particular model was made from 1962 to 1968. Harris then took the glass lenses to an optometrist. The optometrist said that they probably were made in the late 1950s or early 1960s because plastic lenses were common after that. The left lens had a bifocal line and was for a person who was extremely farsighted, while the right lens had no bifocal line and was called a "balance" lens—that is, it had little or no built-in correction and was only for aesthetics. The combination, according to the eye doctor, indicated that the wearer probably had cataracts.

An anthropologist provided more information. In all likelihood, she said, the bones belonged to a Caucasian female who was between five foot one and five foot three in stature and age forty-two or older.

Two weeks after the bones were found, and following a fruitless search of the state Department of Justice's missing-persons database, Harris and another coroner's investigator, Dave Foehner, began doing door-to-door interviews with neighbors in the area. One longtime resident remarked that a woman known as "Mrs. Jones" had disappeared many years earlier. That tip led Harris to go through county archives, which turned up a missing-persons report from 1964. Bruce "B.B." Jones, a longshoreman and union boss in San Francisco, had told authorities that his wife, Gertrude, was missing. They had had a heated argument, he said, in which she refused to add his name to the deeds of several pieces of property she owned. She walked out of the house after that and never was seen again.

With this information, Harris began looking for one of Gertrude Jones's surviving family members to do DNA testing. After much research he located a niece in Florida, and her mitochondrial DNA was compared to a DNA sample of the skeletal remains. (Mitochondrial DNA is passed along the maternal lines of families. A female can pass her mitochondrial DNA on to her children, male or female, but males do not pass along this DNA to their children.) The Department of Justice lab confirmed with a high degree of certainty that the bones found in the shallow grave belonged to Gertrude.

Further evidence of the match was that Gertrude Jones was Caucasian, forty-three years old, five foot three, had poor vision, and had undergone cataract surgery shortly before her disappearance. The place where her remains were found was only a half mile from her home.

The only person who stood to gain from Gertrude's death was her husband. They didn't have any children, and the only close relative was Gertrude's sister, whom Harris managed to track down. She lived in New Jersey and told Harris that she appreciated knowing that Gertrude's remains had been found after all this time. She said she always believed that Gertrude's husband was responsible for her death. He hadn't been in touch with any of Gertrude's relatives after she went missing, and ignored their requests for keepsakes of hers, the sister said. Then she asked Harris a question.

"Would you like me to send you a movie of Gertrude's wedding?"

"You have film from the day she got married?" Harris said.

"I can send it to you."

She did. It was eight-millimeter film shot on the day a half century earlier when Gertrude Kavesh married Bruce Jones.

"Gertrude was in this funky little hat," Holmes says. "She had a 1950s hairdo, glasses, and wore a white dress. Her husband was kind of potbellied and looked aloof."

There was sound, so Holmes and his staff heard both of them talk, too, at the reception. Gertrude's voice was high and excited, like that of a new bride, while Jones's voice was deep and sounded as if he was a little bored.

"It was all a little weird," Holmes says, "because Gertrude's bones were laid out on a piece of brown butcher paper on the conference table in my office."

Anytime Holmes's staff investigated a case involving skeletal remains, the bones were placed in their anatomical positions on the table. This way everyone could see what they had and didn't have.

Gertrude's head, hands, and other missing body parts were never found. Nevertheless, Holmes was confident in ruling that her death was a homicide. The tiny bone in her throat, called the hyoid bone, which enables people to speak, was intact, so she hadn't been strangled, but her first cervical vertebra—the bone closest to the skull—was broken in a manner that wasn't consistent with Gertrude accidentally breaking her neck.

The undersheriff of Marin County took exception to the ruling. By calling it a homicide, Holmes was opening up a case that law enforcement had no desire to handle.

"You're not legally capable of calling it a homicide," he said. "That's my call."

Holmes was surprised. "Surely you know that the coroner is the person who legally rules on the manner of death," he said. "If you don't think it's a homicide, tell me how she dug the grave, got in it, cut off her head and her hands, and buried herself. It's not a suicide, it's not an accident, and it's not a natural death. What would you call it?"

The undersheriff sputtered, then hung up. He didn't have an answer.

Another piece of circumstantial evidence tied B.B. Jones to the crime. From the backyard of the house where he and Gertrude lived, there was a clear view of her burial site. It would have been easy with binoculars to tell whether anyone disturbed it.

Shortly after he reported his wife missing, Jones left the country and settled in Tahiti. When Gertrude was declared legally dead, he inherited her property and returned to Marin, bringing a Tahitian wife with him.

"If he did kill her," Holmes says, "he didn't have long to enjoy what he gained."

Three years later, Jones died of natural causes. Ownership of his belongings passed to his Tahitian wife, who sold it all before returning to her native land.

BABY DOE

In May 1988, the body of an infant washed up on a small beach in Tiburon. Judging by the condition of her body, it was estimated that she had been in the water two or three days. She was wrapped in a white sheet with dark stains, and inside the sheet were a disposable diaper, a woman's blouse, and a woman's black dress. Inscribed on the front of the undershirt the baby was wearing were the words "I'm adorable."

Holmes consulted with a dentist and a forensic anthropologist regarding the child's age. Each estimated it to be sixteen to eighteen months. The Tiburon Police Department issued an all-points bulletin, but it didn't produce any leads. After a week, Holmes contacted local TV stations and asked them to broadcast a poster that the coroner's office created, which included a description of the clothing. They couldn't picture the baby because she had been in the water awhile, but the clothing was distinctive.

The poster said, "Have you seen these items? Do you know this baby?"

Every local station aired the story, but nothing came of it. Holmes didn't receive one response.

Meanwhile, Dr. Jindrich determined during the autopsy that the infant, now being referred to as Baby Jane Doe, had a fractured skull. He speculated that someone dropped her on her head or swung her head against a wall. What confused him, though, was that under the microscope he saw changes in the cell structure of some body tissues, and he couldn't put his finger on what had caused them. He sent copies of the slides to two outside experts, but both of them said that they weren't sure, either.

It wasn't until much later that Holmes learned why no one responded to his news stories, or why Jindrich hadn't understood what he had witnessed under the microscope. As is sometimes the case, the answers, when they came, were the result of chance.

In October 1988, five months after Baby Jane Doe's body washed ashore, a hunter stopped in a remote coastal mountain area in Humboldt County to relieve himself. He was a good distance from any paved road, and three hundred miles north of Marin. Looking down, he saw the skeletal remains of a foot in front of him. The bones were peeking out from underbrush, and he knew immediately that they belonged to a human. Moving aside branches, leaves, and a small amount of dirt, the hunter unearthed a shallow grave and the rest of the body.

The Humboldt County coroner was called to the scene and the body was exhumed. Then the arduous and time-consuming task began of determining who the person was. Three and a half years later, in the middle of 1992, a positive identification was made by matching dental records. The deceased was Renee June, a Berkeley artist who worked at a San Francisco advertising agency. Six years earlier, in August 1986, she had been reported missing. At that time her car had been found abandoned in Berkeley, but she was never seen again.

A brief article appeared shortly thereafter in the *Marin Independent Journal* noting that the remains of a long-missing Berkeley woman had been found and identified. Still missing, according to the article, was the woman's eighteen-month-old daughter, named Marta.

Ray Nichols, one of Holmes's investigators, was off duty and home at the time the article came out. He read it, cut it out, Scotch-taped it to a piece of paper, wrote "Could this be our Baby Jane Doe?" and put it in Holmes's mail slot the next time he was in the office. Holmes came to work, saw the article, and said to himself that it couldn't be. The baby was eighteen months old, but disappeared in 1986. That would make her three and a half in 1988, when Baby Jane Doe was found.

Nevertheless, to cover all bases, Holmes supplied DNA from Baby Jane Doe to the Department of Justice's lab, which compared it with bone samples from Renee June's remains. Much to everyone's surprise, they matched. Baby Jane Doe now had a name, Marta June, as well as a mother. Still unclear, though, was why there was a discrepancy regarding her age. Also unknown, of course, was who killed her and why.

Renee June was married to a Berkeley architect named Arthur Mount. Once her remains were identified, he became the primary suspect in her death. He had moved to Washington State by this time but remained in touch with a longtime lover in the Bay Area named Chan. When the story broke in the *San Francisco Chronicle* about the murders of Renee and Marta June and the suspicion cast on Arthur Mount, Chan contacted Mount and let him know. Three days later, police in Blaine, Washington, found Mount in a hotel room, dead from a gunshot wound to the head. A note signed by Mount said, "I repent my sins. I pray to forgive and to be forgiven." He didn't say what those sins were.

Working backward, Holmes and the police were able to piece together what probably happened, starting with the fact that Arthur Mount was Marta's biological father. A comparison of his DNA with hers confirmed it. His daughter's legal name was Marta June Mount. After killing his wife and daughter in 1986, Mount put their bodies in a chest freezer in his basement. Two years later, when he decided to move to Washington, he didn't want to take the freezer with him so he had to dispose of their remains. He wrapped Renee June's body in several layers of clothing and drove to Humboldt County, where he found an old logging road. A mile or so in, he stopped, dug a shallow grave, laid her wrapped body in it, and covered it with branches and leaves, thinking that she never would be discovered. As for Marta June, it seemed likely that he threw her body in the bay near Berkeley and currents carried it to Tiburon.

It all made sense now. Marta June was two years older than originally thought because her body had been frozen for two years. No
one responded to Holmes's media appeal because no one knew of an
eighteen-month-old infant who went missing recently; Renee June's
friends only knew of a child that age who disappeared two years
earlier, along with her mother. Also, Jindrich had seen evidence of
ice crystals that had been present in Marta's body, but then they had
melted and destroyed various cells.

It was all conjecture—there was nothing concrete that tied Arthur
Mount to the murders—until Mount shot himself. Then everything
fell into place. Mount's girlfriend, Chan, confirmed that he had had
a chest freezer in his basement in Berkeley. No one tracked what
happened to it, and Chan said she didn't know, but it seemed likely
that Mount had it taken to a dump.

As for motive, Tiburon police speculated that Mount killed his
wife and daughter to collect insurance money. Holmes had a different theory, however. He thought it was because Mount wasn't close
to his wife—he and Chan were lovers before Mount married Renee
June, and continued to be lovers after—and he didn't want the added
burden of providing for a child.

"I thought then, and still think now, that Mount killed Renee out
of anger and frustration, then killed Marta because he didn't know
what else to do with her," he says.

When police interviewed Chan, she said that Mount had been
depressed and dealing with financial problems. The two of them
talked about the *Chronicle* article, and Chan said that Mount didn't
deny being involved but also didn't confess to anything. In her mind,
he wouldn't hurt a fly, much less kill anyone. As close as they were,
though, she said there was a lot about his life that he kept from her.
For instance, she didn't know that Mount had married Renee June
until months later. He hadn't told her.

CHAPTER 16

INVESTIGATING ABUSE

The worst injury Holmes incurred in his career was when he wrenched his back helping to carry a two-hundred-pound dead man from a third-floor walk-up in San Rafael. Usually the mortuary that was contacted to pick up the body sent two people, but this time only one person came, a young woman who weighed under one hundred pounds. Holmes took the heavy end of the litter, but before they had even gotten to the stairs the woman dropped her end without warning, unable to hold the weight. Holmes lurched forward, his back gave out, and he went down on his knees. After that, he wasn't able to lift the gurney and had to call the fire department and ask firefighters to take the dead body down the stairs. He managed to drive home, all the while vowing to avoid that situation again.

When Holmes became coroner, local mortuaries said that they no longer could afford to send people out for what the county could pay—three hundred dollars per trip. Holmes understood.

"It's hard to run a removal service," he says, "because you have to have a lot of people available on a moment's notice. I ended up using a special company that was located across the bay, in Richmond. This one contracted with coroner's offices in multiple Bay Area counties and couldn't have been better. They would be in San Rafael in twenty minutes from the time we called them, two guys, shirts and ties, suit coats, shined shoes, perfect gentlemen."

The only time the removal service wasn't contacted was when the deceased was an infant or young child. Then the investigator put the body in the back of his or her car, with as much compassion as possible. Investigators' vehicles weren't big enough to accommodate an adult-sized gurney, but babies and small kids could be laid on the backseat and taken to the mortuary. Given the coroner's tight budget, any opportunity to save money was seized.

Devon Gromer was only seven weeks old when he died. His parents, Katja and Jereme Gromer of San Rafael, told Gary Erickson, the coroner's investigator who responded initially, that their son had had multiple health problems since birth, and had been in and out of various hospitals. When they found him unresponsive at 3:50 A.M. one day in April 2000, they called 911. Paramedics responded, but resuscitation efforts were unsuccessful. The cause of death was unclear, and the case probably wouldn't have gone any further except Holmes was contacted by a relative of one of his closest friends who knew about the baby's medical history.

"Something's not right," Holmes was told. "You need to look into Devon's death further."

Holmes turned to Pam Carter. She was the lone female among his three investigators and had a strong medical background. In her early forties, five foot seven, trim, attractive, with dishwater-blond hair and clear, sparkling eyes, she had worked at Marin General Hospital for more than twenty years before testing for a job in the coroner's office and being hired.

"She would look at lab values," Holmes says, "the printout on blood gases, and go, 'Whoa, the liver is a little high,' or 'Calcium is a little low.' I'd look at it and go, 'Oh, really?' She knew the values, the medicines, the dosages, what was contraindicated. I know most of the regulars that everybody deals with, but she knew them all."

To start, Carter reviewed the write-ups of each of Devon's fifteen visits to the Marin Community Clinic, plus two hospitalizations. The initial clinic visits were to test for a dairy product allergy that Devon's mother thought he had. Later visits and hospitalizations were because there was blood in his stool and he had a prolapsed rectum, meaning his rectum was inverted. It's a condition that occurs at birth on occasion when the mother is pushing hard, but is rare after that. Abdominal X-rays were taken, and nothing else seemed wrong. Devon was treated, ate well, recovered each time, and was released to his parents.

A second set of X-rays told a different story, however. Devon had multiple rib fractures—a red flag for abuse. Fractures of the clavicle can result from physiological problems at birth or an accident of some kind, but anterior and posterior rib fractures in an infant as young as Devon can only come from a squeezing type of injury. A prolapsed rectum also can be evidence of squeezing, of forcing everything out.

Pam Carter interviewed Katja and Jereme Gromer half a dozen times. Holmes participated in all but the first interview, which was three hours and taped by Carter. It included a scene reenactment of Jereme Gromer holding a doll the way he said he held Devon, with Carter taking pictures of it.

Both parents were in their twenties and huge. "Katja was like a linebacker," Holmes says, "and Jereme was even bigger, about 240 pounds."

The Gromers said that they were Devon's only caregivers. Carter asked how Devon got a bruise on his chest, which was discovered during the autopsy. They said it was caused by a Coke glass that fell on him. Carter asked if the Gromers' other child, a three-year-old daughter named Makela, had had any health problems. The Gromers admitted that she had had a couple of broken bones early on, but they were healed now and she had no other problems.

"I'd like you to sign a release form," Carter said, "so that I can review Makela's medical records." The Gromers did.

In subsequent interviews, Carter and Holmes learned that Jereme Gromer worked nights as a security guard. When he came home in the morning, he would lie down on a couch with Devon, then when his wife went to work he would go to bed with the baby. Invariably when she got home, he told her that Devon had been fussy or seemed to have an upset stomach. She either took Devon to the clinic or emergency room to have him checked, or she called an advice nurse. Each episode occurred while her husband was caring for the baby and ended with Katja being the one to seek help or answers. Theories ranged from Devon having colitis or colic to him being lactose intolerant.

Jereme Gromer was with Devon the night he died. When Carter interviewed him, taping the conversation, he was so matter-of-fact that it was chilling.

"I was just about to go to sleep," he said, "when I heard, I don't know how to call it, like whatever was left inside just finally squeezed out, you know, the last breath that came out of his body, and it kind of startled me."

Carter investigated the case for six months and felt that she had established a clear pattern of abuse. In her report she summarized her findings.

"Each time the baby was removed from the parents' custody via hospitalizations, he thrived," she wrote. "It appears, given the symptoms described by the parents and the pattern established in Devon's short life, that he suffered another squeezing event sometime around the day of this death."

Despite her conclusion, which was supported by medical records and the testimony of multiple doctors, the district attorney decided not to charge the Gromers. After the autopsy, Devon's remains were released to his parents. They had him cremated; thus the only evidence of rib fractures was in the second set of X-rays.

Several months passed, then Holmes received another phone call from his informant, who was still in touch with the Gromer family. "Don't give up," Holmes was told. "Katja is pregnant again, and it's going to start all over. Also, Makela has had another broken arm."

The next time Holmes heard from his source was early one morning and the message was alarming. "Just to let you know," the source said, "their new baby was airlifted to Children's Hospital in Oakland with a lacerated liver. He is three weeks old."

Holmes flew out of bed, called Children's Hospital, and told one of the pediatricians about Devon Gromer's history. The pediatrician already had seen the new baby and knew that some kind of child abuse was involved because there were rib fractures on one side. All of the injuries occurred when Jereme Gromer had him, which was most of the time because Jereme wasn't working and his wife was putting in extra hours at her job to compensate.

"It turned out that he didn't like to hear babies cry," Holmes says. "I guess he felt that if he squeezed them long enough and hard enough they would stop."

Jereme Gromer was charged with multiple counts of child abuse and responsibility for Devon's death. He accepted a plea bargain and was sentenced to twenty-one years in state prison. Holmes and Carter attended his sentencing.

In a postscript to the story, Katja Gromer divorced Jereme by the time he was tried. She wanted to keep the new baby, who survived his father's abuse, but Child Protective Services took him from her custody and let him be adopted by a policeman and his wife who couldn't have kids. Makela also was taken from her mother and hasn't had any broken bones since, as far as Holmes knows. Katja eventually remarried, got pregnant, and gave birth. The last time Holmes checked with his source, the baby was healthy and injury-free.

THE FAMILY

Shortly after Holmes discussed the Devon Gromer case with me, he asked, "Have I told you about Ndigo Wright?"

I recognized the name from the file, which actually was labeled "Ndigo Campbell-Bremner–Wilson-Wright." I wondered why a nineteen-month-old boy had four surnames, and Holmes explained. It started when Ndigo's lifeless body was brought into a Kaiser hospital in Marin by three white women, none of whom seemed to have any sense of urgency or emotional attachment to the biracial boy.

"Our child isn't breathing," one woman said. She was older than the other women and seemed to speak for the group.

She told Dr. Tom Meyer that the child's name was Ndigo and he was a year and a half old, but to Meyer the boy looked half that age. His skin was mottled, his belly was distended, and his legs were bow-shaped like the legs of a frog. The woman also told Meyer that they had tried to revive him with a warm bath and CPR prior to bringing him to the hospital.

Meyer said afterward, "It seemed very bizarre to walk up with an obviously dead child and before that not realize that something bad was going on and not call an ambulance."

Odder still, when Meyer informed the women that the child was dead, none of them reacted. Instead, the lead woman asked if the coroner had arrived yet. Meyer said he had.

"Good," the woman said, "because we're ready to go home."

Gary Erickson, Holmes's investigator, viewed Ndigo's body in the hospital's emergency room and noted numerous irregularities. Ndigo's belly was bloated, his back was humped, and there was little or no musculature to his buttocks. All of it pointed to severe malnourishment and neglect.

"Can we get some X-rays?" Erickson asked.

In other settings, the coroner's office paid $200 to $300 to have a mobile X-ray van come and do it, but hospitals had the equipment right there and usually did it for free. When the X-ray technician brought the films to Erickson, he was scratching his head.

"These are really opaque," the tech said. "I can't see much. Let me shoot some more."

A half hour later he returned. "This kid has no bones," he said.

Erickson looked at him. "What do you mean?"

"I mean his bones aren't showing up in X-rays."

"Is there a problem with the machine or the film or the light?"

The technician shook his head. "I took a picture of my arm with the same film and it was clear, so it's not the equipment. There's no density to his bones."

"That doesn't make sense."

"The only possible explanation I can give you is that this kid has never had any vitamin D. He has never been in the sun, and his bones haven't developed."

The autopsy revealed that in addition to being underdeveloped, Ndigo's bones were broken in dozens of places due to a calcium deficiency. He also had rickets, a disease caused by a lack of vitamins, which was prevalent during the 1800s but rare since then.

"Ndigo's arms and legs were Gumby-like," Holmes says. "They could be flexed—not a lot, but a little—because the bones inside them hadn't hardened."

Erickson contacted local police and Child Protective Services and told them about the case. Two cops and a CPS response worker met him at Ndigo's house. It was on a cul-de-sac in the newer part of Marinwood, a subdivision of San Rafael. The older part of Marinwood, where Holmes lived at the time, was middle class and consisted of single-story ranch houses. The newer part was more upscale with larger homes, many of them two stories and valued at $800,000 or more, and featuring expansive, well-maintained yards.

They arrived at seven o'clock on a Wednesday evening. The house was set back from the street, shaded by palm trees and protected by a tall fence with a gate. All of the curtains were drawn, so there was no way to see inside. Only one light appeared to be on.

The police officers went through the gate and rang the doorbell. When no one answered, they knocked loudly on the door. Still there was no response.

Erickson went to talk to the neighbors on one side while the cops went to talk to neighbors on the other side. One set of neighbors told

Erickson that they could hear children every once in a while in the house but never saw any kids. The other set of neighbors said that they had never seen or heard any kids and were fairly certain that no children lived there.

In order to enter the house without permission, the cops needed a search warrant. Getting one usually took several hours, so the CPS worker left. Erickson decided to stay and see if anyone came out of the house. He sat in his car and wrote up his report, keeping an eye on the front door in case anyone emerged. No one did.

With the warrant, police went through the gate again, knocked on the door, and said, "San Rafael Police. We have a search warrant."

A woman opened the door immediately. Nothing prepared the police officers or Erickson for the scene that they encountered.

Inside, in the dark, were twelve children ranging in age from eight months to sixteen years. All were malnourished, and some were deformed. Several children older than Ndigo couldn't walk; they didn't have enough bone structure to stand on their own feet. One two-year-old boy couldn't even sit; he had a huge callus on his forehead because the way he moved was to push his head along the hardwood, linoleum, and tile floors as if he were a wheelbarrow.

All of the children slept on mattresses on the floor in one room, and called each of the four women in the house—Carol Bremner, age forty-five; Mary Campbell and Deirdre Wilson, both thirty-seven; and Kali Polk-Matthews, age twenty—"Mom." There was hardly any food in the refrigerator—no milk or orange juice or anything other than a handful of vegetables—and the kids looked to Erickson as if they had never seen the light of day.

The father wasn't present, but authorities learned that he was an unemployed forty-five-year-old African-American man named Winnfred Wright. Wright had long, graying dreadlocks, smoked crack regularly, and according to one journalist who covered the case, "had convinced the women that they had to pay for the racist sins of their white ancestors by serving him financially, physically, and sexually."

On the walls of the house were bizarre paintings. One was of an African-American man who was holding a rifle over his head and standing on the naked, facedown bodies of white women.

Because Holmes lived nearby, he saw Wright on occasion, walking up and down Lucas Valley Road. Wright was hard to miss. In addition to being a black man in a predominantly white neighborhood, he wore a knitted, multicolored Rastafarian hat, the same kind of tie-dyed shirts favored by Jamaican reggae singer-musician Bob Marley, and tight black pants with wide bell bottoms that started around the knees and had pleats that matched his hat. Still, Holmes didn't think much of him.

"He was just a guy in the neighborhood," he says. "I never actually spoke to him, and of course I had no idea by looking at him what was going on in his world."

What was going on was a small cult that the prosecutors, and subsequently the media, referred to as "The Family," which operated in total seclusion. The children didn't go to school, didn't see a doctor or a dentist, and rarely went outside. They subsisted on a vegan diet and routinely were starved. For punishment, they had to wear tape over their mouths and eat hot chili peppers.

None of the women in the house—three of whom were white, with one (Polk-Matthews) half black—was married to Wright, yet he exerted total mind control over them even though all were intelligent and well educated. Bremner graduated from UC Berkeley. Wilson had attended Wesleyan College; moreover, she was the trust fund granddaughter of the founder of Xerox Corporation. Campbell came from a middle-class Italian-American family in Brooklyn. Polk-Matthews had gone to Lick-Wilmerding, a prestigious private high school in San Francisco. Collectively, the women paid all of the group's living expenses through jobs they had and Wilson's trust fund. In the process they financed Wright's drug habit while suffering quietly from his physical and mental abuse and servicing him sexually. Prosecutors were baffled as to why the women kowtowed to Wright, but he had a powerful presence, preyed on their sense of white guilt, and isolated the women so that they felt dependent on him. When he wasn't meditating, fasting, doing drugs, writing, painting, reading spiritual books, or procreating, Wright was issuing dictums to the women on everything from how they dressed and what food they consumed to how their children were to be raised.

When some of the children began to show bone deformities, Wright insisted that they were due to genetic defects, not illness, and the women took his word for it. They weren't brainwashed zombies, but they had been living with Wright's nonsensical beliefs so long that the beliefs didn't seem strange.

Margaret Singer was a psychology professor at UC Berkeley who specialized in what she called "cults of charisma." In 2002, at the time that Winnfred Wright and his four concubines were arraigned in federal court on a variety of child abuse charges, and a year before Singer herself died, she was interviewed by the *Los Angeles Times* about the case. She said that all of the women who fell under Wright's influence—there had been others previously—were young, naïve, and idealistic.

"Wright first convinced the women that they'd be part of something more spiritual and progressive and wonderful than they could find elsewhere," Singer said, "and then slowly eroded their self-confidence and moral perceptions." He separated them from their families and others who could provide support, instilled fear of physical abuse ("We were terrified of him," Mary Campbell said later), and after impregnating them said that no one would want to help a white woman who had birthed children fathered by a black man.

The fact that "The Family" existed in quiet, affluent, suburban Marin, under everyone's radar, made it that much more sensational. Moreover, it would have continued to exist, with no one aware of it, if little Ndigo hadn't died.

Carol Bremner was the first woman Wright recruited, and she became the de facto leader among them. She bore Wright's two oldest daughters and was instrumental in recruiting other women. The way she recruited them was through the guise of a women's art project.

The project, allegedly, was a mural that celebrated femininity. Photographs of ninety women were needed, Bremner said, as models. Once inside the residence, the women were offered massages, pot, and herbal cigarettes while soft music played in the background. They were told to take off their clothes and slip into a robe because it would make a better picture. If they stayed, Wright had sex with them. If they left, they were replaced by new recruits.

Four months prior to Ndigo's death, Bremner became ill. Wright wouldn't let her see a doctor so she tried to heal herself with herbal remedies. Her condition continued to worsen, however, and Wright finally agreed to take her to a doctor. It turned out that she had leukemia, a fatal form of cancer that attacks a person's bone marrow and blood cells. Wright told her that she had "brought it on herself."

Bremner's diagnosis was received at the same time that Ndigo got sick. Mary Campbell, Ndigo's birth mother, asked Wright to let her take Ndigo for a checkup, but Wright refused. After Ndigo died, he told the four women, "It's Ndigo's time to pass. He doesn't want to live the human life anymore."

Wright was charged with the second-degree murder of Ndigo and accepted a deal in which he pled guilty to felony child abuse instead and was sentenced to seventeen years in prison. Mary Campbell, the mother of five other children by Wright besides Ndigo, was sentenced to ten years in prison for felony child abuse. Deirdre Wilson, the mother of five of Wright's children, was sentenced to seven years for the same offense. Kali Polk-Matthews, the youngest recruit, hadn't birthed a child by Wright yet, and charges of involuntary manslaughter and child endangerment against her ended up being dropped. Carol Bremner, meanwhile, died of leukemia while in judicial custody.

"Do you know what happened to the children?" I asked.

Since the coroner's office wasn't involved in this aspect of the case, because the children were alive, I was worried that Holmes might not know. He followed it, though, as eager as I was to know how everything turned out.

"When workers from Child Protective Services entered the house the night after Ndigo died," Holmes said, "all of the children were removed for their health and protection. None were returned. Each was placed in a new environment, and their health improved once they were nourished, active, and exposed to the sun. Within several months, the boy with the large callus on his forehead was able to stand on his own for the first time in his life, and some of the other children were doing well in school."

It wasn't an out-and-out win, especially considering Ndigo's death and the fact that many if not all of the children were likely to suffer lasting mental health issues. Still, given the situation, it was the most that anyone could hope for. Doctors, police officers, CPS workers, prosecutors, the judge, and Holmes had to be content with that.

Not surprisingly, Mary Campbell and Deirdre Wilson, as well as Winnfred Wright, lost all of their parental rights. They were permanently barred from communicating with any of the children or with each other.

"I had a blessing of being given children," Wilson said afterward. "I aligned with a warped worldview. I gave up my maternal instincts. I squandered my responsibilities. . . . I will cry daily."

Campbell checked out a book from the prison library on grieving, which said that apologizing to the dead can be cathartic. Afterward, she spent hours role-playing with another female inmate who pretended to be Ndigo. Campbell apologized to the substitute Ndigo over and over, weeping all the while. The exercise helped, but only a little.

"The very first thing I'm going to do when I get out of here," she said, "is join a grieving-mothers support group."

Wright wasn't as remorseful. Actually, he wasn't remorseful at all. After he was convicted, he said that the only thing he was guilty of was failing to see that the children got enough vitamin D. He called it an "innocent mistake."

CHAPTER 17

REMEMBRANCES OF OCTOBER

On October 17, 1989, the Loma Prieta Earthquake, magnitude 6.9, struck the San Francisco Bay Area. As memorable as it was, disrupting the third game of the World Series, and as tragic as it was, considering that 69 people were killed, 4,000 others were injured, and 15,000 homes and businesses were destroyed in San Francisco and Santa Cruz County, it was only the second most important event that Ken Holmes had to deal with.

At 6 A.M. the day before, coroner's investigator Bill Thomas was on duty but home when his phone rang. Knowing that it probably was the county Communications Center notifying him of a death, Thomas went into the kitchen to answer it so that he wouldn't disturb his wife or children. He was forty-one years of age, and after years of womanizing he had settled down, married, and become a father.

His intuition was correct; a dispatcher was on the phone relaying details of a death. Thomas was leaning against the kitchen counter talking jovially, as was his way, when he slumped to the floor with spasms and seizures, gagging, coughing, and turning blue. He was having a heart attack, and his young son, who had followed him into the kitchen, saw the whole thing. The son started screaming, waking

Thomas's wife. The Communications Center sent an ambulance right away, but it was too late. Doctors kept Thomas alive for a week; however, he had been brain dead by the time help arrived.

Thomas's funeral service was well attended, as he had many friends and colleagues. The most noticeable contingent was women, who outnumbered men four to one. "Even though Bill was married and had kids by that time," Holmes says, "many women were weeping because they liked him so much."

The other noticeable contingent was law enforcement. They came in uniform and filled one-third of one side of the church. "Total respect for Bill," Holmes says.

As he was sitting there listening to the service, Holmes couldn't help but think of moments over the years when Thomas's humor and charisma had lifted the spirits of everyone around him. Two memories in particular stood out.

The first one occurred early in Holmes's tenure. The investigators in the coroner's office—Thomas, Holmes, and Don Cornish—were required to take a two-week course on fingerprint cartooning at the Department of Justice in Sacramento. Fingerprint cartooning sounds like a comic strip but it's actually making a sketch of an unseen fingerprint that someone is describing over the phone. It's not as necessary today thanks to modern technology that makes it possible to send the image of a fingerprint electronically and receive the results back in seconds, but it was important at that time.

The class was a ninety-minute drive each way from Marin, so the three of them carpooled in the Rambler they shared. They had to leave the county at six thirty each morning, and because he was the junior investigator, Holmes was the designated driver. He didn't mind except that every afternoon, on the way back, Thomas wanted to stop at a topless bar.

Topless bars were just coming into vogue and two of them opened simultaneously on opposite sides of the highway in Dixon, a small town west of Sacramento. The class ended at 4 P.M., and since he was still young and single, Thomas wasn't in a hurry to get home. Cornish and Holmes were older and married, but that didn't matter. Thomas was able to talk people into anything.

When they walked into the bar, it was early enough that they were the only patrons there. It was just them, the bartender, and a forlorn-looking woman who would get up and gyrate halfheartedly on a small elevated platform behind the bar while raucous striptease music blared.

"The woman did her best to look tantalizing," Holmes says, "but the effect was pitiable. The more she took off, the more you wanted her to put something on—a bathrobe, anything."

Typically, Thomas sat between Cornish and Holmes at the bar. He did most of the talking, although the conversation was collegial. Thomas also did most of the drinking, with Cornish matching him on occasion. Holmes didn't drink anything with alcohol because he was driving and didn't want to risk getting pulled over, especially in a county car.

The second week they stopped at the same bar three days in a row, not because it was any less run-down than the other bar but because they realized by then that it didn't matter. Both bars had the same watered-down booze, grating music, and tired-looking, beaten-down women. One bar ended up being frequented more often simply because they didn't have to cross over the highway to get to it.

Each time they were greeted by the same bartender, who never seemed to be aware that he had served them the day before. The fourth day, bored and with nothing else to do, Bill Thomas started ribbing the bartender, but doing it in a fake Middle Eastern accent that sounded genuine (among other skills, Thomas had a gift for mimicry). The bartender shrugged it off at first, thinking that Thomas would let up after a while, but he didn't. The longer Thomas kept at it, the more bothered the bartender became. It was early in his shift and he didn't need this.

"Knock it off," the bartender said finally. "Just enjoy your drink and keep your comments to yourself. If you don't, I'm going to have to eighty-six you."

Thomas looked blankly at Cornish and Holmes. "What that mean, eighty-six me?" he said.

Cornish and Holmes were fighting not to give Thomas away. They stifled their laughter, covered their mouths, and said nothing.

Thomas turned to the bartender. "I no understand. What is eighty-six? What you mean?"

Finally the bartender had had enough. "Get the hell out of here," he said.

Thomas looked at him in astonishment. "Why? I do nothing wrong."

"Out!" the bartender ordered, pointing toward the door.

Cornish and Holmes sat at the bar with their heads bowed as if to say, "We don't know this guy."

Thomas shrugged, then walked out the door. Cornish and Holmes decided to stay another ten minutes so that the bartender wouldn't think the three of them were together, even though they had come into the bar together three days in a row.

After a few minutes a man entered and sat down several stools away from Holmes. Holmes glanced in his direction but gave him no thought until the man ordered a drink. Then Holmes stared at him. The man's voice was all too familiar; it was Thomas. He had gone out to their car, changed into different clothes, including a coat and a hat that had been in his foot locker, and returned, this time without the Middle Eastern accent.

The bartender didn't seem to recognize him. He brought Thomas his drink, and Thomas sat by himself, straight-faced, sipping his drink as if nothing had happened.

The other memory was more recent and concerned a murder in Belvedere. It was the first homicide in the city's history, as far as Holmes knew, and got people's attention for that reason.

Belvedere is one of the most affluent communities in the United

States. It has the highest per capita income—$250,000—of any city in the country with a population over 1,000 (Belvedere's population is 2,000). The average home price is more than $2.5 million. There are no restaurants or stores on Belvedere's two island peninsulas, just jaw-dropping views of San Francisco, Angel Island, Sausalito, the Golden Gate Bridge, and Mount Tamalpais.

The victim was a wealthy antiquities collector who also happened to be a major drug dealer, although neither the police nor Holmes knew it at the time. As far as everyone at the scene was concerned, he was just a middle-age man who was sprawled on the deck of a megamansion with a gunshot wound to his head. Inside the house were Ming vases, statuary behind glass, and other rare Oriental artifacts, many nearly priceless. It was in these artifacts that Chinese heroin was smuggled.

Thomas was the coroner's investigator who was called to the scene. Holmes was assistant coroner at the time, and he instructed the investigators to contact him anytime a case was unusual or likely to attract the media. Given the rarity of a murder in Belvedere, Thomas called Holmes.

When Holmes arrived, Thomas was talking with a young female cop. There was a seven-foot-high grape-stake fence along the street, and the two of them were in front of a gate that led down a path to the house, which had its own dock and panoramic views of the bay. The female cop had a clipboard and was responsible for noting the name and affiliation of every person who entered the crime scene, the time he or she arrived, and the time the person left.

Thomas had been inside already and was just waiting for Holmes. Holmes took one look at him and knew what he was up to.

"Bill was this sage coroner's investigator who was romancing the pants off this woman who was fairly new to the job," Holmes says.

Thomas introduced Holmes to the woman and said, "Ken is my supervisor. He has been at this game much longer than the rest of us, and has seen it all."

Thomas laid it on thick, making up all sorts of stories. Holmes had less experience than Thomas, but the woman would never know it.

After several minutes, Thomas and Holmes went through the gate and down the path to the house. The decedent was still lying on his deck, with police officers milling around him. The officers didn't have anything specific to do but weren't going to miss out on the opportunity to be involved in a homicide in their small, well-to-do community.

There wasn't much for Holmes to see. The man was clearly dead, and it was clearly a homicide, as no weapon was found. The fact that the victim was at the top of the pyramid of an international drug-smuggling ring, without any connections to the people who did the actual dealing, would come out later, long after the coroner's office had put the case to bed.

When they went back through the gate, Thomas resumed his conversation with the female cop. "How long have you been on the force?" he asked.

"Six months," she said.

He nodded as if that was what he expected. "Have they given you bullets yet?" He said it with a perfectly straight face, so she wasn't sure if he was joking.

"Well, yeah."

"Are they real ones or the wooden ones?"

She didn't know what to say before she realized that he was pulling her leg. "Oh, you," she said, and she punched him playfully on the arm.

"That was the epitome of Bill," Holmes says today. "He was the funniest person I ever knew."

Thomas's death left a vacancy that needed to be filled. In the short term, Holmes could handle the added work, but given his other responsibilities he needed to hire a new investigator as soon as possible. He turned to a deputy he knew, Gary Erickson. Erickson had been a tunnel rat in Vietnam, then a longtime cop. He was tired of police work and frustrated that when he arrested someone, more often than not the person was released and back on the street before Erickson had even completed the paperwork. It made him cynical and somewhat bitter, although he was inquisitive and a good thinker.

Because he had been a cop, Erickson was especially good at talking to other cops. "If they tried to bullshit him, he saw through it and didn't accept it," Holmes says. Erickson didn't have Bill Thomas's sense of humor, but then, no one did. Thomas would be missed, and Holmes felt badly for his widow and children, who should have had many more years to enjoy his company.

It wasn't until after Thomas died that Holmes learned something that surprised him. Don Cornish, the other senior investigator, said that Thomas was offended when Dr. Jindrich passed over him five years earlier and chose Holmes to be assistant coroner.

"Bill didn't hold it against you," Cornish told Holmes. "He held it against Doc."

At the time, Thomas had told Holmes that he was fine with the change. Not once in Holmes's presence had Thomas expressed any hard feelings about it.

Holmes couldn't help but ask Cornish, "Did you feel the same way?"

Cornish shrugged. "Basically, yeah. After a while we understood it, though. You were the right person for the job. Besides, you haven't been a jerk."

It was an obvious reference to Keith Craig, Holmes's predecessor, whose prickly personality had been difficult to deal with. In contrast, Holmes had made a point of being open, honest, and fair. The emphasis was on "we," not "I," and they respected that.

KEEPING A COOL HEAD

A year earlier, also in October, Holmes left work at 5 P.M., planning to spend a quiet evening at home watching *Monday Night Football*.

He was divorced by this time and living on his own, and he stopped at a local Safeway store to pick up a couple of TV dinners. As soon as he entered, he noticed a large Halloween display in the front of the store, on the left-hand side. He has always had a special fondness for Halloween—it's his favorite holiday of the year—and he stopped to look at the items that were being featured. As he did, a shopper went out the exit doors near Holmes and a big, muscular African-American man in his twenties charged in through the same doors like a freight train. He was wearing a watch cap and jacket, and his hands were buried in his jacket pockets. Right behind him was a smaller black man wearing a beanie and army peacoat. The smaller man had one hand in his pocket and the other at his side.

The big man looked right at Holmes but was too focused on the rest of the store to see him. Holmes knew immediately that they weren't going shopping, and said to himself, This isn't good.

The big man rolled the watch cap over his face to form a ski mask, pulled out a .45-caliber handgun, held it up in the air, and announced as he walked down the row of check stands, "This is a holdup. Everybody get down."

The small man left his beanie on and followed in his partner's footsteps, giving everyone dirty looks as if to say, He means business. It wasn't necessary; the big man was walking strong and all who saw him knew it. No one was going to challenge him.

Holmes moved around to the back of the display so that he wasn't in their line of sight and considered his options. He was required to carry a gun while on duty, and since he was coming from work he had the gun on him. It was strapped to his waist and concealed by the sport coat he was wearing. When he got home, he would put it in a drawer, but at the moment he was armed.

It wasn't much of a gun, though, a five-shot .38. It was the smallest and lightest gun he could carry within regulations. He didn't want more weight on his hip than absolutely necessary, and wasn't interested in wearing a shoulder strap or ankle holster. More important, he had never fired it at anyone. He had no desire to be a cop, and his attitude was that if he witnessed a crime, he didn't want to draw on somebody because he was at a disadvantage—the other person probably had no qualms about shooting someone, while Holmes did.

Several people were slow to get on the floor and the big man was impatient. "Everybody down!" he said again. For emphasis, he took the butt of his gun and knocked one of the check stand baggers, a slender East Indian teenager, to the ground.

When the robber hit the boy, the gun flew out of his hand. It slid under the steel bar at the check stand and went a couple of feet beyond it. In a flash the man vaulted the bar and retrieved it. Seeing the violence with which he had coldcocked the bagger and the catlike reflexes he displayed getting his gun back, Holmes knew that the man was trouble. He calculated the odds of intervening with his .38 when the man had a much bigger .45 with ten or more shots, and didn't like them.

The better course of action, he decided, was to go to the back of the store and say in a loud voice because there were a lot of shoppers at that time, "Stay here. A holdup is going on in front and the robbers have guns. Someone call 911." After that, he hurried down several aisles to alert other shoppers of the robbery.

After Holmes had told as many people as he could, he walked cautiously toward the front of the store. Everyone but the two robbers was lying on the ground. While Holmes watched, the robbers went from check stand to check stand with the big man pointing his gun at people and the small man taking out trays full of money. The small man also hurriedly scooped up some of the loose bills that had been stashed underneath the trays and stuffed them in his pockets.

"Both of them were stupid as hell," Holmes says. "Hundreds and fifties were on the ground when they left."

He made his way to the end of the store where the two men had come in, thinking that their car had to be in the parking lot. His car was there, too, and was equipped with a police radio. As he started up the last aisle he saw them leaving, the big man still brandishing his gun and the small man carrying a stack of money trays. They hadn't thought to bring bags or pillowcases to put the money into; they just took the whole trays.

Holmes exited a few seconds after they did but couldn't see them. They disappeared around a corner of the building, and when he got there, they were gone. The most he saw was a glimpse of a car speeding away. It was a red Toyota sedan, although some of the paint was worn away, and Holmes thought a woman was driving.

Holmes ran to his car and used the radio to call in the incident. "I just witnessed a 211 with a 245," he said, using the code numbers for armed robbery and assault with a deadly weapon, the latter because the East Indian teen had been knocked out. "The two suspects are African-American. One is at least six foot one, weighs 215 to 225, and is wearing a heavy coat and watch cap. The other is about five eight, weighs 150 to 160, and is wearing an army peacoat and beanie. They might be in a distressed-looking red Toyota with a woman at the wheel."

After that, he went back inside to check on the boy who had been struck. Holmes had requested an ambulance, and it arrived within minutes, along with multiple police cars.

The boy was conscious, but groggy. No one else had been injured or needed assistance.

"Jesus," one cop said to Holmes. "You actually saw the whole thing?"

"Yeah," Holmes said.

"Why didn't you shoot?"

"Because they had bigger guns than me. Besides, this place is packed with women, and if I had let them know I was here, they would have grabbed the first person they saw, and then the situation would have escalated, getting really ugly really quickly. I decided that the best thing to do was get the hell out of their eyesight so they didn't know I was here, then warn others to stay away from the front."

The cop thought about that for a second, then nodded in agreement.

Whenever a crime was committed in Marin, especially a crime in which the suspects were African-American, it was standard practice for the police to position a patrol car at the foot of the Richmond–San Rafael Bridge. Cops didn't think of it as racial profiling; rather, they were just playing the odds. Given the paucity of black residents—except in Marin City—it was likely that the perpetrators lived outside the county. The police car was parked on the off-ramp to San Quentin Prison, where it was easy for the officers to watch every vehicle that passed. It also was easy for motorists to see the stakeout vehicle, which was intended. Law-abiding citizens instinctively slow down when they see a police car, while criminals tend to speed up and, therefore, stand out.

One of Holmes's good friends happened to be in the car that was waiting at San Quentin. He saw a red Toyota race by with a woman at the wheel and an African-American male passenger. Neither of them looked in the cop's direction, which was a tip-off. The cop pulled out quickly and stopped the car, and another police vehicle arrived right behind him. The two occupants, a quivering woman and a small, wiry man, surrendered without incident. When police opened the trunk, they found the trays of stolen money. They also found the big man scrunched up inside.

Police didn't wait to put the trio in a lineup at the station. Instead they were lined up on the side of the road right there. Riding in the front seat of a patrol car, Holmes did a drive-by identification of the two men. They had changed clothes since leaving the grocery store but were unmistakable.

When the case was ready to go to trial, the two men claimed that they were innocent even though they had the trays of stolen money. Police officers informed them that there was a witness to the robbery, a person who was trained in criminal identification and carried a gun but didn't intervene because that might have precipitated the taking of a hostage. When the suspects heard that, they accepted a plea bargain.

"Looking back on it," Holmes says, "a lot of things could have gone wrong in that situation. Fortunately, only the boy was injured, and not seriously. The two idiots were arrested quickly, the money was recovered, and very little court time was needed. Also, I didn't have to use my gun. All things considered, it couldn't have turned out any better."

Holmes still thinks about it, though, every time he sees a Halloween display. It hasn't diminished his appreciation of the holiday, but it does give him pause.

"I guess it's appropriate that it was a Safeway store," he says, drawing out the two syllables. Safe-way. "Although if it had been a Lucky store, that might have been good, too."

CHAPTER 18

CASES IN THE NEWS

The list of well-known musicians and singers who have lived in Marin County is long. It includes Bonnie Raitt, Booker T. Jones, Carlos Santana, David Crosby, Huey Lewis, Janis Joplin, Jesse Colin Young, Maria Muldaur, Peter Tork of the Monkees, Sammy Hagar, and Van Morrison. It also includes various members of the Grateful Dead, Jefferson Airplane, and Metallica, including the lead singers of each of those bands. Bill Champlin (Sons of Champlin), John Cipollina (Quicksilver Messenger Service), and jazz pianist George Duke went to high school in Marin. Concert impresario Bill Graham lived in Marin as well.

As impressive as this list is, a good argument can be made that no one on it has been more influential than the rapper Tupac Shakur, sometimes referred to as 2Pac. Murals bearing his likeness are all over the world, and many current rappers imitate his style and mannerisms.

In 1988, when Shakur was seventeen, his family moved from Harlem to Marin City. It wasn't as dramatic a change as some might think. Although Marin City is only five miles north of San Francisco, and only a mile and a half north of upscale Sausalito, it's on the other side of Highway 101 and is a world apart. Unincorporated and small—it has fewer than three thousand residents—Marin City's racial and socioeconomic composition is closer to Harlem's than to any other place in Marin County. At the time Shakur lived there, Marin City was predominantly African-American. Today, after more than two decades of gentrification, blacks comprise 38 percent of the population—the same percentage as whites. This is in marked contrast to the rest of Marin County, where 80 percent of residents are white and only 3 percent are black. The median income in Marin City is $38,000, versus $91,000 for the county. More than 37 percent of Marin City residents live below the poverty line, compared with 8 percent for the county.

Marin City was developed in 1942 to house World War II shipyard workers, immigrants, and other low-income people. They were crammed into tenement-type buildings of flimsy construction, many of which have since been razed and replaced, although housing remains substandard relative to the rest of the county. The majority of residents are renters who, because of their low incomes, often are forced into crowded living conditions.

In the early days of Holmes's career, Marin City was a hotbed of seething anger. The presence of police was incendiary rather than placating, and served to ignite rather than quell pent-up aggression. When he had to go to Marin City to investigate a death, regardless of the time of day, Holmes usually encountered a crowd of loud, emotional, and sometimes hostile people. As the years went by, the tension subsided considerably and coroner's investigators were accepted. In the beginning, though, their presence was questioned.

"A typical scenario was that Aunt Nellie would die," Holmes says, "and she would be in her seventies. It might be in July, when it was hotter than hell because the air-conditioning in the building didn't work, one o'clock in the morning, and she was on the fourth floor. Despite the late hour and the fact that her death probably was natural, there would be a crowd of people out in front of the building when I arrived, and two or three cops near the entrance, standing back to back because the residents didn't like cops. I came into the building and some folks looked at me skeptically, although I wasn't wearing a uniform with a badge so they knew basically why I was there. They allowed me, sort of, into the fourth-floor hallway, which would be packed, thirty or forty people, all of them talking. I was the only white guy because the cops weren't coming in; that would just make the situation worse."

He pauses. "So I would go in and see Aunt Nellie, and talk to whoever was there that was in the family, tell them what was going to happen, ask them if they had a choice for a mortuary. Then I left. And if it was something like that it was fine, but if there was a homicide, then there were three different factions of people who were mad, and the situation was volatile. I had a gun, but there was no way when I was in the middle of that crowded hallway that it was going to do me any good. Besides, I was pretty sure I wasn't the only person there who was armed right that minute."

One thing Holmes learned was that when he had to go into a building in Marin City, he let his stethoscope hang out of his coat pocket. He didn't make a big deal of it; he just let enough of it hang out so that is was clearly visible. "That way I was perceived as a man of medicine," he says, "rather than a cop. It made a big difference in how I was received."

The most notable case that Holmes investigated in Marin City occurred August 22, 1992. After performing at an outdoor music festival there, Tupac was signing autographs when a fight broke out around him between members of two rival gangs. Reportedly, Tupac drew a legally registered gun, then dropped it. His stepbrother picked up the gun and fired a single shot. He wasn't aiming at anyone, as far as Holmes could tell, but the bullet struck a six-year-old boy named Qa'id Walker-Teal in the forehead. Qa'id was on a school playground one hundred yards away, innocently riding a bicycle. There was no exit wound.

The boy was rushed to Marin General Hospital and placed on life support. He died shortly thereafter. Dr. Jindrich noted in his autopsy report that there was a marked fracture of the skull with excess fluid and bleeding in the brain. Even if Qa'id had survived the shot, which was highly unlikely, so much damage had been done that he would have been in a vegetative state for the rest of his life.

The case never went to trial, so neither Holmes nor Jindrich testified in court regarding it. The stepbrother was arrested for firing the gun, but many people believed that he took the fall in order to protect his famous relative, who hadn't dropped his gun at all and was the real shooter. None of the people who witnessed the event would testify, however, which also was common in Marin City. Qa'id's mother brought a wrongful death suit against Tupac, and there was an out-of-court settlement for an undisclosed amount, thought to be between $300,000 and $500,000. With the settlement, charges were dropped and that was the end of it.

Tupac's own life was cut short when he was gunned down four years later in a drive-by shooting in Las Vegas. Although there was widespread speculation that jealous rival and East Coast rapper Biggie Smalls was behind the shooting, the *Los Angeles Times* reported that Tupac, then twenty-five, was killed by members of the Southside Crips, a Southern California gang, in retaliation for Tupac's involvement several hours earlier in the beating of one of the gang's members.

THE ROCK LEGEND

The death of little Qa'id Walker-Teal and Tupac's alleged role in it drew considerable interest from the media, but it resulted in nowhere near the level of frenzy that followed Jerry Garcia's death three years later, in August 1995. The front man for the Grateful Dead lived in Tiburon and died in a high-end residential drug and alcohol treatment facility in Marin called Serenity Knolls.

On the advice of his physician, Jerry had checked into the facility the previous day, having recently spent two weeks at the Betty Ford Center in Southern California. A night watchman making his rounds heard Jerry snoring at 4 A.M., but when he came by again at

4:23 A.M. the snoring had stopped and Jerry appeared lifeless. A nurse on the premises started CPR and paramedics were summoned. They arrived to find Jerry in asystole—that is, without a heartbeat—and pronounced him dead. He was fifty-three years old.

Holmes went into work that morning only a few hours after Jerry died; nevertheless, word had gotten around quickly that the rock legend was dead. The hallway in front of Holmes's office was jammed with people and cameras and light bars. There were reporters from European news outlets in addition to U.S. print and electronic media. Jerry's body wasn't even there—it had been taken to a local mortuary for autopsy—but that didn't matter to everyone who was eager for any kind of sound bite.

Jane, Holmes's secretary, got there before Holmes, and when she pushed through the throng in order to unlock the door, microphones were pushed in front of her with everyone asking, "What can you tell us about Jerry Garcia?"

Jane was in her seventies and had never heard of Jerry Garcia. "Jerry who?" she said.

"Jerry Garcia of the Grateful Dead," a number of people answered in unison.

She had heard of the Grateful Dead but had no idea what the name referred to. Working in a coroner's office, it could refer to a lot of things.

She shook her head, said, "Sorry," and ducked into the office as quickly as possible, locking the door behind her. When Holmes arrived, everyone clamored around him. He knew that Jerry Garcia had died—his investigator who handled the case, Gary Erickson, had called him at home to let him know—but Holmes didn't have enough information yet to be able to comment publicly about it.

One of the courses that he took years earlier at the police academy provided tips in dealing with the media. As annoying as reporters might be sometimes, the instructor said, they aren't going away. If you try to brush them off, you'll turn them into adversaries and make any situation worse. The trick, he said, is to make them think that they are in your good graces, that they are your confidants. You don't have to tell them much, but if you do it over several sentences it sounds like you're giving them substance. Also, at disaster scenes and car accidents where there are lots of gawkers, the instructor said that investigators shouldn't try to block reporters' access by telling them to stay behind police barricades. They won't do it and instead will sneak up on top of a building or someone's house to try to get a better view. A sounder strategy is to say, "All right, guys, I'm going to take you as close as I can to the area, not just one but all of you together, and I'll answer every question I can, then I'm going to ask you to step back to that second line." If you do that, the instructor said, it gives media people something and they don't feel like you're snowballing them.

Holmes always tried hard to work with the press because there were times when he needed them. He provided as much information as he could without disclosing anything that reporters shouldn't have. What he found was that if he said, "I'll have something for you at two o'clock if you leave me alone now," they would go away, but he needed to be there at two o'clock. If he wasn't, they lost trust in him.

Typically after a death, reporters go to the police first for information. They are told that everything is under investigation pending the outcome of the autopsy, however, which sends them racing to the coroner's office, because each one wants to get "the scoop." In the case of Jerry Garcia's death, there wasn't a lot that Holmes could say other than verify that Jerry was dead and that it appeared he had died from natural causes, although that wouldn't be confirmed until the autopsy was completed in a day or two and the toxicology results were in, which would be several weeks.

Despite having nothing else to report, the media camped outside the coroner's office for the next eight hours. TV reporters filmed live cut-ins from there, which were spliced at the beginning and end of B-roll segments on Jerry and the Grateful Dead, and newspaper reporters wrote articles about Jerry's legacy and speculated on the future of the band. Holmes appeared briefly on film and was quoted in print stories, saying little but trying to sound authoritative while expressing condolences to Jerry's family.

When the autopsy and toxicology reports came back, there were no surprises. Jerry had a history of drug use, of smoking heroin and snorting cocaine, and was in a drug treatment facility, so it was natural to assume that he had drugs his system, and he did. In addition, a small, empty bindle and straws were found in his wallet, typical of cocaine usage.

The medical cause of death was listed as "recent hemorrhage, atherosclerotic coronary artery plaque due to coronary arteriosclerosis with cardiomegaly and multifocal myocardial fibrosis." In other words, a bad heart.

"The reason for the bad heart," Holmes says, "was Jerry's lifestyle, which wasn't just gorging on food or heavy use of drugs and alcohol. It wasn't just the concerts and all the travel that went with them, either. It was all of those things together."

Jerry wasn't old, but years of hard living had caught up with him.

THE PSYCHIATRIST'S WIFE

Early on a cool morning in February 1986, a thirty-eight-year-old woman was found slumped against the steering wheel of her gray BMW sedan. She was wearing a blue sweatsuit, green vest jacket, blue scarf, blue deck shoes, blue leg warmers, white socks, white long underwear, panties, and a bra. In her right hand was a 6.35-millimeter Walther semiautomatic pistol. Her first finger was resting on the trigger, and there was a bullet hole in her head.

It looked like a clear case of suicide, and ultimately Ken Holmes ruled it that way. There were things about the case that prolonged the investigation, though, all of them having to do with the woman's husband.

Elizabeth Blinder wasn't well known, but Martin Blinder certainly was. In fact, he was arguably the best-known psychiatrist in the country. Blinder's fame wasn't due to his academic pedigree, although that was impressive and enabled him to establish a thriving private practice in Marin County. Rather, it was his testimony in a 1979 court case in San Francisco that cemented his reputation.

Dan White was a San Francisco city supervisor and onetime police officer who was charged with two counts of murder after assassinating fellow supervisor Harvey Milk and San Francisco mayor George Moscone in 1978. White's attorneys claimed that their client was depressed and suffered diminished capacity at the time of the crimes, and Blinder, as an expert witness for the defense, vouched for it. He said that a number of factors contributed to White's depression—he had just quit his job, he was estranged from his wife, he had lost interest in exercising, and his clean-cut appearance had become slovenly. It was when Blinder talked about White's diet changing from healthy foods to sugar-laden soft drinks and snacks, however, in particular Coca-Cola and Twinkies, that his testimony became infamous. When the verdict was announced—White was convicted of the lesser charge of voluntary manslaughter—people rioted in the streets of San Francisco and eleven police cars were set on fire outside City Hall. The common misperception was that White's defense team—and Blinder in particular—argued that White's consumption of Twinkies was behind the murders, and the jury bought it, as ludicrous as that seemed. In fact, the defense said that White's newfound proclivity for sweets, including Twinkies, was symptomatic of White's depression, and jurors agreed. (White served five years of a seven-year prison sentence. Two years after he was released, he killed himself.)

Notoriety from the trial didn't bother Blinder. He was confident of his diagnosis, unafraid to take a position that few others shared, and willing to go head-to-head with anyone.

Bill Thomas was the coroner's investigator who was on duty when Elizabeth Blinder's body was found. He notified Dr. Blinder, who said that she left their house at eleven o'clock the previous night in an "angry" mood. She had a history of "crushing problems" he said, which at times overwhelmed her. When this happened, she would leave home for a few days to work them out. When Thomas asked who her doctor was, Blinder said that he was her sole health care provider. In response to Thomas's question about whether Elizabeth Blinder owned a handgun, Blinder said she did, but he didn't know what type.

A week later, Holmes was contacted by an ex-boyfriend of Elizabeth Blinder. He said they lived together for seven years until they broke up and she began living with Blinder. When they met, he said, she was known as Gail Elizabeth "Sunny" Doney and working as a prostitute in Berkeley. Dr. Blinder was one of her johns, the man said, and convinced her to move in with him. Later, Blinder took her to Reno and, after a bout of drinking and drugs, married her. According to the caller, the day after their wedding she told Blinder that she didn't remember much from the previous day and didn't know that she was now married.

The man told Holmes that a week before Elizabeth died, she asked him if he knew the name of a good divorce lawyer. Holmes confirmed this with Elizabeth's mother, who said that her daughter phoned her the day before she died and said she was leaving her husband and getting a divorce. Elizabeth's mother also said that Elizabeth had an argument with her husband the night before she died. When she went out to walk her dog, Blinder locked her out of the house. She and the dog ended up sleeping in her car.

Ten days later, Martin Blinder came into the coroner's office to pick up his wife's personal effects. Holmes asked him if the couple had had any domestic trouble in the days prior to her death. Blinder said no. He also denied that they had been arguing at the time she left the house. Holmes asked for the names of Elizabeth's friends and contact information for her family because he wanted to talk with them. Blinder said his wife didn't have any close friends and was estranged from her family, who lived in Florida. He didn't have phone numbers or addresses for anyone.

After Blinder left, Holmes was called by a woman named Connie. She told him that she was Elizabeth Blinder's best friend. Elizabeth was smart, an artist, and had been widowed from a previous marriage after her husband was killed in a car accident, Connie said. She recounted an incident from two months earlier in which Elizabeth called Connie and said she had just overdosed on medication. Connie and her husband rushed to the Blinders' house in San Anselmo, rang the doorbell, then knocked repeatedly, but no one answered. The front door was unlocked so they entered and went to Elizabeth's bedroom, which was across the hall from Dr. Blinder's bedroom. Connie could hear Blinder in his room but didn't contact him.

Elizabeth was in a stupor, but awake. They got her dressed, packed some clothes, and made several trips to the car before leaving the house. All during this time, Connie said, despite talking and making considerable noise, Martin Blinder didn't come out of his room or look to see who was in his house. They took Elizabeth to Marin General Hospital, where she was treated, recovered, and was released.

Holmes interviewed Dr. Blinder twice. Blinder denied everything and made vague threats of slander. He said his wife had never been a call girl, he had never locked her out of their house, and as far as he knew she had no desire to get a divorce. The years that he and his wife were together "were probably the happiest years of her life," he said.

A reporter for the *San Francisco Chronicle*, writing about the case, talked to Margo St. James, a onetime hooker who founded a nonprofit agency in San Francisco that advocated for decriminalizing prostitution. St. James told him that she introduced Elizabeth Doney when she was a call girl to Martin Blinder. When the reporter asked Blinder about it, Blinder said, "That's preposterous. I met her [Elizabeth] at a Chinese restaurant, Yet Wah, at a fund-raiser."

In response to Holmes's question about Blinder's relationship with his wife, Blinder said, "I was there for her in every possible way. . . . I think we had an extremely loving relationship."

Elizabeth Blinder's mother told Holmes that during an argument with Blinder, Elizabeth said she wanted to shoot herself, and Blinder told her where to put the gun, above and behind her ear. She asked Holmes if that was where she shot herself. Holmes said it was.

Elizabeth's ex-boyfriend told Holmes that during another argument with Blinder, and in his presence, Elizabeth fired the same gun she used to kill herself, this time aiming at a tree. For Blinder to say that he had never seen the gun is a lie, he said.

Several hours after Bill Thomas had gone to the Blinders' house with a San Anselmo cop to notify Blinder of his wife's death, Blinder called the coroner's office. Thomas wasn't in so he talked with Don Cornish instead. Cornish noted in a supplemental report that Blinder "seemed to want to absolve himself from any blame for his wife's anger, frustration, and suicide. . . . I got the feeling he felt he hadn't done too well" when he was first informed "and now had his act together." In this conversation, Blinder placed the blame for his wife's death on her mental problems and said that her leaving their house the previous evening "was in no way marital related."

Meanwhile, Holmes received yet another call pertaining to the case. Martin Blinder's first wife, Dorothy Braco, told Holmes to watch out for Dr. Blinder. "Don't trust him. Don't ever take him at face value," she said.

They had been divorced ten years by this time, and clearly she was still bitter. Holmes knew to take what she said with a certain amount of skepticism. Even so, there were times when ex-spouses were the best judges of character—as well as times when they weren't.

Elizabeth Blinder's relatives believed that her death was a homicide rather than a suicide, and voiced their suspicions to Holmes. If she wasn't planning to leave her husband, they said, why did she have more than $1,400 in cash on her when she died? Why would someone planning to kill herself bring the dog she loved with her in her car? Why would her husband have her body cremated before family members could get to California, which ruled out the possibility of any further tests being done?

Holmes listened with interest but concluded that there wasn't any evidence to support a finding of murder. There was just a lot of supposition.

Before he met Elizabeth Doney, and after his first marriage ended, Martin Blinder dated another prostitute, a woman named Linda Sours. She told the same *Chronicle* reporter that they met when she accompanied Margo St. James on a visit to Blinder's home. Sours and Blinder had a *Pretty Woman* type of relationship, Sours said, referring to the movie in which a wealthy businessman becomes infatuated with a high-class call girl, wining and dining her and buying her a new wardrobe. When the reporter asked Blinder about it, Blinder said it was "news to me" that Sours had been a hooker.

In a postscript to the story, thirteen years after Elizabeth Blinder killed herself, Martin Blinder's first wife did, too. Dorothy Braco, who had warned Holmes about her ex-husband, jumped off the Golden Gate Bridge after Blinder asked—some would say demanded—that she deed back to him her half interest in Blinder's expensive hillside home. They lived there during their marriage, and he continued to reside there after they divorced, but she had retained partial ownership.

Holmes didn't handle Braco's death because her body washed up on a beach in San Mateo County. Her black Volkswagen Jetta was found abandoned at the bridge, though, and her autopsy noted pattern injuries consistent with a fall from a great height, so it was easy to make the connection.

Hours before she jumped, Braco attacked Blinder with a knife, sending him to Marin General Hospital for two hours of emergency room surgery and blood transfusions. It was speculated that her intention was to kill him before killing herself so that their two grown children inherited the house and other assets without him bequeathing them to a current girlfriend. In response to accusations afterward that the noted psychiatrist used his vast intellect and psychological powers to manipulate and control Dorothy Braco, Elizabeth Doney, and others, Blinder said it was merely coincidental that his two wives killed themselves. He had loved both of them very much.

CHILDREN OF THUNDER

Blues guitarist Elvin Bishop is another acclaimed musician with long-standing ties to Marin County. His most famous song, "Fooled Around and Fell in Love," was written about his wife, Jennifer Villarin. After they divorced, she continued to live in Marin, as did their twenty-two-year-old daughter, Selina Bishop.

In 2000, mother and daughter were murdered, along with three other people, in a bizarre plot designed "to speed Christ's return to Earth," according to the perpetrators. As details unfolded in the press, people were horrified, and the story became the subject of a sensationalized book, *Unholy Sacrifice*, by Robert Scott.

Glenn Helzer, age thirty, was a onetime stock broker who went by his middle name, Taylor. His brother, Justin, was two years younger. Both were raised in Northern California by devout Mormon parents and fulfilled their two-year Mormon missions. Upon returning to the Bay Area, Taylor Helzer married and had two daughters before he decided that he had no further interest in being a good Mormon or husband. He was charismatic, gregarious, and fun-loving, and the confines of religion and family wore on him. He took to wearing black clothes and engaging in all of the things that the church prohibited—smoking, drinking, drugs, and sex with whomever he pleased. When he was excommunicated, he didn't care. He believed he was a prophet who could communicate with God directly. Justin, who was more introverted, followed him.

Ironically, considering their future deeds, the brothers met Dawn Godman in 1999 at a murder mystery dinner that was held in a Mormon temple. While everyone ate, the host gave guests clues to a make-believe homicide, which people tried to solve. In their black clothes, the Helzers stood out from everyone else, and Godman gravitated to them. She started dating Justin, but Taylor was the one who fascinated her. He told her that he was starting a group that would defeat Satan and eventually result in Taylor becoming the head of the Mormon Church. For financing, he said, the group would sell drugs, provide prostitutes to wealthy businessmen, and recruit underage girls from Brazil—where Taylor had been a missionary—to seduce married men who would be blackmailed into giving them money.

"He believed that by doing that, he was fulfilling a prophecy from the Book of Mormon," Dawn Godman later said in court, long after she had become the third person in the scheme.

Eventually, Taylor Helzer settled on a simpler plan—he would extort money from one of his former clients, and kill the person or couple afterward. As a stockbroker, he had managed the financial portfolios of well-to-do people, so he had choices in terms of potential victims. The only problem was that he needed someone to launder the money, someone who would open a bank account and deposit extorted checks. That person would be killed, too, of course, so that there were no living witnesses beyond the core three.

Selina Bishop, Elvin Bishop's daughter, was perfect. She was looking for love, met Taylor Helzer at a rave, and fell for the tall, handsome, ponytailed man who said his name was Jordan. She told all her friends about her new boyfriend and refused to heed their warnings. "Jordan" wouldn't tell her his last name or phone number, wouldn't allow her to take pictures of him, and had no interest in meeting anyone in her circle. Nevertheless, she was besotted. When he told her to open a bank account for him under a ruse, she did. The only thing she wanted to know was when his divorce from his estranged wife would be finalized so that he would be unencumbered. He didn't give her an answer because he had more pressing issues on his mind. He had already bought a reciprocating saw at Sears that he would use to cut up the bodies, as well as the duffel bags from Kmart that would hold the remains. All he needed now was to select the victim.

Helzer targeted an elderly couple, Ivan and Annette Stineman, who lived in the East Bay city of Concord—the same city where the Helzers and Godman were renting a house. The Stinemans, ages eighty-five and seventy-eight, knew and trusted him. They were surprised but not alarmed when he and his brother, wearing suits and carrying briefcases, knocked on their door.

Earlier in the day, the Helzers had bought handcuffs and leg irons from an adult bookstore, which they carried in their briefcases along with pistols and Tasers. Once inside, the brothers bound the Stinemans, put them in the couple's van, and drove to the Helzers' house. The Stinemans were forced to call their bank and let the manager there know that several large checks were going to be written on their account. After that, they were given drinks laced with Rohypnol, commonly referred to as the "date rape" drug because it causes people to pass out. The Helzers thought the Rohypnol would kill the Stinemans, but when it didn't they resorted to more violent means. Justin Helzer beat Mr. Stineman's head against a tile floor and Taylor Helzer dragged Mrs. Stineman to the bathroom and slit her throat with a knife. Dawn Godman watched in silent disbelief, testifying later, "The only thing I could do was pray that they [the Stinemans] would die, so it would just be done with."

The next day, in the bathroom, the brothers cut up the bodies with the power saw, then stuffed them in the duffel bags. Meanwhile, Godman practiced forging Annette Stineman's signature, wrote two checks on the couple's account totaling $100,000, and was able to have the funds moved to the account that Selina Bishop had opened.

Once the Helzers had access to the money, Selina Bishop's role was over. So, too, for all practical purposes, was her life.

At the end of their last date, Taylor Helzer offered to give his unwitting girlfriend a massage. While she lay facedown on the carpeted floor in the living room and he rubbed her back, Justin Helzer entered the room behind them, carrying a hammer. Within seconds he had hit Selina over the head multiple times, cracking her skull. Taylor Helzer carried her into the same bathroom where the Stinemans had been dismembered, and for good measure slit her throat. Then Selina's body was cut up as well. Justin Helzer used a toothbrush to scrub every square inch of the bathroom so that, despite all the bloodletting that had occurred, not a single drop of blood from any of the victims was found there.

Taylor Helzer's plan for disposing of the remains of the Stinemans and Selina Bishop, which now were commingled in nine bags, was to rent a personal watercraft and dump the bags in the Sacramento Delta. Stepping-stones from their rented house in Concord were added to the bags to weigh them down. The assumption was that the bags would sink to the bottom and remain there forever, removing all evidence of the murders. It didn't turn out that way, however.

Instead of sinking, the bags slowly bubbled to the surface. A Jet-Skier found the first one after it washed up on a riverbank, and was horrified to find a human torso inside. Other bags were found by police investigators. Dental records and DNA analysis were used to determine the identities of the Stinemans, whose daughter had reported them missing, and of Selina Bishop, but offered no clues as to the identities of their killers. None of the victims had any known enemies; moreover, there was no apparent connection between the elderly couple and Elvin Bishop's daughter. It was the murder in Marin County of Jennifer Villarin that provided the link.

Taylor Helzer had told Selina that he would take her to Yosemite. He had no intention of doing it, knowing that she would be dead before then, but Selina had asked her mother to house-sit for her because she and "Jordan" were going away for a few days. Jennifer Villarin, age forty-five, had been suspicious of Taylor Helzer, and several weeks earlier had tricked her daughter into introducing her to him. Helzer was worried that Jennifer knew too much and could identify him, so he drove to Selina's studio apartment in Marin before dawn, let himself in with the key Selina had given him, crept toward the bed, and from close range fired multiple shots into the bodies of Jennifer Villarin and the man sleeping next to her, James Gamble, fifty-four. An upstairs neighbor heard the gunshots and called the police while Helzer fled.

After police connected the two homicides with that of Selina Bishop, everything became clear. The self-proclaimed "Children of Thunder"—Taylor Helzer, Justin Helzer, and Dawn Godman—were charged with five murders and subject to the death penalty if convicted.

District attorneys and police from the three counties involved in the case—Contra Costa (where the Stinemans and Helzers lived), Sacramento (where the bodies of the Stinemans and Selina Bishop were found), and Marin (where Jennifer Villarin and James Gamble were killed)—agreed that Contra Costa was the appropriate site for the trial. That was fine with Holmes since the court proceedings were expected to be lengthy. He was happy to take a backseat. Gregory Reiber, a forensic pathologist at the UC Davis Medical Center whom Holmes had used on occasion, did the autopsies of all five decedents and was the person who testified regarding the cause and manner of each death. He was straightforward and matter-of-fact, but the details were so grisly that his testimony—particularly regarding the dismembered bodies—couldn't help but be graphic.

During the trial, relatives of the Helzers alluded to a history of mental illness in the family. Another witness, a former girlfriend of Taylor Helzer named Keri Furman, whom he talked into getting breast implants that landed her a spread in *Playboy* magazine under the name Kerrisa Fare, said that she and Taylor drove to Mexico in 1999, the year before the murders, to buy Rohypnol. His plan, she said, was to "involve some girl, make her feel like he was the love of her life."

In exchange for her testimony, Dawn Godman was spared the death penalty and sentenced to thirty-eight years in prison. Justin Helzer pled not guilty by reason of insanity, was convicted of three murders anyway (the Stinemans and Selina Bishop), and sentenced to death. While at San Quentin, he tied a sheet to his cell bars and hanged himself after surviving a previous suicide attempt in which he stabbed a pen in his eyes and was permanently blinded. As for Taylor Helzer, he surprised everyone by confessing to his crimes at the beginning of his trial and pleading guilty. He received five death sentences and remains one of California's 750 male inmates on death row.

CHAPTER 19

THE MITCHELL BROTHERS

In 1964, a twenty-six-year-old waitress and dancer at the Condor Club in San Francisco was given a "monokini" by the club's publicist. It was a new, topless swimsuit, and Carol Doda made international news when she performed wearing it. Five years later, with her natural size thirty-six breasts enlarged through silicone injections to size forty-four and her fame skyrocketing, Doda began dancing fully nude at the Condor, turning the city's North Beach section into a world-famous center for striptease.

That same year, 1969, two brothers from the Central Valley leased and renovated a two-story building on O'Farrell Street in San Francisco's Tenderloin District. It wasn't North Beach, but the rent was cheaper. In addition, the area was home to prostitutes, drug dealers, and liquor stores, which made the brothers' plans to open an adult theater there a fit, of sorts.

Jim Mitchell had been a part-time film student at San Francisco State University who aspired to make a name for himself as a movie director. In school he worked at a cinema that showed brief films with nude actors, and they were extremely popular. He teamed up with his brother, Artie, who was two years younger and had just been discharged from the army, to produce, direct, and show a number of pornographic films at their newly named Mitchell Brothers O'Farrell

Theatre. Their first big success, in 1972, was the movie *Behind the Green Door*, starring Ivory Snow model Marilyn Chambers in her adult movie debut. It cost $60,000 to make and grossed more than $25 million. Subsequently, the Mitchell brothers opened ten other X-rated movie houses in California, amassing a fortune in the process. Along the way they were slapped with dozens of lawsuits on obscenity and related charges, many of them resulting from vice raids on their theaters. With the help of high-priced legal assistance, they successfully defeated each one.

Jim and Artie Mitchell rubbed elbows with many of San Francisco's semi-elite, meaning people who were somewhat well known and didn't mind being seen with the two pornography kings. Underground cartoonists, rock band members, and gonzo journalist Hunter S. Thompson were among their friends. Both brothers had multiple marriages, and between them fathered ten children. They also were into drugs and quarreled with each other frequently.

On a rainy night in February 1991, Jim Mitchell drove to Artie's house in Marin County, believing that he needed to do something about his younger brother. Jim had overcome his own drug addiction for the most part, but Artie's alcoholism and cocaine habit had gotten worse, creating all kinds of business problems. What happened next became the focus of a front-page trial. Jim parked three blocks from Artie's house, and when he got there he kicked in Artie's door. Artie, age forty-five, was in the master bedroom, at the end of a hallway, and was dressed only in sweatpants. Jim brandished a .22-caliber rifle that he had inherited from their father and fired eight shots in Artie's direction. Three of them struck Artie, including one in the head, killing him.

Artie's live-in girlfriend wasn't a witness to the shooting, but she was in the house at the time that the shots were fired and called 911. When police arrived, Jim Mitchell was arrested—he didn't attempt to flee—and the coroner's office was summoned.

Ken Holmes got there shortly after midnight and stayed nearly four hours. As soon as he arrived, he began videotaping. The purpose of the videotape was to capture the layout of the house from the front door, down the hallway, to the master bedroom, where Artie's body lay. Investigators begin making mental notes as soon as they come on the scene but the camera captures things they might miss. Once they leave, they can never view the scene again the way it was when the person died. Even if the scene is sealed, meaning that no one other than the coroner can enter legally, it won't be the same. For one thing, the body will be gone, delivered to a funeral home for autopsy. More important, the scene will have been disturbed by technicians dusting for fingerprints and people trampling through rooms. Photos are taken, but a videotape provides better visual evidence.

It was standard practice for investigators to carry two batteries for the video camera in case one battery died. Holmes was at the scene so long, though, with the camera running most of the time, that well before the end both batteries were used up. One of his best friends, named Andre, was the head investigator in the local police department and happened to be on duty and at Artie Mitchell's house that night. Seeing Holmes's predicament, Andre offered to drive him to the police station and loan him one of the department's cameras. Andre didn't want to do the filming but he was willing to help Holmes do it. The station was a few blocks away, so it would take only a few minutes. Holmes was grateful for the offer and accepted.

At the station, Andre got the camera, took it to his office, and set it up. While he did this, he and Holmes talked, not about the case but about life in general. At one point Holmes said offhandedly, "What's up with the chief?"

It wasn't something he would have said to anyone other than a really good friend who was in the same line of work, and he wouldn't have said it if they were anywhere other than Andre's office with the door closed. What he was referring to was a fact that was known to a few people, but not everyone. The police chief had separated recently from his wife of many years and was showing interest in a woman who was an administrative assistant in the mayor's office.

Andre shrugged. "Some things are hard to figure," he said.

They talked for several minutes about the chief's situation. Neither one said anything derogatory, but it wasn't the sort of gossip that they would have engaged in with others. After a few minutes they went back to the crime scene, finished their work, and forgot about it.

The following morning, Holmes got into the office later than usual because he hadn't had much sleep due to being at Artie Mitchell's house most of the night. Andre went into work later than usual as well, for the same reason. As soon as he was at his desk, though, he called Holmes.

"Sherlock," Andre said, "we're in trouble."

Andre had called Holmes Sherlock practically from the moment they first met. "I had done some funky little thing," Holmes says, "I don't even remember what, and said, 'Well, that's pretty obvious.' Andre said, 'You mean that was elementary?' Both of us laughed, and from that point on I was Sherlock."

When Andre told Holmes they were in trouble, Holmes's immediate response was, "Why? What did we do wrong?"

"You know the conversation we had last night about the chief?" Andre said.

"Yeah?" Holmes said uncertainly. No one could have overheard it.

"Neither of us knew it," Andre said, "but the audio on the camera was on while we were talking. There wasn't any picture, but the audio was on, and—" He hesitated. "And we just played the tape for the entire department, and the chief was there."

The bottom fell out of Holmes's stomach. "Oh shit," he said.

"You probably shouldn't come down today," Andre said. "The chief is mad as hell."

Never one to avoid a problem, Holmes called the chief immediately. He knew him well; in fact, five years earlier the chief had tried to recruit Holmes to be a police investigator. "You won't have to work the street," the chief said. "You won't have to work patrol or worry about drunks. I just want you as an investigator."

It was a flattering offer, but Holmes liked where he was. Now he had just been caught talking about the chief's personal life.

Holmes left a long message on the chief's voice mail. Not surprisingly, he didn't receive a call back. Two days later he went to the chief's office. The chief didn't want to see him, but he let him in anyway. Holmes stood before him and apologized profusely.

"It was wrong, I know it was wrong, and I deeply regret it," Holmes said.

The chief wasn't moved. "It was fucking embarrassing," he said. "All of my investigators were there, some of whom had no idea what was going on. It's none of your goddamn business talking about my private life."

Holmes said, "You're right, you're absolutely right. From the bottom of my heart, I'm sorry."

For the next several years, the chief barely acknowledged him. After a while he got over it, and eventually he married the second woman.

THE TRIAL

Both the coroner, Dr. Jindrich, and Holmes, the assistant coroner, were called as witnesses for the prosecution in Jim Mitchell's trial. Jindrich was there to talk about the autopsy and Holmes was there to talk about the video he shot.

As a medical examiner and forensic pathologist, Jindrich was used to testifying in court, and his qualifications were undeniable. By his count, he had performed more than five thousand autopsies and testified in hundreds of cases. Over the course of several hours of questioning by the district attorney, Jindrich testified as to the number of bullets that struck Artie Mitchell (three), where they struck him (in the head, abdomen, and right arm), the caliber of weapon that they came from (a .22 rifle), the path or angle of each bullet, and the damage that each one caused. He also testified that the shooter had not been close enough to leave a residue of gunpowder—called tattooing—on the decedent. The order of shots couldn't be determined, Jindrich said, although it was likely that the shot to the head was last since it would cause instant collapse, unconsciousness, and probable death.

When asked about the toxicology report that was done on Artie, Jindrich said that Artie's blood alcohol content at the time of his death was .25. No drugs such as cocaine or marijuana were detected in his system.

Holmes was sworn in next, and the district attorney established that he was the assistant coroner of Marin County, had been in that position since 1984, had worked in the coroner's office seventeen years altogether, and had filmed the residence.

"Would you briefly describe what is on the video that you did?" the district attorney said.

Holmes replied that it was a complete walk-through of the house starting from outside the front door and moving through it room by room. The video showed where everything was at the time Holmes arrived at the scene.

The lights in the room were turned low, the video played on a screen, and Holmes was asked to describe what everyone was seeing. He identified each room and where he was standing at the time, referring to a diagram of Artie Mitchell's house that the district attorney had posted in the courtroom. At various times Holmes filmed empty casings from the murder weapon and a bag of marijuana that was found on Artie's bed in the master bedroom. Then the camera focused on Artie's body.

"That's Mr. Mitchell just as he was," Holmes said, "before he was moved. You can barely see, but right in the corner of that eye is where one of the bullet strikes was."

The camera didn't linger over Artie's body. While the prosecution might have preferred it so that jurors developed a strong, visceral reaction to Artie's death, the purpose of the video wasn't to support one side or the other in the court case. It was to provide an accurate representation of the murder scene.

"I believe that's the end," Holmes concluded.

During his testimony, Holmes wasn't asked about an incident that had taken place earlier in the coroner's office. The file on Artie Mitchell's death was nearly one hundred pages, and at one point one of Artie's ex-wives came in and said she wanted to see it. She had that right, and while she was at the counter it was given to her to look at. When she thought no one was observing her, however, the woman slipped the file into an oversized purse.

Holmes's medical transcriber, a woman named Barbara, noticed that the file had disappeared, and without saying a word she walked around behind the woman to the front door and locked it so that she couldn't leave. Then she got Holmes and said that Artie Mitchell's ex-wife was trying to steal the case file, which was one of a kind, with original copies of everything.

Holmes bounded out of his office and confronted the woman. She mumbled an excuse about thinking she could take it home to read. He said that coroner's files never left the office. Without apology, she handed it back to him.

"She was an issue," Holmes says. "Some of the kids were, too."

THE VERDICT AND A NEW MURDER

The same attorney who represented Jim and Artie Mitchell in the obscenity suits against them represented Jim Mitchell in his trial. The lawyer claimed that Artie's death was a tragic mistake, "an intervention gone awry." His argument wasn't helped by a computer-generated video animation of the shooting that the judge ruled could be shown. In the video, an armless, robot-looking figure representing Artie Mitchell was shot three times, the last time in the head. The presumed path of every bullet fired by Jim Mitchell, including the five that missed, was illustrated as a red laser beam against a blue background.

Mitchell's defense attorney objected to the video on the grounds that it was a fabricated account of an event that didn't have any eyewitnesses. Moreover, it purported to show the sequence of Mitchell's shots when this was unknown, according to Dr. Jindrich's testimony. Nevertheless, the judge allowed jurors to see it, making the video one of the first animations to be introduced in a murder trial (similar animations had been introduced in other trials). The only stipulation made by the judge was that in its original form, the video showed Artie's arms at his sides in a seemingly defenseless position when this couldn't be confirmed, thus the figure had to be armless.

A number of prominent people advocated for clemency on Jim Mitchell's behalf. It had an effect because the jury found him guilty of voluntary manslaughter rather than murder, and he was sentenced to six years in prison. In 1997, after serving three years, he was released and resumed running the O'Farrell Theatre, which family members and friends had managed in his absence. He also established the "Artie Fund" to raise money for a local drug rehabilitation center and the San Francisco Fire Department's "Surf Rescue Squad." The latter had intervened in 1990 when Artie was caught in a riptide off Ocean Beach in San Francisco.

The fund did nothing to appease the wrath of Artie Mitchell's children, who denounced it as an attempt by their uncle to whitewash the murder of their father.

"They may have been right," Holmes says, "but there probably wasn't much else Jim Mitchell could have done at that point to make the situation better other than volunteer to serve a longer prison term, which wasn't going to happen."

Artie was dead, Jim was free, and business continued as usual. It wasn't an "only-in-Marin" story, but given the players, the circumstances, and the outcome, it didn't seem that far from it, either. Moreover, it also wasn't the last time that a family member would be in the news.

In 2008, a former stripper, writing under her stage name Simone Corday, self-published a memoir about her ten years at the Mitchell Brothers O'Farrell Theatre and her on-again, off-again romance with the man she called "Party Artie." She claimed to capture his dual personality, the side that was into drugs and alcohol, who would "disappear on binges with a succession of young dancers," and his "affectionate personal and domestic side," which the public rarely saw.

"He was the quintessential bad boy, not the easiest person to figure out or be involved with," Corday recalled. "But I had an unfortunate marriage when I was young, so I wasn't looking for the most secure relationship myself."

One of Artie's daughters, Liberty Bradford Mitchell, forty-three, also wrote about him. In a one-person play titled *The Pornographer's Daughter*, which premiered in San Francisco, she talked about being exposed to rough-cut porn movies as a child and about receiving her first safe-sex talk from her father's girlfriend at the time, who was a porn star. She also talked about being more empathetic toward her own parents after she became a parent herself, and about the fact that when she came of age, AIDS was raging and attitudes about sex had changed considerably.

The same year that the play came out, another one of Artie's daughters, Jasmine Mitchell, thirty-four, was convicted of credit card fraud and identity theft after she used counterfeit cards and a fake driver's license to obtain two thousand dollars for gambling at a casino. When police tried to arrest her at her apartment, she raced off in her Mercedes, striking a deputy's car and a parked car in the process. Six days later police found her outside a hotel in Tiburon. In her defense, an attorney said that her frequent use of methamphetamine the past ten years had "negatively influenced her decision-making," that she had been participating in drug treatment and was "genuinely contrite."

None of that concerned Holmes, but he became part of the story again when Jim Mitchell's twenty-nine-year-old son, James "Rafe" Mitchell, was arrested for the murder of Danielle Keller, also twenty-nine. She was struck multiple times in her Novato backyard with an aluminum baseball bat. A neighbor witnessed the assault and told Holmes afterward that he recognized the son as the assailant because he was the father of Danielle's one-year-old daughter and had threatened her in the past. Rather than attempt to intervene, the neighbor had his wife call

911 while he went to a window and watched Mitchell leave through a side yard holding the daughter and then run down the street to his car.

Police found Mitchell near Sacramento by tracking the signals between his cell phone and various phone towers. In addition to murder, he was charged with kidnapping, child endangerment, child abduction, stalking, and domestic violence. The daughter was unhurt and turned over to Child Protective Services.

In his courtroom trial, Rafe Mitchell recognized Holmes from his father's trial nearly twenty years earlier. Once again Holmes was in court because of a homicide case involving the Mitchell family. The only difference was that he was testifying as the coroner this time rather than as the assistant coroner.

Rafe Mitchell told jurors that when he arrived at Danielle's house, two men were there with a baseball bat and he fought them off before escaping with the young girl. No one bought his story.

In the trial, Danielle's mother wore one of her daughter's dresses and wept as she recounted arriving at the crime scene and being restrained by police officers from approaching Danielle's dead body. "I begged to touch her one last time," she cried.

Unlike his father, the younger Mitchell was convicted of first-degree murder, as well as other charges, and sentenced to thirty-five years to life in prison. He claimed that he was victimized by his father's name and by the fascination that local media had with the family's business. It was a valid point—none of Jim or Artie Mitchell's children had it easy growing up—but it didn't excuse or justify his actions.

"You can love someone and still kill them," Liberty Mitchell said afterward. "It's not pretty, but that reality has always existed. That's why they call it a crime of passion."

Her words were applicable to both deaths, to her cousin's murder of his ex-wife and her uncle's murder of her father. Regarding the latter, after Jim Mitchell died of natural causes in 2007, he was buried next to Artie. The two had had their share of arguments, but they were brothers to the end.

CHAPTER 20

NOTES AND NOTIFICATIONS

The way next of kin are informed of a loved one's death varies from community to community. In many communities it's the responsibility of law enforcement. They knock on someone's door or call the person on the phone and relay the news as quickly as possible, then get out of there or hang up fast. The last thing they want to do is have an extended conversation. It's not that they lack sympathy; it's that it's an uncomfortable situation where cops feel powerless, and they are used to being in control.

In Marin County, throughout Holmes's career, coroner's investigators did most of the death notifications, and always in person if possible. There were multiple reasons for this. First, it was best for the families. They received the information from someone who was caring and not in a hurry to leave. Holmes listened, empathized, and stayed as long as the person needed him to be there. He didn't want someone to be alone after he or she received shocking news and was in a vulnerable state.

Another reason why next of kin were notified in person was to give them important information. Holmes explained the process, including where the person's body had been taken, the steps in claiming it, and how insurance and Social Security benefits could be applied for once the death certificate had been issued. He also answered, to the best of his abilities and based on what he knew at the time, questions regarding the circumstances surrounding someone's death—where and how it happened, who else was present, whether alcohol or drugs appeared to have been involved, and whether death was instantaneous, which in many cases was the hope of families. If death was slow and the person suffered, however, he admitted it, as gently as he could.

"I wish I could tell you that she died quickly, but that wasn't the case."

Were he to say anything else, and family members learned later that they had been misled, the coroner's office would be discredited. Inasmuch as family members often request a copy of a loved one's file, they are likely to learn the truth regardless.

In addition, Holmes provided information about local services. Most communities have free or low-cost bereavement programs operated by a hospital or nonprofit agency. In Marin County it's Marin Counseling and Suicide Prevention. The organization offers no-cost individual and group grief counseling services to people who are mourning the death of a loved one. In the immediate aftermath, the service probably isn't needed because people are too dazed to benefit from it, but later on, when individuals are still hurting and much of their support system has receded, it can be invaluable. The coroner had an arrangement whereby once a month the agency received the names and contact information for people whose loved one had died recently. This enabled the agency to be proactive in contacting families and letting them know about available services.

There was a third reason for doing the notifications in person. Sometimes people literally collapsed upon hearing the news.

A mile from the coroner's office, a young woman was in a car accident right after she visited her mother. The mother lived near the top of a steep hill, and as the daughter was leaving, she turned left at the bottom and reached across the passenger seat in order to grab something that had fallen on the floor. Holmes couldn't figure out what it was because after the crash everything was on the floor.

The daughter was driving a VW bug, and a plumbing truck came from the opposite direction. The driver told Holmes afterward that the woman looked directly at him, then her head disappeared, she veered into his path, and there was no way he could avoid hitting her. Holmes estimated that it was about a thirty-five-mile-per-hour impact—usually not fatal, but the woman was leaning over, the crash broke her neck, and she died.

Forty-five minutes after the woman left her mother's house, Holmes was standing at the mother's door with a San Rafael policeman. There was a reason why he had a cop accompany him.

"If you're a little old lady," he says, "and there's a knock at your door, and you see through the spot hole a guy in a shirt and tie, you probably think he's a salesman or scam artist and don't let him in. If you see a guy in a shirt and tie and another guy with a badge, however, you'll open the door."

After ringing the bell, Holmes thought through the conversation. Finding only one person home, especially a mother or wife, was the worst. At a time like this, people needed someone to hold on to.

The woman opened the door a few inches. "Mrs. Roxbury?" Holmes said.

"Yes," the woman said hesitantly.

"Is your daughter Margery Roxbury?"

"Yes. She just left a few minutes ago. Why? What's wrong?"

Holmes didn't want to have the conversation in the doorway. "Can we come in?"

"No," Mrs. Roxbury said. She wasn't being combative, just cautious.

"It'd really be more comfortable, ma'am, if we could come in and talk," Holmes said.

"I don't understand. Why are you here?"

It looked like he was going to have to tell her while he was standing in her doorway. "When Margery went down your hill," Holmes said, "she made a turn at the bottom and was involved in a head-on crash. She was killed. I'm really sorry."

By this time Holmes had learned to use the person's first name rather than refer to the decedent as "your daughter" or "Ms. So-and-So." Not only was it more respectful but there might be multiple daughters. He also learned to avoid saying something like "she succumbed" or "she didn't survive" or "it was fatal." He had to say the word "dead" or "killed." If he didn't, if he said something like, "Unfortunately, she didn't make it," the next questions were "How bad was it?" "Where is she?" "Can I go talk to her?" because the person didn't hear. It was way too much information coming from a total stranger without any context or preamble. Holmes called it thirty-second psychology. From the time he knocked and heard someone moving behind the door, he had thirty seconds at most to figure out how he was going to deliver terrible news.

Mrs. Roxbury looked at him blankly, then her eyes rolled back in her head and she collapsed. She didn't fall; rather she seemed to melt. In the mortuary business, Holmes had seen people faint. Their knees locked and they fell like a board. In this instance, it was as if Mrs. Roxbury's spine liquefied and she dissolved. He was only a few feet away, yet he couldn't reach out fast enough to catch her.

She hit her head on the tile floor in her entryway. There wasn't any blood, but her head made a hollow sound and Holmes was afraid that she was going to end up with a brain bleed that would kill her in several hours. The cop called an ambulance, and paramedics revived her. She was woozy but aware of what Holmes had told her. Within a few minutes she was sitting up and didn't need to be hospitalized.

If she had been notified over the phone or by someone who left immediately after informing her of her daughter's death, Mrs. Roxbury might have become a second casualty. Instead, she received quick medical care, and Holmes stayed with her until her minister arrived.

PUNCHED IN THE FACE

Late one night, Holmes was contacted by the Communications Center regarding a single-vehicle traffic accident outside Novato. An eighteen-year-old female driver named Drusilla Minor had the top down on her five-year-old Fiat convertible, which she had bought six weeks earlier. Next to her in the passenger seat was her best friend, seventeen-year-old Meyna Sablik. The two were seniors in high school, scheduled to graduate the following week. A third passenger, Tony Galatolo, age sixteen, was perched behind them, his legs straddling the two front seats.

It was a curvy country road that was poorly lit. Drusilla took a turn too fast and lost control; the car shot across the road and into a culvert. Galatolo was thrown from the vehicle and landed hard against a wooden fence, alive but badly bruised. The two girls weren't so lucky. As Galatolo watched in horror, the car hit a utility pole head on. On impact, Meyna was ejected onto the roadway and killed instantly. Drusilla was the only one of the three who was wearing a seat belt. She remained in the car but suffered traumatic head injuries. When the responding police officer arrived at the scene, Galatolo was standing next to the car, in a daze. The officer felt for Drusilla's pulse, found none, and knew that she was dead. He pulled her from the vehicle, laid her on the ground, covered her fully with a blanket, and waited for Holmes.

It was midnight when Holmes arrived. He spoke with the officer, then Galatolo, who told Holmes that the teens were driving to Galatolo's house to finalize plans for the two girls' senior prom the following evening. Galatolo was Drusilla's date. After that, Holmes itemized each girl's visible injuries in a notebook, to be transferred later to his typed investigative report. He also inventoried their clothing, jewelry, and the contents of their purses, including the exact dollar amount in their wallets, all of which was standard protocol.

Ninety minutes later, at 1:30 A.M., Holmes knocked on the door of the house where Drusilla Minor lived. It didn't matter how late it was; notification was made as soon as possible so that loved ones heard the news from the coroner rather than anyone else. A policeman accompanied Holmes.

Drusilla's father answered. He was big—muscular, not fat—and filled the doorway. He also was surly. Seeing the cop he said, "What did she do now?"

At least he was awake. He wasn't half asleep.

"I'm with the county coroner's office," Holmes said. "There has been an accident. I'm sorry to have to tell you, but Drusilla and a friend were killed."

There was no way to sugarcoat the worst kind of news, and Holmes didn't try. It was best to be as simple and straightforward as possible.

Without warning, Mr. Minor punched Holmes hard in the face. Holmes staggered backward, and the cop was on Minor instantly, ready to arrest him. Holmes told him not to. It had been a reflex action; Minor thought he was the victim of a sick joke.

After that Mr. Minor and Holmes talked for a while with Holmes telling him more about the accident. Then Minor asked Holmes if he had been to Meyna Sablik's house yet. Holmes said no, that was his next stop. Minor said, "I wouldn't want your job for anything."

Holmes knew that cops said that sometimes, but he didn't expect to hear it from someone whom he had just notified of a death. "Why is that?" Holmes said.

Minor said that a year earlier Meyna's father had died. Five months ago, Meyna's brother had died. Just recently her mother learned that she had terminal cancer.

Hearing that, the cop who had accompanied Holmes begged off going to Meyna's home. Holmes went alone, oddly grateful for the information. At least he knew what to expect.

PLANE CRASH

Next door to the coroner's office, on the same floor of the Marin Civic Center building, was a restaurant with typical cafeteria food. Many county employees who worked at the civic center ate lunch there because it was convenient. Holmes did, too, on occasion. He lived close enough to work, however, that he could go home for lunch if he wanted to.

One day at noon as he was driving home, he saw a huge plume of black smoke shoot up into the air off to his right. He was on a frontage road that ran parallel to Highway 101, and his first thought was that there wasn't anything in the immediate area to burn—no homes, businesses, or grassy hillsides. Then he realized that it was at Smith Ranch Airport, a small airport on the outskirts of San Rafael with several dozen private planes and no buildings or control tower. Pilots coordinated their takeoffs and landings through an air traffic center in Oakland, thirty miles away.

As soon as he knew it was a plane, Holmes put on his red light and siren to get people out of the way and raced to the airport. He saw the ball of flames on the runway and felt the heat, even though it was impossible to get close. He was the first person on the scene—no one else happened to be there at that time—and reported the crash to the county's Communications Center.

The pilot and sole occupant of the twin-engine Cessna C41 was Earl Pickens II, age thirty-five. He lived in Marin, and Holmes learned that for the past week Earl had been flying back and forth from the county to a family ranch in Cody, Wyoming. The family was having a reunion, and Earl transported one or two people each trip from Marin to the ranch. He was an experienced pilot and had returned home alone a final time to pick up a few things. Immediately after lifting off from the short runway, however, he crashed and was killed.

The plane's log was destroyed in the fire. Holmes checked the airport fuel log, which showed that Earl had purchased 109 gallons of 100-octane airplane fuel the same day. No maintenance was listed at that time. Given the scattered and burned wreckage, it was impossible to know what cargo he had been carrying, but the National Transportation Safety Board determined that the plane was overloaded, and that caused the accident.

After Holmes confirmed Earl's identity, he contacted police in Wyoming and asked them to notify Earl's family. This was standard practice if the victim's next of kin lived out of the area. Police officers didn't like to do it, but invariably they agreed. The officer Holmes talked to balked, however. When he drove up and saw all of the parked cars, he knew he would be walking in on a large family gathering. He called Holmes and said he couldn't go through with it.

"You have to," Holmes said. "They need to know."

"I can't," the officer said. "I just can't. All these people are waiting for him."

Holmes sympathized. Whenever he did a death notification, he knew that he was taking what started out as a normal day for someone and turning it into the worst day of the person's life. Coroners never deliver good news. In this instance, the officer would be ruining a day of celebration that people had been looking forward to for months. Still, it had to be done.

Holmes offered some coaching as well as encouragement. He said that at a party, the person who opens the door may not be the homeowner but rather whoever happens to be closest to the entrance. This means that in the few seconds after the door is opened, you have to look over the person's shoulder and do a quick assessment of the scene to determine which of the adults in the room is the appropriate person to inform of someone's death.

"Do you think you can do that?" Holmes asked.

"I'm not prepared," the officer said. "I'm sorry, but I'm just not. You're going to have to let them know another way."

"You can do it," Holmes said. "Just think that if you were in their shoes, you'd want to hear from someone in person rather than over the phone."

To Holmes's amazement, the officer still refused. In frustration, Holmes called Earl's attorney, who said that he would notify the family. It wasn't a good outcome, but there wasn't another option.

ADVISING THE BEREAVED

On one occasion, Holmes knocked on the front door of a couple whose son was killed in a traffic accident. It was 2:30 A.M. and the man who answered the door was in his pajamas and half asleep. When he saw Holmes standing there with a policeman, his eyes widened.

"I work for the county," Holmes said. "Can we come in for a minute?"

The man opened the door for them, fully awake now. "Is something wrong?"

There was a noise in the hallway behind him, then a woman rushed into the room. "What's wrong?" she practically shouted.

Holmes invited them to sit down, but they ignored him.

"Is it David?" one of them asked. "Is he hurt?"

Holmes said, "David has been in an accident. His car—"

The man interrupted and said in a choked-up voice, "How bad is it?"

Holmes said, "His car was hit by a drunk driver who was going the wrong way on the freeway near Mill Valley. David was taken to the hospital, but the doctors couldn't do anything. He died."

"Oh my God," the woman exclaimed, and started sobbing.

Her husband's face lost all of its color and he looked as if he had aged fifty years. He reached for his wife and they clung to each other as the police officer and Holmes stood by awkwardly.

"It happens sometimes," Holmes says. "They just close you out of their lives for a few minutes. That's when it was uncomfortable for me because they didn't need some stranger there at the moment."

Sometimes when Holmes notified families of a death, people ran screaming from the room. Other times they went into shock and didn't say a word. They couldn't cry or talk. One mother, whose twenty-year-old son was killed in a traffic accident, was divorced and he was her only child. Among his personal effects was his high school class ring. After notification and being given his effects, she put the ring on her finger and stared at it. She didn't say a word, but silent tears streamed down her cheeks.

In many instances, the coroner is the only constant for a family member. When paramedics leave the scene, their work is done. The same is true for police officers, unless a crime has been committed, in which case other police officers become involved. Even friends tend to be less available or less willing to talk about a death after a while. Coroners are the exception.

"I have no problem listening to people talk at length about a dead person," Holmes says, "and I'll say something like, 'You're so lucky you had Fred in your life for all of those years. Look at the things you did, the places you went.' Talking about someone is a way of keeping that person's memory alive."

In his first meeting with families after the notification, whether it was in their home or in his office—but typically in their home—Holmes gave them the same advice for the future. When he became coroner, he instructed his investigators to give it, too, and later on, when he taught classes at the police academy in death notifications, Holmes told officers-in-training to give it as well.

"In the next few days," Holmes said to the family, "everybody is going to gather around you and ask if there's anything they can do. You're not going to know of anything, but try to think of something anyway because they're feeling helpless and don't know what to say or how to act. If you need Kleenex at the grocery store, and someone asks you if there's anything they can do, tell them, 'Would you mind getting me some Kleenex?' Let them help because you're helping them help you. In about three weeks that's going to stop, and you're going to feel like you're on an island. The phone will stop ringing, except maybe your kids. People are uncomfortable talking about Fred's death. There's no easy way to say, 'How are you doing since Fred died?'"

Even so, Holmes would tell them, "Don't let them erase your loved one. Don't let them erase Fred. When you bump into someone at the grocery store or wherever, talk about Fred. Say, 'God, I really miss him.' Remember a time that was fun when you and Fred and the person you're talking to did something together or saw something together. Say, 'Remember when the three of us . . .'"

Another thing Holmes told people, particularly women, was that sometime in the future they would run into a person they hadn't seen in a long time who would ask, "How's Fred?"

"You're going to want to cry," Holmes would say, "and that's okay. Go ahead and cry. It's sad; you've lost Fred, and he's not coming back. Say, 'I know you didn't know, but Fred died.' Don't make it their fault that they didn't know. Don't say, 'You didn't hear?' Instead, use it as an opportunity to talk about and remember Fred."

Many family members told him later that these exact scenarios played out after their loved one died. They were grateful to him for preparing them for it.

"Much of it is just letting people know what to expect," Holmes says. "If you aren't expecting something and it happens, it'll knock you off your feet. With a little guidance, though, you can deal with it. That was my philosophy."

CANDACE

When Manfred Pohl shot himself in front of a beauty salon in Larkspur in 1985, it was the beginning of a case that would consume Holmes for years. The setting wasn't an accident. Pohl, a German national, age forty-six, worked in the salon and, for a while, dated the salon's owner, a pretty woman named Candace. Candace worked in the first chair; a woman named Doris, who was old enough to be Candace's mother but wasn't, worked in the second chair; and Pohl had the third chair.

Candace ended her personal relationship with Pohl because of his instability. He had a volatile personality that got to be too much for her to deal with. Pohl continued to work at the salon after they broke up, but the situation became increasingly uncomfortable for everyone. When Pohl didn't show up to work for several days, there were sighs of relief that maybe he had moved on.

The salon had big glass windows and a glass door facing the street. Near noon on a workday, Doris noticed Pohl drive by, look in the windows, and park down the street. He sat in his car a while, then came walking up to the shop with one hand in a jacket pocket. Doris had a bad feeling, so she went over and locked the front door without saying anything to Candace, who hadn't noticed him. It was only when Pohl reached the salon's front steps that Candace saw him. She discreetly turned her customer's chair in order to avoid looking in his direction.

Pohl started banging on the door, shouting through the glass that he wanted to talk to Candace. She kept her back to him while Doris turned her chair sideways and mouthed an apology. Neither of the women saw Pohl pull a gun out of his jacket pocket, but they heard the explosion. Pohl shot himself in the head on their doorstep.

When Holmes arrived at the shop, the customers had left and Candace and Doris were beside themselves. Blood was splattered all over the glass and brick steps in front.

Holmes talked with Candace for a while and she told him about her relationship with Pohl. Holmes asked if there was anyone he could call on her behalf, and she said that she would call her teenage daughter, but Doris was the best person for her to talk to right now. Holmes told her—as he did all next of kin—that if she needed to talk and there was no one else she could turn to, she could call him.

"I can't make it any different," he said, "but I can help you get through the moment."

Several days later, Candace called. She said she appreciated his offer, and while she didn't need any help, she had some questions. She didn't actually see Pohl shoot himself, but she saw the aftereffects on the front of her building and wanted to understand better what had happened. Holmes talked with her for about twenty minutes.

A few more days passed, then she called again. She said Holmes had a soothing voice and it was easy to talk to him about Pohl's suicide when no one else wanted to discuss it. It wasn't the first time that Holmes had been complimented on his voice—it is melodic—but he thanked her.

"Can I come in and see the photos?" she asked.

The question startled him. "I won't show you photos of the body," Holmes said, "but I can show you photos of your walls and steps if you want."

"I don't need to see those," Candace said. "Why can't I see photos of Manfred?"

"I'm sorry," Holmes said, "but you're not a relation."

Candace came in anyway, and Holmes talked with her in his office. In the following months, she came in half a dozen more times. She said her mother and father didn't like Pohl and didn't want to talk about his death. Neither did her current boyfriend.

Each meeting lasted twenty to thirty minutes, and it started to get to the point where they were interfering with Holmes's work. He enjoyed talking with her—she was attractive, intelligent, and came from a prominent family. For many years her father had been a principal in Halsted & Company, one of the largest mortuaries in San Francisco. Her mother was an accomplished artist whose work had been displayed in museums and galleries. Still, there were only so many hours in the day.

It was obvious that Candace liked Holmes. He was a man of experience and a good listener.

One day Candace invited Holmes to her house for lunch. He accepted and met the older of her two daughters, who was a senior in high school. He also saw firsthand that Candace was a hoarder. So much stuff was piled everywhere that it was nearly impossible to walk around. Holmes had been in the houses of hoarders before, people whose refuse was so deep that there wasn't room to get a gurney through to pick up a body. Sometimes, in order to exit, the gurney had to be turned on its side with the decedent strapped down and Holmes hoping the person didn't slide off. Candace wasn't quite that bad; still, it was a jolt to see that she lived this way. When she invited Holmes to lunch again, he suggested that they meet somewhere close to his office instead.

Four years after Manfred Pohl's suicide, Candace invited Holmes to dinner one night at her parents' house. It was a far cry from Candace's residence.

Hugh and Ann owned ten acres on a ridge in San Anselmo. Theirs was the only house on the ridge, and the views were the best that Holmes had ever seen from a private residence, comparable to the views from the top of Mount Tamalpais. The house was spectacular, too, nearly five thousand square feet and tastefully furnished, with many paintings by Candace's mother hanging on the walls.

Hugh was an old-time duck hunter, and he and Holmes hit it off immediately. He showed Holmes his gun room, then pressed a button and a wall opened up, revealing a walk-in safe. Inside the safe were antique firearms, the likes of which Holmes hadn't seen in a private collection before.

In the ensuing months, Holmes saw Candace's parents frequently. They were interesting people and he enjoyed their company. Then Candace called him one day and said that her mother had liver cancer even though she hadn't consumed a single alcoholic drink in her life. Candace told Holmes that if he wanted to see Ann again he should do it soon because she wouldn't be alive much longer.

Holmes went to the house and sat with Ann, who was now in her early seventies. She was a practical woman who appreciated honesty.

"I want you to tell me," she said. "Is it going to be as painful as I think, because it's painful now." Her liver was enlarged, and she had lost weight.

Holmes knew that a liver death was slow and painful. "I'm afraid it is," he said. "It might be best if you get medications from your doctor."

Holmes isn't an advocate of suicide, but in cases like this he feels that people have a right to make their own end-of-life decisions. If the pain becomes too much to bear, overmedicating is an option.

Candace's mother thanked Holmes profusely. She said she felt at peace now that she knew what her choices were.

The next time Candace called Holmes, it was to tell him that her father wanted to talk with him. Holmes went back to the house.

"Ann told me what the two of you talked about," Hugh said. "I know it's going to be awful for her. She told me about the medicines, but I could just leave a loaded gun in the room."

Holmes was quick to speak. "Don't do that. She's not going to use it, and it wouldn't serve any good purpose. Just leave her be."

Hugh looked Holmes in the eye and said, "You know, when she dies, I'm going to die, too. I don't want to live without her. I'll use the gun."

Holmes was at a loss for words. Hugh was in good health, not struck with an agonizing and fatal illness like his wife. At the same time, Holmes sympathized. To have your spouse die after decades of blissful marriage is one of the hardest losses to endure.

"I can't say that I blame you," Holmes said, "but it wouldn't be my choice. You need to think about Candace, as well as about your two granddaughters. You've got a lot of time left in front of you, and you could be a mentor to each of them."

"I don't want to live without Ann," Hugh said. "I just don't. I'm telling you, as the coroner, that I'm going to kill myself."

Holmes knew it wouldn't do any good to talk about local resources such as suicide counseling or grief counseling. Hugh's mind was made up; he wouldn't reach out for any kind of help.

All Holmes could say was, "Thank you for letting me know."

In the final throes of her mother's life, Candace called Holmes. He raced to the house, which was twenty-five minutes from his office. When he arrived, Candace told him that her mother had died right after she got off the phone with him.

Holmes looked around. "Where's your dad?"

"He's in their room," Candace said. "He ushered everyone out and said he wanted to be alone with her. Then he locked the door and we heard a loud pop, but we couldn't get in."

Holmes swore under his breath. Hugh did what he said he was going to do. "Did he ever talk to you about his plans?" he said.

Candace looked at him. "He said he was going to kill himself. Why? Did he tell you, too?"

Holmes nodded.

"I didn't know that," Candace said.

Holmes jimmied a window from the outside and opened the door to the master bedroom. Hugh was dressed and lying shoulder to shoulder with his wife. She had been in a coma the past forty-eight hours and died in her sleep. The autopsy showed that she hadn't overdosed, because there weren't any medications in her system.

Hugh had shot himself in the head using a small pistol so that it wouldn't make a mess. Holmes pronounced both husband and wife dead and called the county Communications Center. He said that he had come to the house because a woman had passed away in her sleep, after which her husband had killed himself. He said that the family wanted to keep it quiet so just send a patrol unit without sirens.

The house was at the end of a long, gated driveway. Two minutes later, Holmes heard a siren, then saw a fire truck, an ambulance, a patrol car, and a sergeant's car. He walked to the gate and told the firemen that he didn't know why they were there, the wife died of cancer and the husband shot himself after telling him that that was what he was going to do. The gun was still in Hugh's hand.

"If you want to go in and check it out, though, you can," Holmes said.

They said they didn't need to, and left. The ambulance followed.

When Holmes got to the patrol car, he said, "What's with the lights and sirens?"

The officer motioned to the car behind him. "Sergeant ordered it."

The sergeant got out of his car. It was someone Holmes didn't care for, and who didn't care for him.

"Tim," Holmes said, "I specifically told Comm Center no sirens or lights."

Tim said, "I know. I heard dispatch. I told them to roll Code Three." In other words, he sent lights and sirens because Holmes requested them not to.

The deputy went into the house, took a couple of photos, and wrote a brief report. Then he and the sergeant left.

In time, Candace sold her home and moved into her parents' ridgetop house. She closed the salon and began creating artwork of her own. Sadly, she brought all of her clutter with her, and the art projects made it worse. Within three months her parents' large house was filled with half-painted canvases, dried clay, heaping piles of clothing and rags, scattered papers, and much more. The kitchen sink overflowed with dirty dishes, and there were empty containers of food strewn about the pantry. When new bills became buried and weren't paid, assorted services—utilities, water, garbage, and the phone—were cut off.

Candace's two daughters were so upset that they wouldn't have anything to do with her. They didn't know that her hoarding was tied to the growing dementia that was wrecking her mind. When she sold her parents' house, it fetched over $3 million but was worth much more than that. The tract house she moved into was half the size, not nearly big enough to accommodate all of her detritus in addition to the many antiques that her parents had collected, so she rented two enormous storage units and filled them to the brim. When Holmes visited her, he expected to walk in on a mess, but it was far worse than that. There were open bags of rice in the kitchen that had mice nesting at the bottom. There also were mouse nests in the pantry, underneath the refrigerator, and even in the stove and oven.

Holmes was shocked. "Candace," he said, "you can't live like this. You have to get rid of them."

"Why?" Candace asked. "They're not hurting anything."

"Mice bring all kinds of diseases."

"I think they're cute," Candace said. "Besides, I'm healthy."

Holmes shook his head sadly at the depths to which she had fallen. The only salve was that Candace was too far gone to be aware of it.

In her final years, Candace lived in a nursing home. Holmes stopped by every few months to check in on her. Each time she was delighted to see him, and knew that she knew him, but she didn't know his name or how she knew him. She died in 2016 with her two daughters, four grandchildren, and one son-in-law at her bedside. Holmes had left her two hours earlier.

SUICIDE NOTES

In any death that might be a suicide, Holmes looked for a note. The main reason was to shed light on the decedent's intent, but a secondary reason was to help determine whoever should be notified. If there was a note, and it was addressed to a specific individual, Holmes shared the contents with that person only or with someone the person authorized. If it was a general note, along the lines of "Good-bye, world," then he shared it with next of kin.

Few members of the general public have ever seen a suicide note, in part because most suicide victims don't leave one. Even if there is a note, there aren't any rules about what should be in it. Does the person ask for forgiveness from loved ones, cite reasons of rejection and isolation in order to hurt others, or provide general instructions about money and insurance or the disposal of the deceased's remains? In Holmes's experience, the contents of most notes tended to be so meager that they lacked the passion and desperation usually associated with suicide. Mostly, they were just sad.

A fifteen-year-old girl hung herself from a tree in the woods. She used a felt marking pen to write her note in black letters all over her body. "This is the last place I will step, breathe, speak, or cry," she wrote on her left arm.

A nineteen-year-old woman who jumped from the Golden Gate

Bridge wrote, "I really am very sorry to do this to all of you. I know you were rooting for me, but I wasn't rooting for me. Please try to let me go."

Notes were especially important in cases where a husband and wife were found dead together with the weapon at their side. It could be that they had a suicide pact or it could be a murder-suicide.

The bodies of one couple were found in a Sheraton hotel room by staff after the couple failed to check out. In her suicide note, the woman wrote that she had "willfully chosen this," and her husband was "just following my wishes." The husband confirmed this in his note.

Another couple left notes to loved ones in which they apologized for living a lie that they were too embarrassed to share. They had been addicted to painkillers for more than fifteen years, tried to quit many times, and couldn't. "It was our choice and we were stupid," the wife wrote. "Please do not think there was anything that you or anyone could have done."

A thirty-two-year-old woman named Barbara left multiple notes. Holmes found them in her house after he examined her body lying on a morgue table at Marin General Hospital.

Two years earlier, when she and her boyfriend, Steve, had started living together, Barbara took his surname. They weren't married, but she felt married, or wanted to be. After they broke up and he moved out, she kept his name anyway, continuing to hope that he would return to her and to her thirteen-year-old daughter, whom she had borne from a previous marriage. He didn't return, though, and she was devastated. In her mind, there was no reason to go on.

When Steve talked with her by phone at 5:15 P.M., she told him that she was going away for a while and would leave a note for him inside the house, which he could pick up later that evening. He went by her house at 6:40 P.M., didn't see anyone or notice anything amiss, and retrieved the note. After driving a short distance, he stopped and read it, which Barbara had labeled as her last will and testament. It was handwritten and postdated to the following day.

Alarmed, Steve returned to the house, heard a car running in the closed garage, and broke out a window. Barbara had connected a garden hose from the exhaust pipe to inside the car. She was in the front seat, unconscious. He pulled her out and began doing mouth-to-mouth resuscitation. Meanwhile, Barbara's daughter was taking a bath, heard the glass breaking and Steve's shouts, ran outside, and then called 911. Paramedics did CPR en route to the hospital, where resuscitation efforts continued for another thirty minutes before Barbara was declared dead.

When Holmes and a police officer went to Barbara's house, they saw that the hose was still connected to the exhaust pipe with the opposite end lying near the driver's door. Holmes removed it and put it in the backyard, then he and the officer swept up the broken glass and nailed boards to close off the garage window. A rear door was unlocked, and they entered the house to close and lock the windows and turn off the lights. That's when he found the other notes. The one that was addressed to Steve was signed "Your Loving Wife." A note to friends said, "I know I've always had a death wish, and a love wish, and a marriage wish. I've secretly waited all my life for these things. . . . I'm still waiting." A third note was to her brother: "Mom thought I was the healthy and strong one, but look who stayed on the planet." A fourth was to her mother: "I know you're dead, but I love you and I've missed you." A fifth was to her father, whom she entrusted with her daughter's care and of whom she made one request: "Make her know she can make it." The last letter was to her young daughter, asking for forgiveness and promising to be her "guardian angel."

"Barbara's handwriting was so neat and precise," Holmes says, "that she could have taught penmanship classes. No words were crossed out."

As Holmes was leaving, he secured Barbara's house and garage with coroner's seals. The seals were fluorescent orange, had gum backings, and were placed across the frame of any door leading outside. They warned people that breaking the seal was a felony. He wrote the date and time on each seal, then signed them.

"I always thought the seals should be beige," he says, "like a grocery sack, rather than such a bright color. It's hard to miss them, which is the point, but it's also easy for anybody driving down the street to know that nobody's home."

In this instance, not only was nobody home, but nobody was coming back. Barbara's daughter stayed with friends a few days, until Barbara's father could arrive from out of state, handle his daughter's affairs, and take custody. Holmes could only think, as he did after nearly every suicide, that it didn't have to be like that. Suicide is an option for people who are depressed, but it's not the only option. Moreover, suicide doesn't end the pain. It merely transfers it from the dead to the living.

CHAPTER 21

POWER STRUGGLES

In 1998, when his sixth term as the coroner of Marin County ended, Dr. Jindrich decided not to run again. He had accomplished everything he wanted to and was ready to retire. He encouraged Holmes to consider the position, knowing that although he wasn't a forensic pathologist, he could contract for the service, and in every other way he was qualified.

Holmes had never campaigned for public office before. Fortunately for him, there wasn't much campaigning to do. When the deadline came to submit an application, he was the only person to file, meaning that he didn't have an opponent and was certain to be elected. Knowing this, he began thinking about who he wanted to be his assistant.

Don Cornish had worked in the coroner's office even longer than Holmes—twenty-seven years—and was an excellent investigator. He was nearing the end of his career, however, and told Holmes that he planned to retire soon. As for the two junior investigators, neither was the right fit. Gary Erickson had proven to be a good hire, but he was a little too cynical and didn't have the administrative experience that the job required. Ray Nichols, meanwhile, was marginally competent in Holmes's mind—certainly not deserving of a promotion. Holmes's thoughts turned to a man he worked with in the state coroner's association named Gary Tindel.

Tindel was the three-term sheriff-coroner in Yuba County, a small jurisdiction in the Sierra foothills east of Sacramento. He had a degree in civil engineering but never worked a day as an engineer. Just out of college, he couldn't find a job in the field and ended up applying to the Yuba County Sheriff's Office because he had grown up in Yuba City, the county seat, and the sheriff's office had openings. He took the test, was hired, and moved up quickly through the ranks until he was elected county sheriff. He also served as coroner because the coroner's office was part of the sheriff's department.

In meetings of the California State Coroners Association, Tindel was a presence. Part of it was due to his size—six foot one and 350 pounds of mostly muscle. Mainly, though, it was because he was a natural leader and a driving force wherever he went. Being near the state capital, Tindel got to know many state legislators and was a confidant of Governor George Deukmejian and his successor, Pete Wilson. On the walls in his office, Tindel had photos of himself with every major politician in California.

In the coroners association Tindel assumed various leadership positions and twice was elected president. He was a skilled administrator who Holmes knew would be able to handle any personnel issues that came up. Holmes knew something else as well: after three terms as sheriff-coroner, Tindel was being challenged by a female sergeant in Yuba County. Two weeks before the election, Tindel told Holmes that he had underestimated his opponent's chances, hadn't campaigned as hard as he should have, and might end up losing. The vote was close, but Tindel's premonition proved accurate. On the same day that Holmes was elected coroner of Marin County, succeeding Ervin Jindrich, Gary Tindel lost his bid for a fourth term as the sheriff-coroner of Yuba County.

As soon as Holmes heard that, he asked Tindel if he would consider becoming his assistant. Tindel said he appreciated the offer but didn't want to move because his three kids were in Yuba. Pete Wilson had offered him a job, as had a lobbying group, and he was considering other options.

"How about if you come to Marin and just take a look?" Holmes said. "Marin isn't that far from Yuba so it would still be easy to see your kids. The county is slightly bigger, but we don't have many homicides so the work isn't as strenuous."

Holmes knew that while he was sheriff-coroner, Tindel had handled multiple disasters, including the second-worst bus accident in United States history to that time, when a Yuba City school bus overturned and twenty-eight students and an adult advisor were killed. Also, Tindel was in charge of the county's emergency management system and, among other things, dealt with the effect of huge floods one year when cattle drowned and were floating in people's front yards. In addition, Holmes thought—correctly, as it turned out—that Tindel would like Marin's landscape and climate. Yuba is fairly flat and arid, hot during the summer and cold during the winter.

Tindel visited Marin County with his wife, and was sold. In addition to the environment and the weather, he liked the idea of a total change, getting away from local and state politics, as well as all the drama that went with it. He signed on to be the new assistant coroner.

CASTING BITE MARKS

One of Gary Tindel's first cases involved a fifty-five-year-old man who was found dead on the floor in his high-end, two-story duplex in Tiburon. Peter Torrente had been stabbed multiple times and also strangled. In addition, his body had fresh bruises, and chairs and a table in the dining room were upturned and damaged. All of it indicated that Peter had been in a physical fight with his assailant before he was killed. There was something else, though, that caused Tindel to call Holmes and ask him to come to the scene.

"This is a wild one," Tindel said. "There are fresh bite marks on the decedent's nose and one ear. I think the person he was fighting with bit him."

Holmes was intrigued. "I'll be right there," he said.

On the way, Holmes stopped by his dentist's office and picked up forming gel. In other cases he had used plaster of Paris to cast tire impressions, but it wasn't right for this.

When Holmes arrived, the entire Tiburon Police Department—five people—was in the living room. Only one person needed to be there, but murders in Tiburon were rare and all of the officers wanted in on the action. Holmes cast the teeth marks on Peter's ear and nose. Because they were only a couple of hours old, he was able to get good impressions.

There was an obvious suspect in the case—Peter's twenty-seven-year-old son, David. He was in trouble frequently, abused drugs, couldn't hold a job, and browbeat his father constantly for money.

"Up to a point his dad tried to help him," Holmes says, "but there came a time when his father said no, no more money."

David Torrente lived with his father off and on. He wasn't living with him at the time that Peter was killed, but he had come back to the house that day, seeking another handout. He was high on drugs and his father refused, saying that he wasn't going to subsidize his son's wasteful habits anymore. They got into a fight and ended up on the floor.

Peter was somewhat frail and not in good health. At one point as they were fighting, David Torrente bit his father's nose and ear. Eventually he stabbed him with a steak knife and a utility knife, then strangled him before fleeing the scene.

Police were led to the house by Peter's girlfriend, after she couldn't reach him by phone. She used to live with Peter but had moved out because David Torrente scared her.

Over the next two days, David Torrente tried to use his father's credit card to withdraw cash from ATM machines in San Francisco and South San Francisco but was unsuccessful because he didn't use the correct PIN number. Police caught him in the East Bay after a person reported that someone was rustling in the bushes outside his home and eating lemons.

When Holmes heard that David Torrente had been arrested, he encouraged sheriff's detectives, who had been called in by Tiburon police to assist with the case, to get a casting of the son's teeth so that it could be matched against the bite marks he had cast on Peter Torrente. The detectives pooh-poohed the idea, telling Holmes that it wasn't necessary, they already had more than enough evidence for a conviction. Among the items found in David Torrente's possession were two knives that police were confident belonged to his father and had been used in his stabbing.

David Torrente's defense was "I wasn't there." Inasmuch as he had lived with his father periodically, it was natural for his fingerprints to be all over his father's house, including on the knives, which his father could have given him or he had borrowed.

During one of the pretrial conferences, Holmes told the district attorney about his castings. The police had never mentioned them.

"If he bit his dad during this fight," Holmes said, "that's one of the few ways you're going to be able to say he was there at that time. Even if the son said he was in another room when the attack occurred and didn't know anything about it, the teeth marks prove otherwise."

The district attorney got a search warrant, and a jail dentist did a casting of David Torrente's teeth. When the sheriff's detectives heard about the castings, they hired another dentist to race down to the mortuary and get castings of the bite marks on Peter's nose and ear. It was five days after the incident took place, however, and Peter's features were shriveled by this time so the castings were useless. Holmes's castings ended up cinching the case for jurors and led to David Torrente's imprisonment.

A BROKEN NECKLACE

One of Pam Carter's early cases concerned a sixty-seven-year-old woman named Susan King, who died in her bathtub. Her nude body was found submerged in bathwater by her thirty-eight-year-old daughter, Constance Young. Young said that her mother had been ill for several weeks, experiencing vomiting, diarrhea, and weight loss. She had been treated three times at Kaiser, rehydrated, and released. The last time was two weeks earlier.

Carter knew from the moment she arrived that something wasn't right. For one thing, dead bodies float, but Susan King's body was completely underwater. That meant all of the air had been forced out of her lungs prior to or during her death. For another thing, there were three bloody fingerprints on the tub—an antique, clawfoot model—that had dried. The fingerprints looked to be recent, although there wasn't any blood in the water.

The responding police officers decided on their own that Mrs. King had a seizure. When Carter got there, they said they were leaving. Carter tried to convince them to at least consider the possibility of foul play. After all, there was evidence that didn't add up to a natural death.

One of the officers helped Carter lift Mrs. King from the tub with the aid of webbing straps. As they did, Carter noticed a broken, yellow-metal necklace lying directly underneath the body.

"Look," Carter said. "How can you ignore this? You can't account for the fact that she's not floating. She's dead and her lungs are full of water. You can't account for the three bloody fingerprints. There's no blood in the water, and these prints are fresh and dry. Now how are you going to account for this broken necklace?"

The officers downplayed the meaning. There were no bruises or marks on Mrs. King, they said, or other signs of trauma. While they acknowledged that she wasn't taking any serious medications, only Lomotil (for diarrhea) and Flagyl (an antibiotic), that didn't rule out a health problem. Moreover, Constance was quite emotional—appropriately so, in their minds—further convincing the officers that Mrs. King's death was natural.

"We're 10-8," they told Carter. Out of here.

After they left, Carter took lots of photos. She also took a specimen of the bathwater to make sure it was the same water that was in Mrs. King's lungs (it was). There was nothing else Carter could do, though. The bloody prints weren't clear enough to be helpful, and without the police looking into the case further, there was little chance that new information would turn up.

"The curtain came down," Holmes says. "We didn't have anything. The only thing we could do was rule that the manner of death was undetermined because it just didn't feel right."

The rest of the story unfolded over the next several years. Constance Young, Mrs. King's daughter, had been in and out of trouble. She was a meth addict and continually solicited money from her mother to support her habit, much as Peter Torrente's son had done. From time to time, Young and her husband, a onetime inmate at San Quentin, lived in Mrs. King's house, a beautiful, well-maintained mansion in an older part of San Rafael. They weren't living there at the time Mrs. King died—she lived alone—but they had resided in the house in the past. Eventually Mrs. King told her daughter that she wasn't giving her any more money because it just went for drugs. She had had enough.

A short time later, Young and her husband were arrested for breaking into a building at the College of Marin, stealing computer equipment, and trying to sell it at a flea market. The computers still had College of Marin stickers, but the couple was able to avoid a conviction by claiming that somebody gave the equipment to them.

Right after that, Mrs. King died and the Youngs lit out for Montana. Months later, when Mrs. King's estate was settled, they moved back to Marin and into the mother's mansion. The property had deteriorated in the interim, and it became more run-down in the months that followed.

Also living with them was Constance Young's six-year-old son, fathered by a man named Nicklas Stephens. He had married Young several years earlier, then divorced her because of her drug use. Stephens had shared custody, and every time he came to pick up or drop off the boy, it was contentious.

On one occasion, the two ex-spouses got into a loud and vicious argument. In the middle of it Constance bolted up the stairs and their son cried out a warning to Stephens.

"Daddy! Daddy! Mommy's getting the gun."

Young was intoxicated and also high on meth. She came down holding a gun, and she and Stephens scuffled while the boy ran upstairs. Stephens claimed that he was trying to take the gun from her when it went off. The boy gave conflicting accounts, at one point saying that when he left the room his mother was sitting on a couch and his father was standing over her holding the gun.

It was the boy who called police. When officers arrived, they found Constance Young dead on the sofa from a gunshot wound.

Two things came out of it. First, when people in Montana heard that Young was dead and that she had been living in San Rafael, they called the San Rafael Police Department. Young had told friends that she drowned her mother, they said. All she did was put the palm of her hand on her mother's forehead and force her head underwater. That was why there were no bruises. As for the blood on the tub, it was Constance's blood because her mother had bitten her.

Police officers from Marin interviewed people in Montana and were told that Constance Young laughed about killing her mother and inheriting her mother's estate.

"She got the inheritance, she got the house, and she got away with murder," Holmes says. "She thought it was great fun and didn't hide it."

The second development was that police arrested Stephens and charged him with voluntary manslaughter for Young's death. Holmes argued against it.

"Stephens was a straight-arrow, stand-up kind of guy," he says. "Even if it was voluntary, what purpose was served by putting him in jail? Now this kid had no parents, his grandmother was drowned, his mother was shot almost in front of him, and he was placed in foster care. Not that it's okay to kill someone; it's not. But she had the gun, he tried to take it away from her, and she pulled the trigger. The angle of the bullet was absolutely consistent with what he said."

Holmes had examined Constance Young's body, so he knew. He also saw the state to which she had deteriorated in the twelve months since her mother's death.

"She looked like a concentration camp survivor," he says. "She was that skinny. Her teeth were bad and her eyes were sunken. But she was the boy's mother."

The police didn't listen to Holmes, just as they hadn't listened to Pam Carter when she pointed out incongruities in Susan King's death. It might be possible to explain the bloody fingerprints and even the water in Mrs. King's lungs, but the broken necklace was an indication that she didn't have a heart attack or a seizure before she died. For one thing, the necklace wasn't likely to break in that situation unless either the chain or clasp was weak. Carter tested them, and both were solid. More important, though, if the necklace did break accidentally, it would have been on top of Mrs. King's body, not underneath it. That was the real clue.

To Holmes and Carter, it couldn't have been clearer. The problem was they couldn't prove it at the time, and the district attorney didn't think he could get a conviction without a confession.

Nicklas Stephens, meanwhile, was sentenced to seven years in prison. "He was released after three and a half years," Holmes says, "but still . . ."

His voice trails off. Sometimes what's just isn't what's right.

PEDRO AND JOSÉ

Being its own branch of county government, the Marin County Coroner's Office had a level of autonomy during Holmes's career that didn't exist in many other California counties. Dr. Jindrich, Holmes's predecessor, reminded county supervisors of this shortly after he was first elected. Each January the board of supervisors met individually with every department head to talk about how things were going. Heads who were hired by the board—the county administrator, finance director, human resources director, and health and human services director—were told when the meeting would be. With heads who were elected, the board requested a meeting. Jindrich declined to meet with the board, however. In a formal letter, he said that if voters were unhappy with his performance, they would let him know at the ballot box in the next election, but he wasn't obligated to meet with the board or explain himself. Board members were aghast, but there was nothing they could do. For years, Jindrich refused to meet with the board. When Holmes became assistant coroner, Jindrich sent Holmes to sit in for him.

Since it acted autonomously, the coroner's office was an independent supplier of facts. In some cases these facts implicated an individual and in other cases they exonerated someone. Regardless of the outcome, the coroner was on equal footing with the sheriff and district attorney. This was important because at times the three of them disagreed about whether criminal charges should be filed. It wasn't the coroner's place to establish guilt or innocence, but if there was compelling forensic evidence to support criminal charges, Holmes believed that the police and public prosecutor had a responsibility to follow through, that the deceased and next of kin deserved it.

One such occasion concerned two friends, Pedro and José. They were roommates and worked together at a small delicatessen and grocery store in Stinson Beach that was a few miles from their rented house. José owned a pickup truck but his driver's license had been suspended because of past arrests for drunk driving. Pedro had a driver's license but didn't have enough money to buy a vehicle. Thus, when the two of them needed to go somewhere, to work or into town, Pedro drove José's truck.

They started work early in the morning, and generally finished around 2 P.M. At that time their boss often brought out a bottle of red wine and everyone had a drink or two before leaving for the day.

One particular afternoon, Pedro and José didn't make it home from work. Hours after they left, Pedro crawled up a steep hill onto the roadway and hailed a passing car. He was bloody and bruised and his clothes were disheveled.

José's truck was two hundred feet down the embankment, upside down. The embankment was covered with poison oak, and José was lying in the bushes, dead, after being ejected from the vehicle. The police asked Pedro what happened and he said he didn't know. He said José was driving, lost control, and they ended up going over the side.

"José was driving?" the cops said.

"*Sí,*" Pedro said.

The cops checked a database. "José has a suspended license," they said.

"*Lo sé,*" Pedro said. "I know it. That's why I always drive. This time he wanted to drive, though."

Rescue workers brought José's body up to the roadway. There was no blood, just evidence of trauma from the crash and its aftermath. A winch was used to haul up the truck. Its roof was caved in, the doors were jammed, and there was blood in the top of the window track on the driver's side.

After the pathologist did the autopsy on José, he called Holmes. "This guy wasn't driving," the pathologist said. "He has a seat belt mark from his right shoulder down his chest."

Photos were taken, then Holmes called the police officer who was handling the case and suggested that photos be taken of Pedro. Pedro had a seat belt mark from his left shoulder to his right hip. Police talked to people at the restaurant who said that when they left, Pedro was driving and José was in the passenger seat. When confronted with this information, Pedro told police that after they went a short distance, José said he wanted to drive so they switched seats and José was driving.

Holmes didn't believe it, and neither did the police. Both thought that Pedro should be charged with manslaughter. When the case reached the district attorney's office, however, a female prosecutor said she wasn't going to pursue it.

"The evidence is insufficient," she said.

Hearing that, the police officer asked her to talk to Holmes. Holmes laid the photos he had and the photos that CHP had taken of the accident on a table in front of the woman, lining them up as if she were looking through the front windshield of the pickup. The seat belt marks matched those of the driver and passenger exactly.

She wasn't impressed. "It's a 'he said, she said' kind of case," she said.

The coroner's office tested the blood on the driver's side of the truck, and it turned out to be the same type as Pedro's blood. He had crawled out through the broken window. José's blood was a different type. The woman still wouldn't prosecute, so Holmes asked for another meeting with her to try to understand why.

"It's vehicular homicide," he said. "Maybe not intentional, but that's not my job to decide."

She said, "You can call it anything you want, but there's not enough information."

Holmes knew from experience that oftentimes in a traffic accident, the person who survives is the driver. He or she has half a second before everyone else in the vehicle to understand that something bad is going to happen and prepare for it. Also the driver has something to hold on to—the steering wheel—which can reduce the level of bodily injury if the vehicle is hit from the side. This fact didn't convince the district attorney, either, however.

Pedro wasn't charged. It still bothers Holmes to think about it.

DISASTER PLANNING

When it comes to county government, the coroner's office often is the forgotten stepchild. People don't want to think about it, and they definitely don't want to know any details of how it operates. Nowhere is this more apparent than in county disaster planning.

Because Marin is surrounded on three sides by water, any large-scale disaster has the potential to leave county residents isolated. A major earthquake on the San Andreas Fault, for instance, which runs through Marin, or heavy flooding in low-lying areas such as the Canal District in central San Rafael, could stop all automotive traffic into and out of the county. The two primary access points—the Golden Gate Bridge to the south and Richmond–San Rafael Bridge to the east—will close if they suffer any significant damage. West is the Pacific Ocean, so the only direction people in Marin can travel without crossing a bridge is north.

"Everyone remembers the aerial photos of traffic after Hurricane Katrina," Holmes says. "There were twelve lanes heading out of town, and cars were backed up for miles. There are only four northbound lanes on Highway 101 from Marin, and just one lane north on Highway 1. The only way to bring in supplies will be by boat."

County officials weren't interested in hearing about it, though, nor did they think in the beginning to even have a representative of the coroner's office present in the county's emergency operations center during planning meetings. It was only when someone said, "What happens to the dead bodies?" and another person said, "They go to the coroner," that people realized Holmes needed to be there. Even so, no one was eager to hear what he had to say.

"I'd ask about having contracts with tugboat and barge companies," Holmes says, "and with businesses that had large refrigeration units, and people would look at me blankly, barely stifling a yawn."

Holmes's questions grew out of a relationship he developed with people in the Los Angeles County Coroner's Office. It began in February 2000 after Alaskan Airlines Flight 261, en route from Puerto Vallarta, Mexico, to Seattle, Washington, crashed into the Pacific Ocean several miles off the coast of Ventura. Everyone on board—eighty-three passengers and five crew members—was killed. Holmes was part of the federal disaster mortuary response team that assisted in retrieving and identifying the remains, and because the wreckage was spread out and most of the bodies were torn apart, three thousand body bags ended up being used.

Six years later Holmes was back in Southern California, helping out after another aviation disaster. A DC-9 passenger plane from Mexico City was descending into Los Angeles International Airport when it collided with a family-owned Piper aircraft that had just taken off. All sixty-four passengers and crew members in the DC-9 and the three people in the Piper were killed. In addition, the DC-9 crashed into a residential neighborhood in Cerritos, a suburb of Los Angeles, destroying five houses, damaging four others, and killing fifteen people on the ground (the Piper fell onto an empty playground in Cerritos). Ironically, the street the DC-9 landed on was Holmes Avenue.

The remains were brought back to a large, makeshift tented area that was fully enclosed and refrigerated. It was on a scale that Holmes would have had a hard time imagining prior to seeing it.

"The L.A. coroner was really well prepared and had the total support of his board of supervisors," Holmes says. "That made all the difference."

Afterward, his contact gave him advice. "As soon as you go back to Marin, begin making formal agreements with people who have large refrigeration units. That's where you can put the bodies after a disaster until you've had a chance to examine and identify them. Tell the county that you'll only be using the units temporarily, even though the fact is that once they've had dead people in them, no one will use them for any other purpose again. The county will have to buy them."

Holmes didn't go that far, but he did visit and establish agreements with three large suppliers of cold storage. All were beer distributors. One had a two-story refrigerated building and another had a three-story one.

"Even if Marin had a morgue," Holmes says, "it couldn't have accommodated more than seven or eight bodies. In identifying places, I used the number four hundred. Could it hold four hundred dead bodies?"

It was an arbitrary number but conveyed the potential magnitude of what the county—and the coroner's office—might be dealing with. If the unit had that kind of capacity, then Holmes's next question was simple: "How soon can you empty the place if I need it?"

These were large, warehouse-type operations, and beer in cases was stacked on pallets, sometimes to the ceiling.

"A day," he was told.

"That's all?" Holmes said.

"We have big forklifts and are used to moving product quickly."

That solved the refrigeration problem. There was still the issue of water transportation.

"In a major disaster, we won't be able to transport anything into or out of the county by road," Holmes told county planners. "Marin doesn't have any rail lines, and we're too suburban to have access to large helicopters—they'll be deployed in metropolitan areas. Tugboats pulling barges are the only answer, or ferries. Look at all of our landing points—Stinson Beach, Drake's Bay, Larkspur Landing, Richardson Bay, Tomales Bay, even the Petaluma River."

County administrators believed that the possibility of all three major land routes—two bridges and a federal highway—being impassable simultaneously was too remote to consider. They listened to Holmes but didn't act on what he said. He could only hope that if there was a major disaster in the future, he would be proven wrong in his assumptions or at least would be retired by that time.

CHAPTER 22

A SUPERVISOR'S WRATH

The suicide of a seventeen-year-old boy named Brett wasn't the last case Holmes handled, but it contributed to the end of his career. He just didn't know it at the time.

By most accounts, Brett was an average teenage boy. He had a pretty, sixteen-year-old girlfriend, four good friends he hung out with, and a part-time job, and was scheduled to graduate from high school in four months. When he didn't show up for work, one of his friends who worked with him became alarmed. He knew that Brett had tried to kill himself twice before, and just two days earlier Brett had said that if he should die, don't be sad but rather be happy for him because he finally had done it. That night the friend tried to phone Brett but couldn't reach him. The next morning Brett's mother called the friend to say that Brett hadn't come home the previous night. The friend rounded up five other boys and they started looking for Brett. They knew some of the places where he liked to go hiking, one of which was near a water tower on a fire road not far from Brett's house. That's where they found Brett's body, hanging by a rope from a pipe that protruded from the tower. Laid out neatly on the cement foundation were Brett's backpack, wallet, and cell phone. In the wallet were two letters. One was a good-bye letter addressed to "Boo," his girlfriend. The other was addressed to

"Everyone" and said that Brett had never been happy, and this was the best thing for him.

It seemed like another tragic case of a despondent youth who took his life and left everyone who loved him reeling. Holmes had seen far too many cases like it. This time, though, there was a twist, and it would have repercussions that he couldn't have imagined.

Brett's birth mother had been a drug addict who wasn't capable of raising him or his sister. When Brett was a baby, his maternal grandmother applied for and received legal custody of him, while another family adopted his young sister.

From the outset, Brett's grandmother, a woman named Tabitha, told all of her friends, neighbors, and people in the community that Brett was her biological son, not her grandson, despite the fact that it was highly unusual for a woman her age to birth a child. Once Brett was old enough to talk, Tabitha insisted that he refer to her as his mother, not as his grandmother. As Brett grew older, she told him that when his sister came to visit, he was to introduce her to people as his cousin, not as his sister. Also, at no time was he to mention or try to talk to his birth mother, Tabitha said.

Gary Tindel, Holmes's assistant, was the investigator on the case. He was summoned after Brett's friends called 911 and police officers confirmed Brett's death. Tindel saw that Brett's body was cut down and removed to a local mortuary for an autopsy, then he wrote up his report.

Holmes had the case file on his desk the next morning and was looking at it when he was phoned by a local reporter. People already knew about Brett's suicide—word had gotten around—and the reporter asked Holmes where Brett's family resided. Reading off the report, Holmes said that Brett had a grandmother in San Rafael who was his adoptive mother. The next day, the *Marin Independent Journal* ran a brief story that said Brett was survived by his grandmother. As soon as it appeared, Tabitha called Holmes. She was irate and said she wasn't Brett's grandmother, she was his mother, and she wanted him to print a retraction in the newspaper.

Holmes was confused. "You're his mother's mother, correct?" he said.

"Yes," Tabitha said as if it hardly mattered, "but I'm his adoptive mother, and I demand that you print a retraction."

Holmes tried to reason with her, saying that any kind of retraction would bring more attention to the case, which he didn't think she wanted. Besides, she was his blood grandmother.

"All my friends think I'm his mother," Tabitha said. "I've never told anybody that I'm his grandmother."

"Let me get this straight," Holmes said. "You're asking me to change my story, which is true, in order to match your story, which isn't true?"

Tabitha practically spit out the words. "Who's your supervisor?"

"You are," Holmes said, "because I'm elected."

"Don't go anywhere," Tabitha said. "I'm on my way down there to talk to you."

She showed up at the front counter of the coroner's office with her husband in tow. He wasn't Brett's grandfather, but he went along with the ruse and didn't say a word throughout the conversation.

"I insist that you print a retraction and an apology," Tabitha said. "I'm Brett's legal mother."

Holmes could have been accommodating, and under other circumstances he would have been. Tabitha's assertiveness and sense of entitlement rubbed him the wrong way, though.

"I'm not going to print a retraction of something that's true," he said, "nor am I going to apologize for saying it."

They went back and forth for several minutes, neither one giving ground. Then Tabitha said, "I heard Brett left a note. I want it."

Holmes said, "He left two notes. One is addressed to 'Everyone' and I can give you a copy of it. The other one isn't addressed to you, so I can't let you have that."

Tabitha was incensed. "Who's it addressed to?"

"I can't tell you that."

"I'm his mother," Tabitha snapped.

Holmes said, "I'm sorry, but the law prevents me from letting you see it."

Tabitha could barely restrain herself. "Can you tell me what's in it?"

"No, because it's a private letter from one person to another."

Tabitha huffed that she was going to get an attorney. Holmes told her she was welcome to do that, or she could go upstairs and talk to one of the attorneys at county counsel. This wasn't the first time a situation like this had come up, he said.

For several seconds she stared hard at him. Then, her jaw set tight, she said, "We'll see about this. I want that letter."

A short time later, Holmes received a call from an attorney who said he was acting on Tabitha's behalf. He asked Holmes whom the letter was addressed to.

"It's not addressed to anyone in the family," Holmes said, "so I don't know whether I can tell you. I need to talk to my attorney first."

Holmes's attorney was a woman in the county counsel office named Jennifer. She told him that there was no harm in saying that the letter was addressed to Brett's girlfriend.

"Can you tell her attorney that?" Holmes said. "I don't want to be involved in that part of it."

"Sure," Jennifer said.

Within hours, Tabitha was on the phone again with Holmes. "Where is that little— Where is she?" she sputtered, referring to Boo.

"I have no idea where she is," Holmes said. "She hasn't come in to get the letter. I don't even know if she knows that we have a letter."

Once a case was closed, the coroner's office informed someone if the decedent had left that person a note or letter, but usually not before.

"I'll tell her!" Tabitha said. "I'll tell her!"

Holmes had barely gotten off the phone with Tabitha before she was in his office again, this time with Brett's girlfriend. "The girl was as pretty as a picture," he says, "as timid as could be, and clearly frightened of this overbearing woman."

Tabitha's husband was there, too, and once again was silent.

"Give her the note," Tabitha said to Holmes. "She's going to give it to me."

Holmes looked at Boo, who seemed terrified. "Is it your preference after you've read the note to give it to her?" he said, motioning in Tabitha's direction.

Boo bowed her head and said softly, "No, it's not my preference. She's telling me I have to."

"If you don't want to, you don't have to," he said.

Tabitha erupted. "You asshole! You can't prevent her from giving it to me."

Holmes nodded. "No, I can't. But she can." Then he turned to Boo. "You need legal representation here. You can't be bullied by somebody who's not related to you."

"I'm not a bully!" Tabitha said through clenched teeth. "That note is my property!"

"It's not," he said. "It's her property."

Before Tabitha could say anything further, Holmes said to Boo, "Do you want to read it?"

Near tears, Boo nodded.

Holmes took her into a private room, leaving Tabitha and her husband at the counter. With the door closed behind them, he gave Boo the letter that Brett had written to her.

"You can have the original after I make a copy for our files," Holmes said. "You don't have to show it to her."

Boo said, "If I have it when I walk out of here, she'll take it from me."

Holmes said, "Well, then read it and don't take it out of here."

He left the room so that Boo would have privacy, then told Tabitha that Boo was reading the note and probably would need time to herself afterward. Tabitha was nearly apoplectic, but there was nothing she could do.

When Holmes's secretary told him that Boo had finished and was ready to leave, he went to talk with her again. "Would you like me to walk you out?" he said.

Boo said, tears streaming down her face, "Would you walk me to my car?" She and Tabitha had come separately and met in the parking lot.

Holmes approached Tabitha at the counter and told her that Boo had read the letter and decided to leave it there. Tabitha lit into Boo. "You told me you were going to let me have it. What kind of a girlfriend are you, you cheap little . . ."

She never actually called her any names, just kept repeating the words "cheap" and "little."

Boo was sobbing, partly because her boyfriend was dead and partly because she was being browbeaten by Tabitha.

"The part of the letter about Boo was sweet," Holmes says, "but in the middle Brett vented about Tabitha, about how controlling she was and how she forced him to deny his sister and birth mother."

A month later, Holmes received a call from one of the five members of the Marin County Board of Supervisors. She happened to represent his district and he had supported her campaign, displaying her signs in his front yard, although that wasn't why she was calling him now.

"I was contacted by one of my constituents," she said. "There was a death and a suicide note, and apparently you made a misstatement in the paper. Can you and I meet to talk about it?"

Holmes said, "There's really nothing to meet about. It wasn't a mistake. The lady has been lying to her entire community for something like fifteen years and wants me to cover for her."

"What!" the supervisor exclaimed.

He told her some of the details. "It's his blood grandmother. She adopted him legally, and she demands to be called his mother. She's told her friends that she's his mother. She's a sixty-five-year-old woman with a seventeen-year-old son? It's possible, but it means she was close to fifty when he was born. I, unknowingly, put the truth in the paper."

"Okay," the supervisor said. "That makes a different story."

Only it didn't. The following week the supervisor called Holmes again. Tabitha continued to complain to her about being referred to as Brett's grandmother rather than his mother.

"It'd be a lot easier if you went ahead and put an apology in the newspaper," the supervisor told Holmes. He was shocked.

"I can't believe you're asking me to do that," he said. "This woman has lived a lie for years and wants us to support her for the sake of her face in the community. Admittedly, I got my back up in the beginning because she came into my office with an attitude, but the bottom line is I didn't say anything wrong, and I'm going to stand with that. I'm not going to write a retraction or apology."

Holmes thought that was the end of it, but the supervisor's secretary contacted him shortly thereafter and said the supervisor wanted to meet with him. When he went to the supervisor's office, which was on a different floor of the Marin Civic Center building than Holmes's office, she had an attorney with her, another person in the county counsel's office.

Holmes looked at him uneasily. "Do I need my attorney?"

The man nodded. "It'd probably be good."

Jennifer, Holmes's attorney, came in and got a quick update. Then the supervisor said, "For the good of the community, and to keep peace with everyone, it would be best if you issued an apology and we're all done with it."

"What is this woman to you?" Holmes said. "Why are you carrying her banner?"

"I keep hearing from her."

"I keep hearing from her, too, and I just told her no. I'm not going to write a letter of apology. At this point it's the principle of the thing."

Holmes turned to Jennifer for support. She said, "It's totally up to you."

The supervisor glared at Holmes. It was the first time they had had a serious disagreement, and she was perturbed. "I'm elected," she said, "and I'm telling you to write this letter."

It was an astonishing thing to say, and Holmes gaped at her in disbelief. He was elected, too, and she knew that. He wasn't her underling.

Holmes couldn't help but reply, "You're elected by one-fifth of the people who elected me."

It was true. There were five supervisorial districts in Marin, and people in each district elected their supervisor. In contrast, everyone in the county voted to elect the coroner.

The supervisor didn't understand why Holmes was fighting her. In her mind it wasn't a big deal, just a letter. If it stopped Tabitha from hounding her, it was worth it.

She couldn't make Holmes write it, though, and he never did. Tabitha didn't get the retraction or public apology she wanted. She also didn't get to see Brett's letter to Boo. Tabitha did exact a measure of revenge, though.

To start with, neither Brett's birth mother nor his sister—Tabitha's daughter and granddaughter—was invited to Brett's funeral service. Holmes learned this later from Lisa, Brett's birth mother. The two of them struck up a friendship after Lisa came to Holmes's office and poured her heart out to him. She had cleaned up years earlier, remarried, and owned a small business in San Francisco with her new husband. She told Holmes that when she was young she did a lot of stupid things to try to get away from her mother. She also said that Tabitha forbade Brett from seeing her and was livid when she found out that he was in contact with her.

Holmes's stubbornness had consequences for him as well. Within months the supervisor mounted a quiet campaign to get rid of the coroner's office by merging it with the sheriff's department. Holmes couldn't be fired for dereliction of duty, and he didn't have any health problems, so the only way to get him out of office was to consolidate his department with the sheriff's.

To be fair, the supervisor wasn't the first person to consider a merger. The county administrator had asked Holmes previously when he planned to retire because combining the two offices made sense to him. He didn't want to do it while Holmes was still in office, though. Holmes said that he didn't have any immediate plans to retire and expected to serve one more four-year term, through 2014.

Soon after the incident with Tabitha, the supervisor began lobbying her fellow supervisors. A merger would save the county money, she maintained, and place the operation of the coroner's office under the sheriff the way it was in most other California counties. Sheriff Robert Doyle was in favor of the merger—it increased his power— and the triumvirate of an influential county supervisor, the county administrator, and the sheriff was formidable.

Holmes pointed out the advantages of having the coroner's office separate from the sheriff. Death investigators came into the job already trained in medicine and forensics while police officers lacked this knowledge. An independent coroner paid greater attention to accident victims, suicides, and individuals who died from natural causes than did cops, whose focus was on homicides. Families also received more and better support because investigators were willing to spend time with them and help them deal with their grief rather than move quickly to the next case.

Unsaid but implied was that the outcome of many cases would have been different if the coroner's office hadn't devoted considerable time and resources to them. Gertrude Jones's remains wouldn't have been identified forty-four years after she disappeared, and the cause of her death—murder—wouldn't be known. Little Devon Gromer's death would have been attributed to natural causes when, in fact, his father killed him. A foot and shoe found in San Francisco Bay wouldn't be connected to a specific person, and the cause of death—a jump from the Golden Gate Bridge—would be a mystery to next of kin and others.

There were so many instances when coroner's investigators, working independently from law enforcement, unveiled the truth in cases that would have been dropped if they hadn't been given the freedom to pursue them. Sammie Marshall died in the course of being removed from his cell at San Quentin, but the cause of his death wasn't natural, despite what prison officials said. Wolfram Fischer, whose body was found without any identification beneath the Golden Gate Bridge, would have died in anonymity if Holmes had been less determined and if Wolfram's body had been cremated rather than buried, making future DNA testing impossible. Peter Torrente's son might have gotten away with murdering his father—much the same way that Constance Young got away with murdering her mother in her bathtub—if Holmes hadn't cast the bite marks he left behind.

This wasn't a slap at law enforcement. Rather, Holmes noted that police officers had different responsibilities and priorities than coroners, and keeping the offices separate benefited the county in several ways.

Despite his efforts, Holmes knew well before the issue was voted on that it was a done deal. There was no opposition except his, and barely any discussion.

In November 2009, the county board of supervisors approved the merger of the coroner's office with the sheriff's department effective January 1, 2011. The vote was unanimous.

CHAPTER 23

ENDING AND BEGINNING

After the merger was announced, Holmes considered his options. By the time it occurred, he would be sixty-eight and have spent more than half his life working in the coroner's office, including the past twelve years as coroner. It was a good run, and he had a lot to be proud of, in particular the positive relationships forged over the years between his office and thousands of families who had lost loved ones. He could collect his pension and just walk away. That was what most people would do.

Holmes wasn't ready to retire, however. While he had many interests outside of work, which he looked forward to pursuing when he had the time, he continued to be energized by the job and felt that he had more to give still.

In June 2010, elections were held for several county positions, including, for the first time, that of sheriff-coroner. If the merger hadn't taken place, the coroner would have been a separate item on the ballot with Holmes seeking a fourth term. Instead, beginning in 2011 Sheriff Doyle would be the coroner and would appoint a staff person to oversee the coroner's function. Already he had indicated that he had a sergeant in mind, so Holmes would be out of a job.

Two months before the election, Holmes filed papers to run against Doyle. The chances of Holmes winning were slim since there were no serious black marks against the sheriff and the majority of voters would assume, given concerns about safety, that it was better to have a sheriff who was also the coroner rather than a coroner who was also the sheriff. Holmes knew he was a long shot, especially with only two months to campaign, but decided to try anyway.

Doyle was sixty-two and had spent his entire career—forty years— in the sheriff's department, starting as a court bailiff. He had been sheriff fourteen years and, like Holmes, had never faced a contested election. He was experienced, savvy, and had a solid base of community support. In addition, he was in charge of 316 employees and managed a budget that was nearly fifty times larger than the coroner's budget. Holmes matched him in tenure, but his office was much smaller. Doyle emphasized the disparity of their respective departments by featuring in his campaign literature the image of a minnow trying to devour a much larger bass.

"Someone who's been managing a $1 million budget, I don't think he can have any comprehension of what a $50 million budget is like," Doyle said.

Holmes countered by saying that he had always managed a balanced budget, whereas the sheriff's department frequently had overruns. In addition, Holmes had advanced certificates from the state's Commission on Peace Officer Standards and Training, making him qualified, he felt, to assume the sheriff's duties, while Doyle wasn't qualified to be the coroner because he had no training in medicine or forensics.

Doyle garnered more endorsements than Holmes and raised a lot more money—$100,000, a large amount given Marin's small size and the fact that little funding had been spent on sheriff's elections in the past. The results were predictable. Doyle received 63 percent of the 39,500 votes that were cast, while Holmes received 37 percent. In the same election, the supervisor who wanted Holmes to issue a public apology to Tabitha received 52 percent of the votes in her district to earn another term as supervisor.

Holmes began making plans to retire on December 31, 2010, the last day that the coroner's office would operate independently. One thing he did was send all of the coroner's case files from earlier than 2000 to the Marin County library to be archived. It was the policy of the sheriff's office to destroy most records that were ten years old or older, and Holmes didn't want that to happen with his records.

"Coroners' records are different than arrest records," he says. "To destroy them isn't just about the legal implications of a homicide, accidental death, or car wreck. Coroners have information about families that goes back generations. Every week we had people coming to us with questions about genealogy because there was no place else for them to get the information. Mortuaries don't have it all; cemeteries don't have it all; families seldom have it all. Many of the things that come to bear on a person's life are in the coroner's records."

At one time Holmes and his staff tried to microfiche inquest records from the 1800s and early 1900s. The records were on onionskin paper, however, which started to dissolve in the process. After they put the first ten pages in a scanner, they stopped. The heat was taking the ink out of the onionskin. Some of the inquests were fifteen pages long, recorded in calligraphy—"Difficult to read, but absolutely beautiful," Holmes says. "We had hundreds of them because every single one since 1853 was kept, and I was afraid that the sheriff's office would either try to find a way to minimize them or get rid of them."

In the olden days, an inquest was held whenever someone died. The coroner had the power, by law, to go into the hallway of whatever building he was in and pick six people for the jury. He didn't need a subpoena, and the people had to come immediately, unless they had a compelling reason why they couldn't. That is still true today, incidentally, although no one does it that way. When Holmes held an inquest, he would go to the regular court jury pool, take forty people off the roll, and sort through them just like any other jury trial. The only difference was that the process would be completed in one day whereas jury selections in courtroom trials can take several days or longer.

Holmes was told that the only records older than ten years that the Marin County Sheriff's Office kept now were the original report pertaining to a criminal case and the case's disposition. The hand-written notes taken by deputies during interviews weren't retained, which alarmed him since they contained many details. He thought that if similar information in coroners' records was discarded, it would constitute an enormous loss. In addition to a one-page summary, each coroner's file included an investigative report, supplemental findings, pathology and toxicology reports, police reports, and sui-cide notes if found. Some files had fifty pages or more. In addition, there were photographs taken at the scene and during autopsies, as well as all of the negatives. The latter were kept so that if copies were requested by the district attorney, defense attorneys, or insurance companies, the coroner could provide them. Holmes believed that if he ever supplied an original print or negative, there was a risk that it wouldn't be returned.

The Marin County Library was two floors above the coroner's office in the Frank Lloyd Wright–designed Civic Center building; nevertheless, moving all of the files there was a chore. Dozens of large, four-drawer file cabinets, each one filled with paper records of cases that collectively went back nearly 150 years, were loaded onto dollies and taken upstairs by elevator. Library staff weren't quite sure what to do with them but recognized their historical value and made plans to house the collection.

As with other facets of the coroner's work that people in the sheriff's office didn't fully understand or appreciate prior to taking over, the realization was slow in coming that everything would need to be kept. There were too many instances when law enforcement personnel had to access old information because it had bearing on an open case. As a result, over time all files ended up being moved out of the library and into a big storage area used by the sheriff.

THE AXE FALLS

Because Sheriff Doyle had promised the board of supervisors that merging the coroner's office with his department would save money, there had to be funding cuts. The cuts wouldn't be in the sheriff's budget but in the coroner's. The first one was the assistant coroner position. Gary Tindel, the former sheriff-coroner of Yuba County, represented the old regime and also posed a perceived threat to the newly appointed coroner because Tindel had far more knowledge and experience in death investigations than the sergeant did. Abolishing the position reduced costs as well as removed any fears. It didn't leave anyone to train or supervise the three investigators, but the thinking was that new investigators would come into the job already trained, and the sergeant could do the supervising. As for other responsibilities of the job, they would be spread out or eliminated.

Another cost-cutting move was to reduce the number of autopsies that were performed in the county. The stated rationale was that they weren't necessary, but the real reason, Holmes believed, was that autopsies are expensive and, from the sheriff's point of view, only worth doing in homicide cases. That's not surprising, although Holmes had cases where police officers were quick to attribute someone's death to a manner other than homicide so that they didn't have to investigate.

"In the 1980s," Holmes says, "we were called to a house where a man was found dead on the floor of his kitchen. He had been stabbed three times in the heart, once in the lung, and once in the belly. Police found the knife that had been used. It had been washed off in the sink—there were small drops of blood there—then put back on a magnetic knife rack. Three cops were at the scene, and they discussed at length the angle of the knife for each piercing. They dusted the knife for fingerprints, but it had been wiped clean. The blood in the sink proved to be that of the decedent. The police couldn't develop any other scenarios or a suspect, so they decided that he must have stabbed himself, wiped the knife, returned it to its holder, cleaned the sink, then laid on the floor and died. They concluded in their report that it was a suicide even though we said it was undetermined and a probable homicide."

Over the years, one of the police officers involved in the case and Holmes shared a bemused laugh over it. Sometimes it's not easy to determine what happened, but at least you make an effort to find out. Next of kin deserve it.

"In today's world," Holmes says, "the police would never do that. City chiefs and sheriffs wouldn't allow it. A man stabs himself five times, then has the wherewithal to rinse the knife, dry it, and hang it back on the rack before he staggers around and dies? It's not impossible. He could have had a really solid heart, and the knife went in cleanly and came out cleanly so there was only a little blood. Similarly, you can puncture one lung and your other lung will keep functioning, at least for a short period of time. It's not likely, though."

With the merger, the Coroner Division of the Marin County Sheriff's Office, as it was now known, stopped doing autopsies on most suicides, including Golden Gate Bridge jumpers. Autopsies stopped being done on most hospital deaths, too, where a person died during the course of receiving treatment or while undergoing surgery. Instead, the new coroner accepted the explanation of medical staff concerning a patient's demise. This was problematic, though, since doctors and nurses have a vested interest in deflecting blame. In the vast majority of cases, they are competent, and when there is a poor outcome it's usually for reasons beyond their control. That was why Holmes referred to deaths in hospitals that ended up in court as "medical misadventures" rather than medical malpractice cases. There were isolated instances, however, where someone made a preventable mistake and a person died as a result.

"In one case," Holmes says, "an anesthesiologist didn't use the right combination of gases, and a patient died. The decedent was an old man, and there probably were a lot of things wrong with him. Moreover, he needed the surgery; it wasn't elective. Still, he was given the wrong anesthesia, plain and simple. When Dr. Jindrich finished the autopsy and reviewed the surgical notes in hospital records, he saw that there had been an inappropriate mixture of gases. The anesthesiologist's jaw hit the floor when we told him; he didn't realize what he had done. It was an accident, in no way intentional. Even so, it was his fault."

In time, Holmes's successor resumed the practice of doing autopsies on people who died in hospitals and clinics, but not for suicides from the Golden Gate Bridge. If families of bridge jumpers wanted an autopsy or toxicology test done, they had to pay for it.

Related to autopsies, the part-time position of the person who transcribed audio accounts of physicians' pathology findings into written reports was also cut. He or she was paid only fourteen dollars per hour, so the savings weren't significant, however, the impact was big. During Holmes's tenure, dictated autopsy reports were transcribed the following day, making it possible for the coroner to issue death certificates promptly. After the change, the pathologist who did the autopsy was expected to transcribe his or her own notes and provide them to the coroner. It's an onerous task and at the bottom of every physician's to-do list. As a result, death certificates stopped being produced in the same timely manner.

GOING IN DIFFERENT DIRECTIONS

Following the election, Holmes's three investigators began receiving calls from coroners in other areas wanting to recruit them. Dave Foehner, the last investigator Holmes hired, left December 31, 2010— the same day as Holmes—to take a job as a coroner's investigator in the Maryland Office of the Chief Medical Examiner. In short order he was promoted to supervisor, then to assistant coroner. There were so many cases, however, that he became frustrated by the inability of investigators to follow through on many of them and ended up leaving.

The situation was different for Pam Carter. She wanted to continue but had a bitter history with the sergeant, before he became the new coroner and her boss.

"He married one of Pam's best friends," Holmes says, "and his authoritative and arrogant personality ruined their friendship."

Carter ended up leaving and today is the founder, president, and principal owner of a company that developed, manufactures, and markets an aerial fitness program for home use.

Darrell Harris was the only one of the three investigators who stayed. In 2008, the *Marin Independent Journal* reported that he had been named investigator of the year by the California State Coroners Association. Since he was the only person left in the office with experience in death investigations, he ended up training the two cops who replaced Foehner and Carter. Five years after Holmes retired, in October 2015, the sergeant who succeeded him was reassigned and Harris was named the new deputy chief coroner under Sheriff-Coroner Robert Doyle.

As for Holmes, when San Francisco's chief medical examiner stepped down in 2014, Holmes was asked if he would be interested in the job temporarily. While he wasn't a physician, Holmes knew how to run a coroner's office and that was what people in San Francisco needed. There was a six-month backlog of more than eight hundred cases—far more than in most other parts of the country. Holmes said thanks, but no thanks. A job that in essence was sixteen hours a day, seven days per week, held no appeal at this stage in his life. Besides, he had other interests he wanted to pursue.

One of the things he had dreamed about since adolescence was owning a hunting ranch. In 2002, after a divorce, Holmes sold the house in Fresno that he had inherited from his grandparents and bought a 360-acre hunting ranch in Colusa County, about 120 miles northeast of Marin. There, on days off, he led commercial hunts for deer, wild pigs, turkeys, and doves.

When he remarried, his new wife liked to hunt, but not at the ranch. It was too hot in the summer and too muddy in the winter.

They talked about owning property at Clear Lake, north of Marin, and ended up buying a place there. From that point on the ranch started going to seed. Six years after he bought it, Holmes sold the ranch and decided to scratch another item off his bucket list—he bought a Ferrari. For more than two decades he had built and driven cars in circle track auto racing, and ever since he saw his first Ferrari at a racetrack when he was a teenager he had dreamed of owning one.

On Sunday mornings, while everyone else in his household was asleep, he drove his new toy to the coast "just to stretch its legs." Twice he took it to Sears Point–Infineon Raceway.

"Because of the way the track is configured, I could only get it up to 135 miles per hour," he says. "There were several other places where I had it up to 150, though, on Highway 280 by Stanford. If you go there late at night or early in the morning on weekends, you can open it up a little."

As much as he loved the car, Holmes found that it was sitting in his garage most of the time. He didn't drive it to work, and he was so busy on his days off that he had relatively few opportunities to take it out then. Reluctantly, in September 2014, six years after he bought the car, he sold it.

Currently, Holmes and his wife are completing renovations on their place in Clear Lake. Reporters still contact him on occasion, wanting his take on a case, and he stays in touch with many of his former colleagues, retired coroners and investigators in Marin and elsewhere whom he got to know through cases that crossed county lines or through his years with the California State Coroners Association.

Holmes also continues to hunt, accompanied by his two black Labrador retrievers—Quincy (named after the medical examiner in the TV show of the same name) and Mia. He loves to camp, too, has a motorboat that he takes out frequently, is an enthusiastic dancer, and enjoys rooting for local sports teams, particularly the San Francisco 49ers and Giants. He also operates an estate liquidation service and does some consulting in forensics.

LESSONS LEARNED

It's natural at the end of a long career to look back and reflect on what one has learned. In one of our last conversations prior to submitting the final draft of this book, I ask Holmes what he has learned about life, death, and human nature.

"Death knows no keeper," he says. "It's a great leveler. The rich and famous are touched the same as your average Joe. I have seen members of the Hells Angels—scary dudes—on their knees weeping at a roadside where one of their members was killed and his wife was seriously injured in a motorcycle accident. I have talked with homeless people after another homeless person died and they were beside themselves with grief. I have also met with celebrities—Jane Russell and her husband Bob Waterfield, Norton Buffalo, Elvin Bishop, Klaus Kinski—after a loved one died. All of them had to face it alone because grief is a personal thing. Even in a roomful of people, you are by yourself. There's lots of advice out there, and some might apply, but in the end we go through it alone."

Holmes had retired by the time Robin Williams died in 2014, but thirteen years earlier, in 2001, he was called to the scene following the death of Robin's mother, Laurie Williams, from natural causes. It was the same house in Marin County where Robin later killed himself—Robin bought the house for his mother, and moved into it after she died—and Holmes explained the next steps to the actor-comedian. Robin listened silently and dutifully, like any grieving family member. There were no jokes, funny faces, or affected accents—only profound sadness.

"I have a hard time when I hear someone say that another person isn't grieving 'appropriately,'" Holmes says. "Just what is appropriate for a young mother whose five-year-old daughter drowned in their pool because Mom went into the house 'for a moment'? How does an eighty-year-old man grieve for his wife of sixty-one years? How does a doctor grieve when his next-door neighbor, who happens to be his patient, dies because the doctor's diagnosis was incorrect? How do police and fire personnel grieve when they are bombarded constantly with every imaginable kind of death? How do they grieve for one of their own, whether a family member or another person who wore the badge?"

The questions are rhetorical; Holmes doesn't expect answers.

"I firmly believe that we never have 'closure' following a death of someone close to us," he says. "We may find some peace, we may 'get through it' and our lives continue, but true closure is elusive at best and probably nonexistent."

"Have there been any instances where your thinking has changed dramatically over the years?" I ask. "Where you felt strongly about something early in your career and over time shifted 180 degrees in the other direction?"

Holmes says, without hesitation, "I have experienced two prominent changes in my personal attitude. The biggest is my attitude toward suicide. When I first became a death investigator, I had little regard for people who jumped off the Golden Gate Bridge or killed themselves another way. After years of meeting with families of suicide victims, however, and reading the heartbreaking notes left behind, notes that explained the person's troubles and formidable barriers to a healthy life, my view changed completely. I became aware of the whole mess we have in this country regarding mental health, and of the urgent need as a society to address it.

"The second change has been in the area of crime and, therefore, punishment. As a young adult I knew there were good guys and bad guys. The good guys wore the white hat and the bad guys needed to go to jail for as long as possible. After investigating hundreds of homicides, however, I have come to understand that a large number of them didn't start out that way. An argument or grievance escalated, fed by the liquid fuel any of us can buy in liquor stores or the powder we can buy on street corners, and if a suitable weapon was within easy reach—a gun, a knife, even a sharp pencil—the situation suddenly became deadly. Male ego or pride often enters into it, too. The machismo that believes, 'If I can't have you, no one can,' is at the root of many female murders. In my entire professional career, I cannot recall a single instance where a woman took a man's life under the same premise."

He shakes his head. "That said, I have seen our court system fail in so many different ways—fail the victim, fail the aggressor, and fail our society. Do we really need to put a soccer mom in a penitentiary for fifteen years because she fell while intoxicated and dropped her infant, who then died? Why do we continually release sexual predators until they kill a victim? Why are small-time marijuana growers sentenced to twenty to thirty years and the shooter of San Francisco's mayor and a city supervisor is given six years with time off for 'good behavior'? Was his behavior good before he was tried?"

He's referring to the assassinations of George Moscone and Harvey Milk by Dan White.

"I have learned that plea bargains are horrible, yet necessary," he says. "I have learned that when it comes to justice, the poor have the worst of it. I have learned that there are no quick fixes; moreover, any proposed changes are so steeped in politics that they have little chance of being implemented, much less the right way."

"It's odd for me to hear you say that," I say. "You're usually optimistic."

Holmes smiles. "I'm the first to admit that our system is flawed. It's still the best system on this good, green earth, though."

Both of us are silent for a minute, then Holmes says, "Throughout my career, I've been continually reminded how fragile life is, how quickly it can be snatched from us. My grandfather used to say, 'Ain't nobody getting out of here alive.' From that I learned to cherish those who are important to me, and not just my family—teachers, coworkers, honest friends—because death can grab us at any time, in many silent and not-so-silent ways."

He goes on. "I have learned, and preach, that it's okay to talk about death, and about a loved one who dies. Talk about them in the present if you want. We don't have to hide the loss of a parent, or speak of them in hushed tones. Call them by name. I know now that it's healthy to be angry at a dead person, to blame them if they contributed to their own death passively or aggressively."

Holmes lets out a laugh. "Do you want to know a coroner's dilemma? If your doctor tells you that you'll certainly die if you don't quit drinking a quart of whiskey every day, and you continue to drink a quart of whiskey every day anyway, when you die is that suicide?"

"I suppose the same can be said for smoking," I say, "or using drugs or engaging in other high-risk behaviors like mountain climbing and skydiving. There are trade-offs with nearly everything people do, and one of them is knowing that, in some instances, in exchange for doing something desirable—whether it's self-medicating or experiencing an adrenaline rush—we risk shortening our life."

Holmes says, "Another thing I've learned is that lack of preparation for end-of-life considerations can compound the devastation for those left behind. Write your will, damn it. Write it as soon as you have something to leave to someone. A twenty-two-year-old father needs a will the same as his grandfather does. A single, thirtysomething mom who owns a home needs a trust the same as Warren Buffett."

I know—or strongly sense—Holmes's answer to my next question, but ask it anyway. "Have you been surprised sometimes by people's resilience?"

"I have," Holmes says. "Many people, I've found, are able to endure the worst tragedy and find reasons to go on even when they don't think that's possible. It's a cliché to say that time is a great healer, but also true. Having a strong support system and a positive attitude help a lot, too."

I ask Holmes if he has given much thought to his own death. At the time of this writing he is seventy-three and in good health, so death seems far-off still. Even so, the older we get the more natural it is to contemplate our mortality.

"I've thought about it," he says. "I haven't gone so far as to think about my obituary, what it might say, but I do know that I'm not afraid of dying. I'm not in any hurry—like most everyone I want my remaining life to be active and mobile—but when my time comes I'll be content knowing that I did some good things and left a meaningful example for my children, stepchildren, grandchildren, and great-grandchildren. In addition to helping some people deal with their darkest days, I've spent a good part of my adult life teaching. Some of it has been as a coach in youth sports and Scouts, but I've also mentored many high school and college-age students in the world of forensics. Six of them have gone on to earn medical degrees, and two earned PhDs."

"I know this may sound morbid," I say, "but after reviewing eight hundred case files and reading all the information in them, I wonder if you've thought about the contents of your own case file. I mean, just going over these I can't help but think that someday my death will be recorded in a coroner's office, and I imagine that at some time or another you've had a similar thought."

Holmes surprises me. "I really haven't," he says. "The more time you spend around death, the more you appreciate life. That's where my mind has always been."

I find myself nodding in agreement. "Is there anything you would have done differently?"

Holmes thinks about it before saying, "Little things, sure, but no big things. I guess I've been fortunate that way. I've had the career I always wanted, the family I always wanted, trusted friends, good health, lots of interests that I've been able to pursue, and on top of that have witnessed the incomparable beauty of nature. What else is there?"

"I think that covers it," I say.

He says, "There's one other thing I'm proud of professionally, which is that in all my years in the coroner's office, not a single employee quit to take another job. Every person stayed until he or she retired, or in Bill Thomas's case, until he died. If you're in a position of authority, the most important thing you can do, I think, is hire good people and create an environment where they excel. If you do that, the rest takes care of itself."

"I believe that, too," I say.

Holmes adds a final thought. "Every death has a story, just like every life. Coroners are privy to it in ways that other professions are not. That's what draws people like me to it, the chance to be present, understand, and help others deal with something that usually is awful, at a time when people tend to feel most alone."

It's an unusual calling, one that most of us can't imagine doing. For a select few, though, it's a lure. No two cases are exactly the same, which means that every day is different. A variety of skills are needed, and being able to think fast is a must. At the same time, one can't jump to conclusions or fail to notice details that, at first glance, might not add up.

If there's a lesson in this it's that the education of a coroner reflects our own educations about life and death. The two are inseparable, and while we celebrate one and mourn the other, both comprise our world—and always will.

ACKNOWLEDGMENTS

Obviously, this book could not have been written without the participation of Ken Holmes. I'm thankful for his trust in allowing me to tell stories from his career, none of which he shared in any sort of boastful way but always with great respect and compassion for the deceased and their loved ones. Ken read each draft of the manuscript and noted factual errors, which have been corrected. If any errors still exist, they are my doing.

Early on I made a decision not to interview any of Ken's colleagues, current or past, but rather to base perceptions of them through his eyes. Even so, I want to acknowledge several people: Ervin Jindrich, the late Bill Thomas, Don Cornish, Pam Carter, Gary Tindel, Gary Erickson, and Darrell Harris. Each one helped make the Marin County Coroner's Office exemplary in many ways.

In terms of this book's publication, a big debt of gratitude is owed to Scribner and to my editor, Colin Harrison. From the outset, he championed the book, and I can't thank him enough. Many other talented people contributed as well—in particular Liese Mayer, whose editing was masterful, and John Glynn, who took over after Liese left Scribner—and I appreciate their efforts.

Lastly, I want to thank my wife, Suzan, and our four adult children. Their encouragement and support are the greatest gifts I could receive.

BIBLIOGRAPHY

INTERVIEWS

Half-day and full-day interviews between the author and Ken Holmes were conducted on June 13, 2014, August 27, 2014, October 16, 2014, November 18, 2014, January 16, 2015, and February 6, 2015. The locations varied. In addition, we communicated numerous times during this period and afterward by phone, email, and in person over lunch until the final draft of the manuscript was submitted.

BOOKS

Bateson, John. *The Final Leap: Suicide on the Golden Gate Bridge*. Berkeley: University of California Press, 2012.

Cataldie, Louis. *Coroner's Journal: Stalking Death in Louisiana*. New York: G. P. Putnam Sons, 2006.

Colt, George Howe. *November of the Soul: The Enigma of Suicide*. New York: Scribner, 2006.

Daly, Erin Marie. *Generation Rx: A Story of Dope, Death, and America's Opiate Crisis*. Berkeley, CA: Counterpoint, 2014.

Joiner, Thomas. *Myths of Suicide*. Cambridge, MA: Harvard University Press, 2010.

———. *The Perversion of Virtue*. New York: Oxford University Press, 2014.

Levine, Richard M. *Bad Blood: A Family Murder in Marin County*. New York: Signet Books, 1982.

Linde, Paul R. *Danger to Self: On the Front Line with an ER Psychiatrist.* Berkeley: University of California Press, 2010.

Melinek, Judy, and T. J. Mitchell. *Working Stiff: Two Years, 262 Bodies, and the Making of a Medical Examiner.* New York: Scribner, 2014.

Noguchi, Thomas T., with Joseph DiMona. *Coroner.* New York: Simon & Schuster, 1983.

Roach, Mary. *Stiff: The Curious Lives of Human Cadavers.* New York: Norton, 2003.

Scott, Robert. *Unholy Sacrifice: Brothers by Blood, Killers by Choice.* New York: Pinnacle Books, 2005.

Temple, John. *Deadhouse: Life in a Coroner's Office.* Jackson: University Press of Mississippi, 2005.

West, Robert S. *It Can (and Does) Happen Here! One Physician's Four-Decades-Long Journey as Coroner in Rural North Idaho.* Bloomington, IN: Abbott Press, 2014.

ARTICLES AND REPORTS

ABC News. "Marin County Sheriff Robert Doyle Re-elected." June 9, 2010.

Allen, Teresa, and Erik Ingram. "Murder Shakes Up Bolinas." *Marin Independent Journal,* February 1, 1983.

Anderson, Lessley. "Death in the Family." *SF Weekly,* October 13, 2004.

Angle, Pat. "Ladd Deaths Blamed on County Agencies." *Marin Independent Journal,* August 19, 1975.

———. "'Worst Job': Picking Up Pieces." *Marin Independent Journal,* February 10, 1981.

Associated Press. "Baby Linked to Murders." March 2, 1993.

———. "Girl Regains Baby after Murder of Adoptive Parents." January 6, 1989.

———. "Murder Conviction Overturned in 'Pendragon' Plot." September 18, 2007.

Bard, Bonnie, Spencer Silas, and Nels Johnson. "Slain Teenagers Mourned." *Marin Independent Journal,* December 2, 1980.

Bay City News. "16 Years for Man Who Killed Pregnant Lover." February 20, 2008.

Becker, Ingrid. "Jurors See Video of Slaying Site." *Marin Independent Journal,* May 15, 1992.

———. "Life Term for Ex-saloon Owner." *Marin Independent Journal,* August 19, 1992.

Berton, Justin. "James Mitchell Gets 35 to Life for Killing His Ex." *San Francisco Chronicle,* August 16, 2011.

Breithaupt, Brad. "Brutal Marin Murder." *Marin Independent Journal*, February 10, 1983.

———. "Woman Killed in Blaze." *Marin Independent Journal*, February 1, 1983.

Brewer, Jim, and Kevin Lowry. "How Cops Learned of Grisly Killing." *Marin Independent Journal*, July 3, 1975.

Brewer, Jim, and George Williamson. "Youths Held in Grisly Murders." *Marin Independent Journal*, July 2, 1975.

California Department of Corrections and Rehabilitation. Condemned Inmates List, February 6, 2015.

———. "Monthly Report of Population as of October 30, 2013."

California Department of General Services. "Preliminary Analysis of Potential Reuse and Relocation of San Quentin Prison." June 2001.

Callaghan, Catherine. *Bodega Miwok Dictionary*. University of California Publication in Linguistics, vol. 60, December 1970.

Cane, Paul. " 'Olive Family Quiet, Gentle.' " *Marin Independent Journal*, July 2, 1975.

CBS News. "Marin Ranked as Healthiest County in California for 5th Year Running." March 26, 2014.

Centers for Disease Control and Prevention. "Suicides in National Parks—United States, 2003–2009." December 3, 2010.

CNN. "California Lawmaker Proposes Selling San Quentin Prison." March 31, 2009.

Connell, Mary. " 'Delightful Cynic' Finds a Way to Mix Sensitivity with Forensic Expertise." *Marin Independent Journal*, March 15, 2000.

Corwin, Miles. "Woman Is Killed in Courthouse Hallway; Bailiff Then Shoots Her Alleged Attacker." *Los Angeles Times*, December 5, 1987.

Craig, Pat. "Porn Moguls Mitchell Brothers' Story Told by Daughter." *Marin Independent Journal*, January 27, 2014.

Curtis, Kim. "Jury Urges Death in Marin Slayings." Associated Press, December 18, 2004.

Daily Mail. "Notorious Killer Who Murdered Five People in Bizarre Plot 'to Speed Christ's Return to Earth' Hangs Himself on Death Row." April 16, 2013.

Davis, Gregory J., and Randy L. Hanzlick. "The Medical Examiner and Coroner Systems." *Medscape*, May 20, 2013.

Dougan, Michael. "Trail Led to Son in Tiburon Man's Slaying." *San Francisco Chronicle*, May 18, 1999.

Doyle, Jim. "Settlement in Rapper's Trial for Boy's Death." *San Francisco Chronicle*, November 8, 1995.

Fernandez, Elizabeth. "Killer to Be Freed After 23 Years." *San Francisco Chronicle*, December 23, 2003.

Fierro, Marcella. "Comparing Medical Examiner and Coroner Systems." National Academies of Sciences, Engineering, and Medicine, 2015.

Fimrite, Peter. "Farewell to a Porn King." *San Francisco Chronicle*, July 20, 2007.

Frontline. "Post Mortem: Death Investigation in America." February 1, 2011.

Frueh, Sara. " 'Badly Fragmented' Forensic Science System Needs Overhaul." Press release from the National Academies of Sciences, Engineering, and Medicine, February 18, 2009.

Garretson, Con. "Guilty Plea Deal in San Rafael Killing." *Marin Independent Journal*, October 29, 2003.

———. "Guilty Verdict in Novato Motel Murder." *Marin Independent Journal*, December 11, 2003.

———. "Human Bones Found at Novato Construction Site." *Marin Independent Journal*, May 10, 2005.

———. "Was Killing Rage or Deliberate?" *Marin Independent Journal*, November 25, 2003.

Gladstone, Mark. "San Quentin 'Decrepit.' " *San Jose Mercury News*, April 14, 2005.

Glionna, John M. "Guards on Death Row Face Escalating Dangers." *Los Angeles Times*, April 21, 2001.

Golden Gate Bridge, Highway, and Transportation District. "Highlights, Facts, and Figures." 6th ed., July 2009.

Greer, Jeff. "Pet Not the Best Bodyguard." *Marin Independent Journal*, March 13, 1980.

Guthrie, Julian. "Porn King's Daughter Could Go Prime Time." *San Francisco Chronicle*, December 2, 2014.

Halstead, Richard. "Marin Parents Who Lost Children to Prescription Drug Abuse Join New Task Force." *Marin Independent Journal*, March 23, 2014.

———. "Syringes Found Near Body at Hospital." *Marin Independent Journal*, December 4, 2004.

———. "White's Hill Roadway Plagued by Accidents." *Marin Independent Journal*, September 24, 1996.

Hanzlick, Randy. "An Overview of Medical Examiner/Coroner Systems in the United States." Presentation to the National Academies of Sciences, Engineering, and Medicine, not dated.

Harris, Ron. "Blues Guitarist's Daughter Killed." ABC News, August 10, 2000.

Hatfield, Larry D., and Donna Horowitz. "Four Dead in Novato Shooting Rampage." *San Francisco Chronicle*, April 4, 1995.

Haupt, Angela. "America's 50 Healthiest Counties for Kids." *U.S. News & World Report*, June 16, 2014.

Hickman, Matthew J., Kristen A. Hughes, Keven J. Strom, and Jeri D. Ropero-Miller. "Medical Examiners and Coroners' Offices, 2004." Bureau of Justice Statistics, 2007.

Hill, Angela. "Grim History Displayed at San Quentin." *Contra Costa Times*, January 11, 2015.

Horowitz, Donna. "Houseboater Slain in Drug Dispute." *Marin Independent Journal*, March 5, 1980.

———. "Marin Suicide Center Busy." *Marin Independent Journal*, May 20, 1983.

———. "No Progress in Identifying Brutally Murdered Woman." *Marin Independent Journal*, September 28, 1977.

———. "Women Won't Stay Away from Tam." *Marin Independent Journal*, October 17, 1980.

Horowitz, Donna, and Alex Neill. "FBI Agent Key to Old Murder Cases." *Marin Independent Journal*, April 5, 1991.

Ingram, Erik. "Artist Found Shot to Death." *Marin Independent Journal*, August 4, 1980.

———. "Ban Bodies as Evidence, Lawyer Asks." *Marin Independent Journal*, February 27, 1981.

———. "Caller Says He's Slaying Suspect—Intends to Kill." *Marin Independent Journal*, October 22, 1980.

———. "Falling Branch Kills Woman." *Marin Independent Journal*, July 6, 1981.

———. "'Frightened' Suspect's Letter to Sheriff." *Marin Independent Journal*, October 21, 1980.

———. "Guilty Plea in Slaying of Optician." *Marin Independent Journal*, October 14, 1980.

———. "Gun Lists Checked in Kane Case." *Marin Independent Journal*, October 26, 1977.

———. "Investigators Still Baffled on a Motive for Slayings." *Marin Independent Journal*, October 29, 1980.

———. "Man's Dumped Body Discovered." *Marin Independent Journal*, May 12, 1983.

———. "McDermand Profile Drawn." *Marin Independent Journal*, October 24, 1980.

———. "Mrs. Wickersham Is Sentenced." *Marin Independent Journal*, February 29, 1980.

———. "Murder Case Focuses on One Suspect." *Marin Independent Journal*, February 16, 1981.

———. "Navy Deserter Linked to Two Cases." *Marin Independent Journal*, November 7, 1980.

———. "Possible Link in Mount Tam Slayings." *Marin Independent Journal*, October 18, 1980.

———. "Probers Optimistic in Search for Killer." *Marin Independent Journal*, March 25, 1980.

———. "Sailor Admits Slaying Woman." *Marin Independent Journal*, February 13, 1981.

———. "17,000 for Eight-Hour Week? It's Possible in Marin County." *Marin Independent Journal*, February 25, 1974.

———. "Sheriff Lines Up Group to Patrol Mount Tam." *Marin Independent Journal*, March 12, 1980.

———. "Slaying Probe Focuses on Weapon." *Marin Independent Journal*, March 13, 1980.

———. "Slayings Suspect Calls Sheriff Again." *Marin Independent Journal*, October 27, 1980.

———. "Suspect on Spending Spree?" *Marin Independent Journal*, April 25, 1980.

———. "Tam Valley Slaying Suspect Calls Sheriff; Says He's OK." *Marin Independent Journal*, October 25, 1980.

———. "Tam Valley Suspect Pleads Not Guilty." *Marin Independent Journal*, October 31, 1980.

———. "Tam Valley Woman, Son Slain." *Marin Independent Journal*, October 17, 1980.

———. "Two Convicted in Drug Murder." *Marin Independent Journal*, August 20, 1980.

———. "Two Face Trial in Houseboat Shooting." *Marin Independent Journal*, April 4, 1980.

———. "Youths Find Bloody Knife Near Site of Murder." *Marin Independent Journal*, March 11, 1980.

Ingram, Erik, and Nels Johnson. "Could Slayings Have Been Averted?" *Marin Independent Journal*, December 2, 1980.

———. "Detectives Take Another Look at 1977 Slaying on Mountain." *Marin Independent Journal*, January 9, 1981.

———. "San Anselmo Slaying Remains Unsolved." *Marin Independent Journal*, January 8, 1981.

———. "Tam Valley Suspect Surrenders." *Marin Independent Journal*, October 28, 1980.

Ingram, Erik, and Jeff Levine. "Double Killing Clues Studied." *Marin Independent Journal*, October 20, 1980.

Ioffee, Karina. "Deadly Jump in Opiate Abuse." *Contra Costa Times*, September 7, 2014.

Johnson, John. "Tragedy Leaves Troubling Questions." *Los Angeles Times*, March 17, 2002.

Johnson, Nels. "Barbecue Murders Revisited." *Marin Independent Journal*, September 3, 1995.

———. "Cameras Film Tam Valley Slaying Arraignment." *Marin Independent Journal*, October 29, 1980.

———. "Marin County's Murder Mysteries." *Marin Independent Journal*, April 7, 1991.

———. "Marin's Coroner Sees His Office as One Requiring High Degree of Professionalism." *Marin Independent Journal*, February 7, 1976.

———. "Report: Marin Coroner/Sheriff's Office Merger Will Save Big Bucks." *Marin Independent Journal*, November 4, 2010.

———. "Two Teenagers Held in Couple's Slaying." *Marin Independent Journal*, July 2, 1975.

Johnson, Nels, and Brad Breithaupt. "Murder, Drug Link Probed." *Marin Independent Journal*, February 11, 1983.

Johnson, Nels, and Erik Ingram. "Marin's Grim List of Unsolved Murders." *Marin Independent Journal*, January 5, 1981.

———. "1976 Slayings Tied to Global Drug Trade." *Marin Independent Journal*, January 7, 1980.

Journal of the American Medical Association. "SAMHSA: Pain Medication Abuse a Common Path to Heroin." October 9, 2013.

Keown, Don. "What Does a Pathologist Do?" *Marin Independent Journal*, May 13, 1983.

Klien, Gary. " 'Barbecue' Killer Riley Won't Be Paroled." *Marin Independent Journal*, May 17, 2005.

———. "DA Won't Fight Ruling in Murder Case." *Marin Independent Journal*, September 20, 2005.

———. "Dad Gets Prison in San Rafael Baby Killing." *Marin Independent Journal*, July 29, 2009.

———. "Daughter of Porn King Artie Mitchell Sentenced in Federal Fraud Case." *Marin Independent Journal*, October 15, 2014.

———. "Evidence Suggests Novato Victim Died in Violent Struggle." *Marin Independent Journal*, December 21, 2006.

———. "Girl's Remains a Mystery." *Marin Independent Journal*, May 12, 2003.

———. "Helzer Gets Death in Bishop Case." *Marin Independent Journal*, August 4, 2004.

———. "Marin Library Builds Database of Old Coroners' Files." *Marin Independent Journal*, January 1, 2011.

———. "MGH Workers Overdosed on Same Drug." *Marin Independent Journal*, November 20, 2004.

———. "Novato Killer Rocks Court, Takes Back Confession." *San Jose Mercury News*, February 15, 2008.

———. "'70 Civic Center Gunman Denied Parole." *Marin Independent Journal*, September 9, 2005.

———. "Sheriff, Coroner Lock Horns in Historic Election." *Marin Independent Journal*, June 5, 2010.

———. "Sheriff Defeats Coroner for Marin Sheriff-Coroner." *Marin Independent Journal*, June 8, 2010.

———. "Tips on Unsolved Murders Come in; Reward Offered." *Marin Independent Journal*, May 15, 2005.

Klinger, Karen. "Slain Hub Woman Found by Fireman." *Marin Independent Journal*, January 28, 1977.

———. "Student Found Slain." *Marin Independent Journal*, February 7, 1976.

Knight, Heather. "S.F. Hires New Chief Medical Examiner." *San Francisco Chronicle*, January 21, 2015.

Kroll, Michael. "San Quentin Investigating Odd Death of Psychotic Spared Execution." *Albion Monitor*, July 16, 1997.

KTVU News. "Court Restores Murder Conviction of Man in Marin Pendragon Cult." January 6, 2009.

Lagos, Marisa. "Novato Man Won't Face Extra Charges in Death of Pregnant Woman." *San Francisco Chronicle*, April 25, 2007.

Larsen, Rebecca. "Suspect Left Jail Two Weeks Before Girl's Death." *Marin Independent Journal*, October 2, 1976.

Leader, Lewis. "The Woman Who Pleased Everyone but Herself." *San Francisco Examiner*, July 11, 1980.

Lee, Henry K. "DUI Killer from Marin Is Killed in Prison." *Crime*, July 28, 2010.

———. "Justin Helzer Hangs Himself in Prison." *San Francisco Chronicle*, April 16, 2013.

Levine, Jeff. "The Grim Process of Identifying Decomposed Bodies." *Marin Independent Journal*, December 1, 1980.

———. "Guarding Against a Riot." *Marin Independent Journal*, March 4, 1981.

———. "How Search Teams Tracked Down Bodies in Difficult Terrain." *Marin Independent Journal*, December 1, 1980.

———. "Protecting Prisoners from Other Inmates." *Marin Independent Journal*, March 4, 1981.

———. "Screening Inmates Helps Cut Violence." *Marin Independent Journal*, March 3, 1981.

———. "Suspect Asked for Early Paycheck." *Marin Independent Journal*, October 18, 1980.

Levine, Jeff, and Spencer Sias. "Murder Toll: 61 Since 1970." *Marin Independent Journal*, March 2, 1981.

Leydecker, Mary. "Canal Man Slain in His Apartment." *Marin Independent Journal*, April 7, 1980.

———. "Charles Riley Said He Was High on LSD." *Marin Independent Journal*, November 17, 1975.

———. "Contractor's Confession to Jail Mate Bared." *Marin Independent Journal*, January 9, 1976.

———. "Death and Surrender End West Marin Robbers' Chase." *Marin Independent Journal*, September 5, 1975.

———. "'Grinning Cat' Testimony at Murder Trial." *Marin Independent Journal*, January 5, 1976.

———. "Hypnosis Expert Says Riley an Unusually Easy Subject." *Marin Independent Journal*, December 1, 1975.

———. "Hypnotic Voice of Riley Heard." *Marin Independent Journal*, December 5, 1975.

———. "Jury Will Hear Riley Tapes Telling of Olive Slayings." *Marin Independent Journal*, November 18, 1975.

———. "Keeping Peace Inside the Prison." *Marin Independent Journal*, March 4, 1981.

———. "Lambson Killing Still a Mystery." *Marin Independent Journal*, November 12, 1977.

———. "'A Lovely Young Lady.'" *Marin Independent Journal*, March 10, 1980.

———. "Mill Valley Man Bludgeoned to Death." *Marin Independent Journal*, March 24, 1983.

———. "Mrs. Olive's Death Denied as Riley Doing." *Marin Independent Journal*, November 21, 1975.

———. "Novato Murder Suspect Found." *Marin Independent Journal*, May 19, 1976.

———. "Pair Slain in Tam Valley." *Marin Independent Journal*, May 27, 1976.

———. "Parent Killer Pleads Guilty to Forgery." *Marin Independent Journal*, August 1, 1987.

———. "Poisonous Mushroom Victim Died." *Marin Independent Journal*, December 22, 1981.

————. "Prosecution Claims Evidence Proves That Riley Is Guilty." *Marin Independent Journal*, December 15, 1975.

————. "San Rafael Invalid Kills Wife, Himself." *Marin Independent Journal*, August 10, 1981.

————. "San Rafael Woman Slain." *Marin Independent Journal*, May 8–9, 1976.

————. "Sister Sees Slaying as a Voluntary Job." *Marin Independent Journal*, January 8, 1976.

————. "Slain Man Pilgrim Descent." *Marin Independent Journal*, May 28, 1976.

————. "Three Die in Quentin Racial Strife." *Marin Independent Journal*, July 13, 1977.

————. "Tragedy Strikes Anew for Mill Valley Woman." *Marin Independent Journal*, July 15, 1981.

————. "Woman's Siege Ends: Ex-Boyfriend Dead." *Marin Independent Journal*, July 15, 1981.

————. "Youth, Evasiveness Trip Marlene Olive." *Marin Independent Journal*, July 21, 1979.

Leydecker, Mary, and Jeff Levine. "A Violent World Behind the Walls." *Marin Independent Journal*, March 2, 1981.

Leydecker, Mary, and Ed Smith. "Siege in San Anselmo." *Marin Independent Journal*, July 14, 1981.

Leydecker, Mary, Spencer Sias, and Jeff Levine. "Getting Tough Proves Expensive, Dangerous." *Marin Independent Journal*, March 4, 1981.

Liberatore, Paul. "Delivery Boy Tells Girl's Hold on Riley." *Marin Independent Journal*, November 15, 1975.

————. "Former Stripper Recalls Her Time as Artie Mitchell's Sometime Lover." *San Francisco Chronicle*, January 29, 2008.

————. "A Grandmother's Pain." *Marin Independent Journal*, December 25, 2004.

————. "Key Witness Changes Her Story in Testimony on Olive Slayings." *Marin Independent Journal*, November 11, 1975.

————. "Marlene Olive's Relationship with Riley Termed 'Bizarre.'" *Marin Independent Journal,* November 13, 1975.

Ludlow, Lynn. "Marin Sheriff's 'Scientific' Hunt for Tam Killer." *San Francisco Examiner*, March 15, 1981.

Marin County Grand Jury Report. "Gangs of Marin: A Tale of Two Counties." May 18, 2011.

————. "The Marin Youth Alcohol Crisis: One City's Response." June 12, 2012.

Marin Independent Journal. "Air Crash Kills San Rafael Flier." July 8, 1977.

———. "Attorney's Death Seen as Foul Play." August 2, 1977.

———. "Author's Body Found in Tide." September 5, 1975.

———. "Auto Death Probe Takes a New Turn." September 13, 1978.

———. "Autopsy Due in Marin Slaying." August 3, 1977.

———. "Battered Body Found in Tiburon." September 27, 1977.

———. "Body Found in Marin Identified." August 9, 1975.

———. "Body Identified as that of Lake Tahoe Woman." February 2, 1980.

———. "Body Is Identified as German Student." January 13, 1976.

———. "Body of a Murder Victim Is Found in West Marin." May 23, 1977.

———. "Body of a Woman Found by Roadside." August 8, 1975.

———. "Boy Found Dead in Room." July 24, 1975.

———. "Boy, 4, Dies in Auto Accident." March 9, 1976.

———. "Bridge Jumper's Body Recovered." No date [death recorded May 2014].

———. "Car Owner Sues to Get Cash Returned." January 27, 1976.

———. "Cash Released to Suspected Drug Figure's Estate." January 26, 1981.

———. "Cell Topped 1,000 Degrees." June 4, 1981.

———. "Coroner's Office Won by Jindrich." June 5, 1974.

———. "Corte Madera Woman Found Dead." April 15, 1980.

———. "Courtroom Escape Foiled." May 21, 1980.

———. "Dead Body Identified as Daly City Woman." August 31, 1976.

———. "Death of Woman Apparently Suicide." August 8, 1978.

———. "Deserter Sought in Novato Slaying." November 5, 1980.

———. "Dr. Ervin Jindrich Enters Coroner Race." February 28, 1974.

———. "Driver Convicted in Woman's Death." July 19, 1977.

———. "Driver on Bridge Dies in Wrong-Way Accident." January 5, 1977.

———. "Drug Death Is Accidental." December 30, 1975.

———. "Fairfax Woman Found Dead." May 14, 1975.

———. "Fatal Crash Driver Gets Six Months." August 9, 1977.

———. "Few Clues at Tam Murder Site." October 17, 1980.

———. "Filipino Relatives Identified as Bridge Victims." October 4, 1977.

———. "507 Coroner's Cases in Marin." July 11, 1977.

———. "Fourth Inmate Slain in a Month's Time." August 27, 1976.

———. "Girl Won't Get Money of Murdered Parents." October 19, 1976.

———. "Greenbrae Couple Found Shot to Death." January 4, 1980.

———. "Hallinan Appointed Marlene's Attorney." December 8, 1975.

———. "Headless, Handless Body Is Found in Fort Baker." November 25, 1976.

———. "High School Haunted by Violent Death." June 1, 1975.

———. "How Fatal Crash Occurred." August 11, 1980.

———. "Identity Sought of Woman's Body on Beach." September 12, 1977.

————. "Ingenuous, Crude, and Dangerous." November 2, 1974.

————. "Insurance Man Is Found Dead." June 18, 1975.

————. "Investigation Due in Death of Woman, 32." August 9, 1978.

————. "Jennings Trial Heads into Final Arguments." February 6, 1976.

————. "Jumper's Body Identified." July 12, 1980.

————. "Juvenile Hall Suspends Marlene's Benefactor." December 2, 1975.

————. "Leads Pursued in Canal Slaying." April 9, 1980.

————. "Marin County Coroner: Cooke or Jindrich?" May 24, 1974.

————. "Marinite Dies in Bridge Leap." May 7, 1975.

————. "Marin Woman Killed in Crash." January 21, 1981.

————. "Marlene After Parents' Insurance." March 24, 1976.

————. "Marlene Makes an Offer for Defense by Hallinan." November 27, 1975.

————. "Marlene Olive Is Named in Slain Parents' Wills." July 24, 1975.

————. "Marlene Sheds Tears as Sentence Is Read." March 23, 1976.

————. "Murder Indictment for Convict." May 23, 1976.

————. "Murder Victim Identified; Car Found." October 31, 1980.

————. "Murder Victim's Identity Is Established by FBI." May 28, 1977.

————. "Novato Man Is Found Dead." August 4, 1980.

————. "Novato Man Killed as Car Lands in Ditch." June 9, 1975.

————. "Novato Man, 20, Dies in Shooting." July 1, 1975.

————. "Novato Police Seek Suspect in Slaying." November 3, 1980.

————. "Novato Woman Guilty of Slaying Husband." January 25, 1980.

————. "Novato Woman Out on Bail." March 3, 1980.

————. "Novato Woman's Death Is Probed." May 5, 1975.

————. Obituary for Amy G. Niman, December 27, 1976.

————. Obituary for Doris Schuster, May 5, 1975.

————. "$100,000 Turns Up in Fatal Crash." July 17, 1980.

————. "Pair Arraigned in Slaying Case." March 7, 1980.

————. "Petaluma Woman Is Killed in Car Wreck." October 10, 1977.

————. "Pianist Dies of Injuries from Crash." July 24, 1980.

————. "Poetic Note in Lovers' Deaths." October 3, 1977.

————. "Police Probe Shooting Death." April 19, 1980.

————. "Police Say Bomb Victim Apparently Blew Himself Up." October 28, 1980.

————. "Prison Guard Kills Inmate at San Quentin." May 27, 1975.

————. "Prison Worker Dies of Injuries from Assault." April 2, 1981.

————. "Probers Virtually Sure Woman Causes Own Death." March 17, 1978.

————. "Riley Indicted by Grand Jury." July 10, 1975.

———. "Riley Reveals Dream that Triggered Doubt." November 22, 1975.

———. "Rohnert Park Woman Seriously Hurt in Car Crash." November 10, 1980.

———. "San Anselmo Woman Is Found Dead at Home." March 14, 1978.

———. "San Quentin Inmate Killed in Savage Stabbing Attack." April 11, 1977.

———. "San Quentin Prisoner Is Slain." August 11, 1975.

———. "San Rafael Man Dies after Revised Try Fails." February 24, 1981.

———. "San Rafael Police Sift New Killing." June 14, 1975.

———. "San Rafael Woman Dies in Blaze." April 12, 1977.

———. "Slayer Marlene Olive Escapes." September 10, 1978.

———. "Slaying Is Still a Mystery." June 16, 1975.

———. "Some Slang Originated Behind Bars." March 2, 1981.

———. "Suspected Killer's Newest Warning." October 23, 1980.

———. "Tamalpais Man Held in Shooting Death." July 18, 1979.

———. "Third Aide Appointed by Coroner." May 14, 1975.

———. "Three Burglaries at Home of Cash-Carrying Crash Victim." July 21, 1980.

———. "Three Killed in Bridge Crashes." December 15, 1979.

———. "Tiburon Lawyer Found Dead." February 23, 1981.

———. "Tiburon Nurse Found Dead in Bolinas." May 5, 1975.

———. "Tiburon Woman Killed in Car Crash." August 9, 1980.

———. "Timeline of 1979 Tiburon Murder Case." September 30, 2007.

———. "Traffic Signal Failure Probed in Fatal Crash." September 14, 1978.

———. "22-Year-Old Woman Slain in San Rafael." March 6, 1978.

———. "Two Ignacio Students Killed in Auto Crash." May 31, 1975.

———. "Two Killed in Tiburon Boulevard Crash." June 25, 1976.

———. "Two Novato Teenagers Dead in Warehouse Blaze." May 15, 1975.

———. "Unsolved Murders Still Haunting Us." Editorial, May 13, 2005.

———. "Victim Identified in Marin Crash." July 18, 1980.

———. "Waitress Said Killed with Blunt Object." January 29, 1977.

———. "Warrant Issued in Canal Slaying." April 21, 1980.

———. "Woman Collapses, Dies After a Swim." July 16, 1980.

———. "Woman Dies the Day Before Her Marriage." August 29, 1981.

———. "Woman Fatally Shot, Suspect Stabs Himself." April 18, 1980.

———. "Woman Found Dead in Motel." May 6, 1981.

———. "Woman Found Slain in Marin Headlands." July 24, 1977.

———. "Woman Killed in Bridge Crash." November 22, 1979.

———. "Woman Killed in Fairfax Crash." March 6, 1980.

———. "Woman Missing; on Mount Tam." October 15, 1980.

———. "Wrong-Way Cyclist, 21, Killed in 101 Collision." February 27, 1980.

Mullane, Nancy. "The Adjustment Center: Where No One Wants to Go." KALW Radio, October 22, 2012.

———. "Reporter on Death Row." *Life of the Law*, March 12, 2013.

———. "San Quentin's North Segregation—the 'Penthouse' of Death Row." KALW Radio, November 5, 2012.

———. "Walking Death Row at San Quentin State Prison." KALW Radio, October 29, 2012.

Nation, Nancy Isles. "Attorneys Give 2 Portrayals of Murder Suspect." *Marin Independent Journal*, June 24, 1992.

———. "DA Challenges Murder Retrial." *Marin Independent Journal*, September 16, 2005.

———. "Father Charged in Death of Marin Infant." *San Jose Mercury News*, April 27, 2008.

———. "Guilty Plea in Death of Ex-Wife." *Marin Independent Journal*, July 6, 2005.

———. "Helzer Shocks Court: 'I Just Want to Die.'" *Marin Independent Journal*, July 22, 2004.

———. "Judge: Schizophrenic Not Fully Recovered." *Marin Independent Journal*, November 15, 1990.

———. "Marin Drug Slayings Recounted." *Marin Independent Journal*, April 4, 1991.

———. "Marin Killer to Stay Locked Up." *Marin Independent Journal*, February 1, 2005.

———. "Marin Man Jailed in 3 Murders." *Marin Independent Journal*, April 4, 1991.

———. "Mitchell Not the Only Slaying in Marin." *Marin Independent Journal*, January 19, 1992.

———. "Murder in Marin." *Marin Independent Journal*, April 6, 1991.

———. "Murder Trial Set in Grisly 1976 Marin Slayings." *Marin Independent Journal*, May 3, 1991.

———. "New Murder Charge Added in Slaying." *San Jose Mercury News*, January 11, 2007.

———. "Suspect Pleads Innocent to Murder Charges." *Marin Independent Journal*, April 17, 1991.

———. "3 Murder Verdicts in '76 Slayings." *Marin Independent Journal*, July 1, 1992.

———. "Witness Recounts Slayings." *Marin Independent Journal*, May 20, 1992.

Nevin, George. "Ex-Convict Still Missing: Murder Warrant Is Issued." *Marin Independent Journal*, May 30, 1975.

———. "Fresno Contractor Is Held in Corte Madera Slaying." *Marin Independent Journal*, July 24, 1974.

———. "Jindrich Will Make Some Coroner's Office Changes." *Marin Independent Journal*, January 13, 1975.

Nevin, George, Erik Ingram, and Mary Leydecker. "Slain Girl's Body Found in Novato Trailer Park." *Marin Independent Journal*, May 29, 1975.

News-Pointer. "Murder Suspect Caught." September 10, 1980.

———. "San Rafael Hill Body Still Unidentified." December 5, 1979.

Nieves, Evelyn. "Rash of Violence Disrupts San Quentin's Death Row." *New York Times*, May 22, 2001.

Noe, Dennis. "The Mitchell Family's Murders." Crime Library, March 6, 2014.

Opatrny, Dennis. "Prominent UCSF Researcher Slain." *San Francisco Examiner*, February 15, 1981.

Peterzell, Paul. "Camera to Search for Bodies." *Marin Independent Journal*, December 2, 1980.

———. "Many Oppose Parole for Sex Murderer." *Marin Independent Journal*, July 20, 1996.

———. "Marin County Shootout 25 Years Later." *Marin Independent Journal*, August 7, 1995.

———. "Marin Man, 39, Found Murdered." *Marin Independent Journal*, May 31, 1975.

———. "San Rafael Brothers Die; Mother Held." *Marin Independent Journal*, August 18, 1975.

———. "Santa Venetia Girl Is Murdered." *Marin Independent Journal*, October 1, 1976.

Phillips, Chuck. "Who Killed Tupac Shakur?" *Los Angeles Times*, September 6 and September 7, 2002.

Pogash, Carol. "Instead of a Day of Great Joy, a Day of Sadness." *San Francisco Examiner*, August 30, 1981.

———. "The Strange Death of a Talented Singer." *San Francisco Examiner*, May 10, 1981.

Polito, Richard. "Writer Looks Back." *Marin Independent Journal*, August 2, 1996.

Ramsland, Katherine. "The Trailside Killer of San Francisco." Crime Library, accessed February 5, 2015.

Read, Simon. "Court Records Indicate Glenn Helzer Had Plans to Escape." *Tri-Valley Herald*, December 3, 2004.

———. "Helzer's Ex-wife: Execution Would Devastate Daughters." *Tri-Valley Herald*, December 14, 2004.

Robert Wood Johnson Foundation. "County Health Rankings and Roadmaps." 2014.

Robert Wood Johnson Foundation and the University of Wisconsin Population Health Institute. "2014 Rankings." http://countyhealthrankings.org/app /california/2014/county/snapshots/041.

St. John, Kelly. "Lifelike Sculpture Created to ID Jane Doe." *San Francisco Chronicle*, August 18, 2005.

San Francisco Chronicle. "Man Dies in Leap from Gate Bridge." June 14, 1980.

Sanger-Katz, Margot. "The Science Behind Suicide Contagion." *New York Times*, August 13, 2014.

Scheeres, Julia. "Children of Thunder: The Helzer Brothers." Crime Library. http://www.crimelibrary.com/notorious_murders/classics/helzer_brothers .html.

———. "The Family of Winnfred Wright." Crime Library. http://www.crime library.com/notorious_murders/family.winnfred_wright/15.html.

Schwab, Peter. "Police Car Kills Novato Woman." *Marin Independent Journal*, September 12, 1978.

Shallwani, Pervaiz, and Mark Martin. "Ex-Wife of 'Twinkie Defense' Doctor Found Dead." *San Francisco Chronicle*, October 9, 2000.

Sias, Spencer. "All Types of Street Drugs Available Inside Prison." *Marin Independent Journal*, March 4, 1981.

———. "Behind the Scenes Look at an Investigation—Police Hear Murder Suspect Confess." *Marin Independent Journal*, April 23, 1981.

———. "Campers Stunned as They Hear the Chilling News." *Marin Independent Journal*, December 1, 1980.

———. "Digging for Clues: How Detectives Begin the Painstaking Investigation." *Marin Independent Journal*, April 20, 1981.

———. "Police Finally Put Pieces of Murder Puzzle Together." *Marin Independent Journal*, April 22, 1981.

———. "Man Buys Gun, Is Found Dead." *Marin Independent Journal*, November 10, 1981.

———. "Man Held in Novato Slaying." *Marin Independent Journal*, November 6, 1980.

———. "Massive Search Uncovers Body of Mount Tam Hiker." *Marin Independent Journal*, August 21, 1977.

———. "Mount Tam Hiker Shot to Death." *Marin Independent Journal*, August 22, 1977.

———. "Murky Kent Lake Fails to Yield Pilot's Body." *Marin Independent Journal*, January 29, 1982.

———. "Novato Man Shoots, Kills Stepdaughter, Himself." *Marin Independent Journal*, August 29, 1980.

———. "Search Dog Leads to Hiker's Body." *Marin Independent Journal*, August 21, 1979.

———. "Slaying Victim Is Identified as Novato Mother." *Marin Independent Journal*, October 30, 1980.

Sias, Spencer, and Jeff Levine. "Fires Kill Woman, Destroy Home." *Marin Independent Journal*, December 24, 1980.

Sias, Spencer, and Mary Leydecker. "Sharing of Cells Adds to Prison Tension." *Marin Independent Journal*, March 3, 1981.

Sias, Spencer, Jeff Levine, and Mary Leydecker. "Prison Gangs Have History of Bloodshed." *Marin Independent Journal*, March 4, 1981.

Simon, Dan, and Scott Thompson. "California Lawmaker Proposes Selling San Quentin Prison." CNN, March 31, 2009.

Smith, Ed. "Cell Fire Kills Two at Quentin." *Marin Independent Journal*, May 30, 1981.

———. "Fatal Crash Is Linked to Storm." *Marin Independent Journal*, December 16, 1980.

———. "Holiday Tragedy on 101." *Marin Independent Journal*, November 27, 1981.

———. "Love and Memories Along the Waterfront." *Marin Independent Journal*, January 23, 1983.

———. "Slaying Brings Anger, Sadness." *Marin Independent Journal*, March 12, 1980.

Smith, Ed, and Bonnie Bard. "Woman Killed in Novato Accident." *Marin Independent Journal*, November 17, 1980.

Southall, Mary. "Girl's 1989 Slaying Shocked Novato." *Marin Scope*, April 1, 2009.

Staats, Jim. "'Somber' Terra Linda High Dealing with Senior's Suicide." *Marin Independent Journal*, March 4, 2008.

Stack, Peter. "New Version of Parent Killings." *San Francisco Chronicle*, November 21, 1975.

Stein, Mark A. "Woman, 67, Kills Former Son-in-Law in Courtroom, then Turns Gun on Herself." *Los Angeles Times*, May 24, 1986.

Stephenson, Ed. "Marin's Quincy." *Pacific Sun*, March 25–31, 1983.

Sward, Susan. "Porn King Jim Mitchell Walks Out of Prison Today." *San Francisco Chronicle*, October 3, 1997.

Thompson, A. C. "Medical Examiners in America: A Dysfunctional System." *Huffington Post*, May 25, 2011.

United Press International. "Two Plead Innocent in Slayings of Couple." *Los Angeles Times*, January 5, 1989.

Upshaw, Jennifer, and Gary Klien. "Two Victims of Fatal Crash in Novato Identified as Santa Rosa Residents." *Marin Independent Journal*, December 22, 2004.

Van Derbeken, Jaxon. "Winnfred Wright Prosecutors Want Supervised Parole." *San Francisco Chronicle*, November 17, 2010.

Viets, Jack. "A Psychological Autopsy for Apparent Suicides." *Marin Independent Journal*, July 5, 1976.

———. "Suspect Gives Up in Marin Slayings." *San Francisco Chronicle*, October 28, 1980.

Warren, Jenifer. "Inmate Lauded, Parole Doubtful." *Los Angeles Times*, October 18, 2002.

Watson, Kendall. "Murder Charge Dropped for Fetus." *Marin Scope*, April 25, 2007.

———. "Novato Man Pleas Not Guilty: Second Murder Charge Raises Stakes." *Marin Scope*, January 18, 2007.

Weiss, Mike. "Marital Troubles Dogged Noted Family Therapist." *San Francisco Chronicle*, May 21, 2001.

———. "Mayhem Shadowed Therapist's Life." *Marin Independent Journal*, May 22, 2001.

———. "Psychiatrist's Work Echoes in Personal Life." *Marin Independent Journal*, May 20, 2001.

Welte, Jim. "James Mitchell Jr. Had a Tragic Childhood." *Marin Independent Journal*, July 13, 2009.

Whitaker, Tad. "Young Marin Crash Victims Mourned." *Marin Independent Journal*, November 19, 2003.

White, Ryan. "Half-Century Later, Cold Case Solved." *Mill Valley Herald*, April 16, 2008.

Whitely, Peyton. "Detective Work in 2 States Identifies '79 Slaying Victim." *Seattle Times*, September 30, 2007.

Whittington, Mark. "Writer Slays His Ailing Wife, Self." *Marin Independent Journal*, October 24, 1977.

Whittington, Mark, and Mary Leydecker. "Scientist Found Shot to Death." *Marin Independent Journal*, February 14, 1981.

Wides, Laura. "Lawyer Says Jury Swayed in Choosing Death Sentence." Associated Press, December 30, 2004.

Winokur, Scott. "Pepper Spray Blamed in Prisoner's Death." *San Francisco Examiner*, December 2, 1997.

Wolfcale, John. "28 Vehicles Crash, 2 Killed in Waldo Grado Snowstorm." *Marin Independent Journal*, March 12, 2006.

————. "Victim in 1979 Tiburon Murder Finally Identified." *Marin Independent Journal*, September 29, 2007.

Wood, Jim. "A Local Murder: Terra Linda Was the Setting for a Real-Life 1975 Crime." *Marin Magazine*, November 2008.

MARIN COUNTY CORONER'S OFFICE CASES

#70280, homicide of 65-year-old male, August 7, 1970.

#70282, homicide of 17-year-old male, August 7, 1970.

#71307, homicide of 52-year-old male, August 21, 1971.

#71309, homicide of 29-year-old male, August 21, 1971.

#74291, homicide of 52-year-old female, August 27, 1974.

#74296, suicide of 25-year-old female, September 6, 1974.

#75130, suicide of 42-year-old female, May 2, 1975.

#75131, undetermined death of 29-year-old female, May 3, 1975.

#75138, suicide of 50-year-old female, May 6, 1975.

#75141, suicide of 32-year-old female, May 9, 1975.

#75142, suicide of 33-year-old female, May 13, 1975.

#75162, homicide of 19-year-old female, May 28, 1975.

#75166, homicide of 39-year-old male, May 30, 1975.

#75167, accidental death of 18-year-old female, May 30, 1975.

#75168, accidental death of 17-year-old female, May 30, 1975.

#75173, accidental death of 28-year-old male, June 8, 1975.

#75174, accidental death of 25-year-old female, June 9, 1975.

#75175, undetermined death of 25-year-old male, June 9, 1975.

#75183, homicide of 63-year-old male, June 14, 1975.

#75186, suicide of 52-year-old male, June 16, 1975.

#75205, homicide of 52-year-old female, June 30, 1975.

#75206, homicide of 59-year-old male, June 30, 1975.

#75207, suicide of 20-year-old female, July 1, 1975.

#75216, natural death of 74-year-old male, July 7, 1975.

#75218, accidental death of 21-year-old female, July 12, 1975.

#75224, accidental death of 46-year-old male, July 20, 1975.

#75227, accidental death of 22-year-old male, July 22, 1975.

#75243, undetermined death of 22-year-old female, August 8, 1975.

#75250, homicide of 18-year-old male, August 16, 1975.

#75251, homicide of 19-year-old male, August 16, 1975.

#75257, accidental death of 48-year-old female, August 24, 1975.

#75265, suicide of 51-year-old male, September 4, 1975.

#75266, suicide of 26-year-old male, September 4, 1975.

#75282, accidental death of 24-year-old male, September 24, 1975.

#75292, homicide of 21-year-old female, October 5, 1975.

#75299, homicide of 20-year-old female, October 13, 1975.

#75339, undetermined death of 21-year-old female, December 6, 1975.

#75342, homicide of 26-year-old male, December 9, 1975.

#75360, accidental death of 26-year-old male, December 27, 1975.

#75366, undetermined death of 30-year-old female, December 29, 1975.

#75369, natural death of 14-year-old female, December 31, 1975.

#76007, accidental death of 29-year-old female, January 8, 1976.

#76008, accidental death of 30-year-old male, January 8, 1976.

#76013, suicide of 31-year-old male, January 11, 1976.

#76016, undetermined death of unknown male, January 15, 1976.

#76031, suicide of 36-year-old male, January 27, 1976.

#76038, accidental death of 21-year-old female, February 3, 1976.

#76039, accidental death of 31-year-old male, February 4, 1976.

#76042, homicide of 23-year-old female, February 6, 1976.

#76054, suicide of 31-year-old female, February 6, 1976.

#76067, accidental death of 4-year-old male, March 8, 1976.

#76096, accidental death of 24-year-old male, April 10, 1976.

#76107, homicide of 34-year-old female, April 16, 1976.

#76113, homicide of 39-year-old male, April 26, 1976.

#76124, undetermined death of 22-year-old female, May 7, 1976.

#76125, homicide of 39-year-old female, May 7, 1976.

#76129, suicide of 41-year-old female, May 14, 1976.

#76133, suicide of 52-year-old female, May 14, 1976.

#76152, accidental death of 24-year-old female, June 8, 1976.

#76159, homicide of 23-year-old male, June 10, 1976.

#76165, accidental death of 17-year-old male, June 15, 1976.

#76166, accidental death of 36-year-old male, June 16, 1976.

#76177, accidental death of 51-year-old female, June 25, 1976.

#76178, accidental death of 67-year-old male, June 25, 1976.

#76187, suicide of 56-year-old female, July 2, 1976.

#76211, undetermined death of 13-year-old male, July 16, 1976.

#76216, undetermined death of 82-year-old female, July 23, 1976.

#76238, homicide of 51-year-old male, August 14, 1976.

#76255, undetermined death of 19-year-old female, August 29, 1976.

#76259, accidental death of 30-year-old male, September 5, 1976.

#76283, undetermined death of 29-year-old male, September 29, 1976.

#76284, homicide of 5-year-old female, October 1, 1976.

#76292, natural death of 37-year-old female, October 17, 1976.

#76305, accidental death of 45-year-old male, October 31, 1976.

#76306, accidental death of 36-year-old male, October 31, 1976.

#76313, suicide of 23-year-old female, November 5, 1976.

#76335, homicide of unidentified male, November 24, 1976.

#76341, suicide of 40-year-old male, December 2, 1976.

#76361, accidental death of 33-year-old female, December 25, 1976.

#77002, homicide of 19-year-old female, January 1, 1977.

#77006, undetermined death of 27-year-old female, January 2, 1977.

#77009, accidental death of 31-year-old female, January 5, 1977.

#77012, undetermined death of 55-year-old female, January 7, 1977.

#77019, homicide of 18-year-old female, January 11, 1977.

#77026, accidental death of 42-year-old male, January 18, 1977.

#77036, homicide of 29-year-old female, January 27, 1977.

#77037, suicide of 44-year-old female, January 28, 1977.

#77038, suicide of 34-year-old female, January 30, 1977.

#77051, natural death of 29-year-old female, February 8, 1977.

#77065, accidental death of 52-year-old male, February 17, 1977.

#77067, suicide of 41-year-old female, February 21, 1977.

#77073, accidental death of 16-year-old female, March 3, 1977.

#77106, homicide of 27-year-old male, April 10, 1977.

#77107, accidental death of 63-year-old female, April 11, 1977.

#77126, undetermined death of 3-year-old male, April 29, 1977.

#77144, homicide of 26-year-old female, May 21, 1977.

#77175, accidental death of 83-year-old female, June 26, 1977.

#77187, accidental death of 35-year-old male, July 7, 1977.

#77219, homicide of 45-year-old male, August 2, 1977.

#77275, undetermined death of 22-year-old female, September 24, 1977.

#77276, undetermined death of 41-year-old female, September 25, 1977.

#77290, suicide of 23-year-old woman, October 1, 1977.

#77291, suicide of 28-year-old male, October 1, 1977.

#77300, accidental death of 18-year-old female, October 9, 1977.

#77304, homicide of 19-year-old female, October 9, 1977.

#77361, undetermined death of 22-year-old female, December 14, 1977.

#78012, suicide of 33-year-old female, January 10, 1978.

#78017, suicide of 32-year-old female, January 18, 1978.

#78021, undetermined death of 26-year-old female, January 24, 1978.

#78046, undetermined death of 45-year-old male, February 20, 1978.

#78050, suicide of 37-year-old female, February 22, 1978.

#78062, homicide of 22-year-old female, March 4, 1978.

#78069, suicide of 48-year-old woman, March 9, 1978.

#78072, homicide of 23-year-old woman, March 12, 1978.

#78077, suicide of 33-year-old female, March 15, 1978.

#78080, accidental death of 19-year-old female, March 17, 1978.

#78085, accidental death of 15-year-old female, March 21, 1978.

#78109, homicide of 26-year-old female, April 14, 1978.

#78114, undetermined death of 23-year-old female, April 19, 1978.

#78132, accidental death of 28-year-old male, May 5, 1978.

#78155, accidental death of 31-year-old female, June 5, 1978.

#78181, undetermined death of 18-year-old female, June 19, 1978.

#78200, accidental death of 43-year-old female, July 21, 1978.

#78209, undetermined death of 27-year-old male, July 31, 1978.

#78215, suicide of 32-year-old female, August 8, 1978.

#78217, accidental death of 16-year-old female, August 11, 1978.

#78231, accidental death of 34-year-old female, August 26, 1978.

#78235, undetermined death of 36-year-old female, August 29, 1978.

#78243, accidental death of 32-year-old female, September 11, 1978.

#78249, suicide of 32-year-old male, September 19, 1978.

#78264, suicide of 42-year-old female, October 9, 1978.

#78277, undetermined death of 39-year-old female, October 25, 1978.

#78289, accidental death of 20-year-old male, November 9, 1978.

#78301, accidental death of 11-year-old female, November 14, 1978.

#78313, suicide of 28-year-old female, November 26, 1978.

#78332, suicide of 29-year-old female, December 22, 1978.

#78337, undetermined death of 49-year-old male, December 27, 1978.

#78345, undetermined death of 33-year-old female, December 31, 1978.

#79036, undetermined death of 30-year-old female, February 17, 1979.

#79045, suicide of 38-year-old female, February 26, 1979.

#79048, suicide of 27-year-old female, March 1, 1979.

#79070, accidental death of 32-year-old female, March 21, 1979.

#79071, accidental death of 26-year-old male, March 21, 1979.

#79078, suicide of 27-year-old woman, March 28, 1979.

#79112, accidental death of 19-year-old male, May 11, 1979.

#79113, accidental death of 17-year-old male, May 12, 1979.

#79125, undetermined death of 15-year-old female, May 26, 1979.

#79170, homicide of 32-year-old male, July 17, 1979.

#79178, homicide of 26-year-old female, July 23, 1979.

#79186, accidental death of 22-year-old male, August 1, 1979.

#79187, accidental death of 28-year-old male, August 1, 1979.

#79190, suicide of 30-year-old female, August 5, 1979.

#79206, homicide of 44-year-old woman, August 20, 1979.

#79226, accidental death of 23-year-old female, September 19, 1979.

#79233, homicide of 17-year-old female, September 26, 1979.

#79255, homicide of 83-year-old woman, October 23, 1979.

#79256, suicide of 81-year-old male, October 23, 1979.

#79281, accidental death of 22-year-old female, November 21, 1979.

#79286, undetermined death of unidentified male, November 25, 1979.

#79301, suicide of 28-year-old female, December 10, 1979.

#79303, accidental death of 31-year-old male, December 15, 1979.

#79304, accidental death of 28-year-old male, December 15, 1979.

#79305, accidental death of 19-year-old female, December 15, 1979.

#80003, suicide of 38-year-old male, January 2, 1980.

#80005, homicide of 62-year-old female, January 3, 1980.

#80006, suicide of 68-year-old male, January 3, 1980.

#80017, undetermined death of 85-year-old female, January 14, 1980.

#80020, suicide of 74-year-old male, January 22, 1980.

#80030, suicide of 22-year-old male, February 3, 1980.

#80040, accidental death of 38-year-old male, February 18, 1980.

#80048, accidental death of 21-year-old male, February 26, 1980.

#80051, suicide of 42-year-old male, March 1, 1980.

#80052, homicide of 36-year-old male, March 4, 1980.

#80055, accidental death of 32-year-old female, March 6, 1980.

#80058, homicide of 23-year-old female, March 8, 1980.

#80069, suicide of 20-year-old male, March 23, 1980.

#80088, suicide of 79-year-old female, April 14, 1980.

#80091, homicide of 21-year-old female, April 17, 1980.

#80092, undetermined death of 31-year-old male, April 18, 1980.

#80101, suicide of 33-year-old female, April 26, 1980.

#80105, suicide of 43-year-old male, May 1, 1980.

#80127, suicide of 39-year-old male, May 20, 1980.

#80129, undetermined death of 45-year-old female, May 26, 1980.

#80130, suicide of 34-year-old male, May 27, 1980.

#80148, suicide of 43-year-old male, June 13, 1980.

#80155, accidental death of 21-year-old female, June 21, 1980.

#80156, undetermined death of 49-year-old female, June 21, 1980.

#80164, suicide of 37-year-old female, June 27, 1980.

#80174, suicide of 33-year-old female, July 9, 1980.

#80179, natural death of 21-year-old female, July 15, 1980.

#80206, suicide of 30-year-old male, August 4, 1980.

#80208, accidental death of 15-year-old female, August 5, 1980.

#80209, accidental death of 36-year-old male, August 5, 1980.

#80211, accidental death of 24-year-old female, August 8, 1980.

#80227, homicide of 14-year-old female, August 29, 1980.

#80228, suicide of 39-year-old male, August 29, 1980.

#80233, accidental death of 58-year-old male, September 3, 1980.

#80241, accidental death of 20-year-old male, September 13, 1980.

#80243, undetermined death of 39-year-old male, September 16, 1980.

#80259, accidental death of 37-year-old male, October 7, 1980.

#80265, homicide of 26-year-old female, October 15, 1980.

#80268, homicide of 40-year-old male, October 16, 1980.

#80269, homicide of 74-year-old female, October 16, 1980.

#80276, suicide of 19-year-old male, October 27, 1980.

#80277, homicide of 27-year-old female, October 29, 1980.

#80279, undetermined death of 58-year-old female, November 3, 1980.

#80285, undetermined death of 31-year-old female, November 8, 1980.

#80292, accidental death of 18-year-old female, November 16, 1980.

#80296, accidental death of 22-year-old female, November 18, 1980.

#80301, accidental death of 20-year-old male, November 21, 1980.

#80308, homicide of 19-year-old male, November 29, 1980.

#80309, homicide of 18-year-old female, November 29, 1980.

#80310, homicide of 22-year-old female, November 29, 1980.

#80311, homicide of 23-year-old female, November 29, 1980.

#80322, accidental death of 65-year-old male, December 12, 1980.

#80338, accidental death of 26-year-old female, December 21, 1980.

#80340, undetermined death of 34-year-old female, December 23, 1980.

#81016, homicide of 56-year-old female, January 14, 1981.

#81020, accidental death of 26-year-old female, January 21, 1981.

#81045, accidental death of 38-year-old male, February 14, 1981.

#81047, undetermined death of 35-year-old female, February 14, 1981.

#81052, suicide of 42-year-old male, February 20, 1981.

#81054, suicide of 19-year-old male, February 21, 1981.

#81073, accidental death of 18-year-old female, March 12, 1981.

#81086, natural death of 38-year-old female, March 26, 1981.

#81102, accidental death of 28-year-old male, April 28, 1981.

#81113, natural death of 34-year-old female, April 28, 1981.

#81120, accidental death of 25-year-old female, May 5, 1981.

#81121, homicide of 62-year-old male, May 6, 1981.

#81136, suicide of 21-year-old male, May 28, 1981.

#81137, accidental death of 28-year-old male, May 30, 1981.

#81138, accidental death of 25-year-old male, May 30, 1981.

#81141, suicide of 39-year-old female, June 4, 1981.

#81150, suicide of 69-year-old female, June 12, 1981.

#81154, accidental death of 23-year-old female, June 21, 1981.

#81158, undetermined death of 56-year-old female, June 25, 1981.

#81167, accidental death of 35-year-old female, July 3, 1981.

#81165, accidental death of 18-year-old female, July 7, 1981.

#81171, undetermined death of 30-year-old female, July 13, 1981.

#81173, homicide of 32-year-old male, July 13, 1981.

#81174, suicide of 40-year-old female, July 14, 1981.

#81175, undetermined death of 42-year-old male, July 16, 1981.

#81177, accidental death of 20-year-old female, July 17, 1981.

#81184, accidental death of 28-year-old male, July 25, 1981.

#81186, accidental death of 18-year-old female, July 26, 1981.

#81193, undetermined death of 36-year-old female, July 31, 1981.

#81197, suicide of 55-year-old female, August 2, 1981.

#81206, homicide of 59-year-old female, August 9, 1981.

#81207, suicide of 60-year-old male, August 9, 1981.

#81213, suicide of 28-year-old female, August 13, 1981.

#81217, natural death of 23-year-old female, August 28, 1981.

#81225, natural death of 43-year-old female, September 6, 1981.

#81227, suicide of 32-year-old female, September 9, 1981.

#81236, suicide of 43-year-old female, September 24, 1981.

#81249, accidental death of 34-year-old male, October 10, 1981.

#81253, homicide of 50-year-old female, October 12, 1981.

#81254, suicide of 64-year-old male, October 12, 1981.

#81271, accidental death of 45-year-old male, November 9, 1981.

#81285, natural death of 30-year-old female, November 30, 1981.

#81295, accidental death of 29-year-old male, December 11, 1981.

#81314, suicide of 27-year-old female, December 27, 1981.

#82005, accidental death of 39-year-old female, January 4, 1982.

#82008, accidental death of 39-year-old female, January 5, 1982.

#82024, accidental death of 27-year-old male, January 16, 1982.

#82027, accidental death of 21-year-old male, January 20, 1982.

#82036, undetermined death of 28-year-old female, January 29, 1982.

#82090, suicide of 43-year-old female, March 29, 1982.

#82091, natural death of 44-year-old female, March 30, 1982.

#82096, accidental death of 37-year-old female, April 3, 1982.

#82101, undetermined death of 34-year-old female, April 10, 1982.

#82113, suicide of 13-year-old male, April 20, 1982.

#82114, accidental death of 31-year-old female, April 20, 1982.

#82126, accidental death of 24-year-old male, May 13, 1982.

#82152, undetermined death of 21-year-old female, June 8, 1982.

#82164, undetermined death of 37-year-old female, June 21, 1982.

#82167, undetermined death of 25-year-old female, June 23, 1982.

#82170, accidental death of 17-year-old female, June 25, 1982.

#82189, undetermined death of 34-year-old female, July 19, 1982.

#82204, suicide of 34-year-old female, August 12, 1982.

#82205, undetermined death of 55-year-old female, August 14, 1982.

#82212, undetermined death of 45-year-old male, August 26, 1982.

#82247, suicide of 30-year-old female, October 11, 1982.

#82250, undetermined death of 30-year-old female, October 15, 1982.

#82255, natural death of 28-year-old female, October 19, 1982.

#82258, accidental death of 36-year-old female, October 21, 1982.

#82259, suicide of 34-year-old male, October 24, 1982.

#82260, suicide of 49-year-old female, October 23, 1982.

#82275, accidental death of 24-year-old female, November 6, 1982.

#82289, undetermined death of 25-year-old female, December 5, 1982.

#82306, homicide of 30-year-old male, December 19, 1982.

#82315, homicide of 43-year-old male, December 24, 1982.

#82321, accidental death of 27-year-old male, December 29, 1982.

#83001, accidental death of 32-year-old male, January 1, 1983.

#83015, suicide of 60-year-old male, January 12, 1983.

#83034, homicide of 32-year-old male, January 22, 1983.

#83050, homicide of 27-year-old female, February 9, 1983.

#83062, suicide of 36-year-old female, February 23, 1983.

#83078, accidental death of 59-year-old male, March 16, 1983.

#83081, accidental death of 21-year-old female, March 20, 1983.

#83085, suicide of 26-year-old female, March 26, 1983.

#83106, undetermined death of 61-year-old male, April 8, 1983.

#83133, homicide of 42-year-old female, May 15, 1983.

#83150, suicide of 53-year-old male, June 5, 1983.

#83156, natural death of 34-year-old female, June 15, 1983.

#83162, accidental death of 26-year-old male, June 21, 1983.

#83178, homicide of 41-year-old male, July 8, 1983.

#83225, undetermined death of 23-year-old female, August 31, 1983.

#83229, undetermined death of 32-year-old female, September 4, 1983.

#83239, accidental death of 37-year-old female, September 18, 1983.

#83246, homicide of 39-year-old female, September 28, 1983.

#83247, suicide of 33-year-old female, October 6, 1983.

#83253, accidental death of 24-year-old female, October 8, 1983.

#83255, suicide of 37-year-old female, October 9, 1983.

#83284, suicide of 17-year-old female, November 3, 1983.

#84005, natural death of 33-year-old female, January 8, 1984.

#84039, homicide of 41-year-old female, February 14, 1984.

#84049, undetermined death of 23-year-old female, February 26, 1984.

#84059, suicide of 76-year-old male, March 9, 1984.

#84081, accidental death of 32-year-old female, March 31, 1984.

#84083, homicide of 48-year-old female, April 2, 1984.

#84096, undetermined death of 38-year-old female, April 21, 1984.

#84098, suicide of 22-year-old female, April 25, 1984.

#84115, homicide of 24-year-old female, May 11, 1984.

#84149, accidental death of 22-year-old female, June 19, 1984.

#84176, homicide of 34-year-old female, July 11, 1984.

#84214, accidental death of 18-year-old female, August 12, 1984.

#84219, undetermined death of 30-year-old female, August 14, 1984.

#84267, suicide of 46-year-old female, September 23, 1984.

#84274, homicide of 19-year-old male, October 2, 1984.

#84277, suicide of 38-year-old female, October 6, 1984.

#84279, undetermined death of 34-year-old female, October 7, 1984.

#84281, suicide of 27-year-old female, October 8, 1984.

#84287, accidental death of 21-year-old female, October 10, 1984.

#84321, undetermined death of 15-year-old female, November 8, 1984.

#84357, homicide of 41-year-old male, December 16, 1984.

#85003, undetermined death of 42-year-old female, January 4, 1985.

#85004, homicide of 29-year-old female, January 4, 1985.

#85028, homicide of 45-year-old male, January 23, 1985.

#85036, suicide of 46-year-old male, January 26, 1985.

#85044, accidental death of 40-year-old female, February 5, 1985.

#85049, accidental death of 18-year-old female, February 9, 1985.
#85052, suicide of 38-year-old female, February 10, 1985.
#85055, suicide of 24-year-old female, February 14, 1985.
#85086, accidental death of 35-year-old female, March 23, 1985.
#85091, homicide of 44-year-old male, April 5, 1985.
#85095, undetermined death of 37-year-old female, April 13, 1985.
#85102, natural death of 36-year-old female, April 22, 1985.
#85103, undetermined death of 18-year-old female, April 23, 1985.
#85115, homicide of 26-year-old male, May 6, 1985.
#85154, homicide of 19-year-old female, June 18, 1985.
#85170, accidental death of 23-year-old female, June 29, 1985.
#85173, suicide of 36-year-old female, June 29, 1985.
#85216, suicide of 41-year-old female, August 17, 1985.
#85219, suicide of 33-year-old female, August 20, 1985.
#85228, natural death of 38-year-old female, September 4, 1985.
#85242, natural death of 31-year-old female, September 19, 1985.
#85244, accidental death of 18-year-old female, September 21, 1985.
#85251, suicide of 28-year-old female, September 29, 1985.
#85275, homicide of 24-year-old male, October 28, 1985.
#85281, undetermined death of 40-year-old female, November 1, 1985.
#85309, natural death of 32-year-old female, December 3, 1985.
#85320, accidental death of 30-year-old female, December 21, 1985.
#85329, undetermined death of 29-year-old female, December 28, 1985.
#86009, suicide of 23-year-old female, January 1, 1986.
#86031, suicide of 38-year-old female, February 4, 1986.
#86131, natural death of 25-year-old female, May 20, 1986.
#86136, homicide of 36-year-old male, May 23, 1986.
#86137, suicide of 67-year-old female, May 23, 1986.
#86148, accidental death of 39-year-old female, June 7, 1986.
#86150, undetermined death of 33-year-old female, June 10, 1986.
#86156, accidental death of 20-year-old female, June 15, 1986.
#86189, undetermined death of 37-year-old female, July 25, 1986.
#86194, accidental death of 30-year-old female, August 1, 1986.
#86214, homicide of 15-year-old female, August 17, 1986.
#86215, suicide of male in his 20s, August 17, 1986.
#86244, homicide of 70-year-old female, September 22, 1986.
#86245, accidental death of 23-year-old female, September 23, 1986.
#86246, accidental death of 46-year-old female, September 24, 1986.
#86260, suicide of 20-year-old female, October 14, 1986.

#86269, undetermined death of 39-year-old female, October 24, 1986.

#86280, undetermined death of 41-year-old female, November 10, 1986.

#86284, suicide of 35-year-old female, November 12, 1986.

#86297, homicide of 66-year-old male, November 18, 1986.

#86298, suicide of 72-year-old male, November 18, 1986.

#86301, natural death of 35-year-old female, November 25, 1986.

#86318, undetermined death of 46-year-old female, December 17, 1986.

#87001, homicide of 31-year-old female, January 1, 1987.

#87027, natural death of 14-year-old female, January 18, 1987.

#87042, suicide of 29-year-old female, February 17, 1987.

#87047, suicide of 39-year-old female, February 18, 1987.

#87048, accidental death of 27-year-old female, February 19, 1987.

#87071, undetermined death of 31-year-old male, March 17, 1987.

#87140, undetermined death of 33-year-old female, June 6, 1987.

#87176, suicide of 38-year-old female, July 30, 1987.

#87196, accidental death of 38-year-old female, August 17, 1987.

#87213, accidental death of 38-year-old female, September 8, 1987.

#87254, suicide of 27-year-old female, October 23, 1987.

#87283, suicide of 29-year-old female, November 27, 1987.

#87292, undetermined death of 42-year-old female, December 10, 1987.

#87296, undetermined death of 36-year-old female, December 17, 1987.

#87297, natural death of 19-year-old female, December 18, 1987.

#88038, undetermined death of 22-year-old female, February 26, 1988.

#88048, suicide of 38-year-old female, March 10, 1988.

#88071, accidental death of 54-year-old male, April 16, 1988.

#88102, homicide of 3-year-old female, May 24, 1988.

#88107, suicide of 30-year-old female, May 30, 1988.

#88115, homicide of 4-year-old male, June 11, 1988.

#88145, accidental death of 16-year-old female, July 19, 1988.

#88177, suicide of 31-year-old female, August 21, 1988.

#88196, accidental death of 31-year-old female, September 25, 1988.

#88198, undetermined death of 38-year-old female, September 26, 1988.

#88199, suicide of 30-year-old female, September 30, 1988.

#88201, suicide of 45-year-old female, October 2, 1988.

#88207, suicide of 36-year-old female, October 9, 1988.

#88226, undetermined death of 33-year-old female, November 6, 1988.

#88229, homicide of 11-year-old male, November 7, 1988.

#88230, undetermined death of 35-year-old female, November 8, 1988.

#88233, homicide of 42-year-old male, November 14, 1988.

#88236, suicide of 54-year-old female, November 17, 1988.

#88257, homicide of 45-year-old male, December 14, 1988.

#88258, homicide of 43-year-old female, December 14, 1988.

#88261, undetermined death of 27-year-old female, December 17, 1988.

#89020, suicide of 26-year-old male, January 29, 1989.

#89054, natural death of 32-year-old female, March 9, 1989.

#89058, natural death of 27-year-old female, March 15, 1989.

#89068, undetermined death of 35-year-old female, March 29, 1989.

#89077, undetermined death of 41-year-old female, April 7, 1989.

#89085, homicide of 13-year-old female, April 17, 1989.

#89098, accidental death of 22-year-old female, May 6, 1989.

#89106, homicide of 26-year-old female, May 18, 1989.

#89138, homicide of 82-year-old female, June 22, 1989.

#89143, homicide of 24-year-old male, June 30, 1989.

#89174, accidental death of 46-year-old female, August 13, 1989.

#89178, undetermined death of 47-year-old female, August 16, 1989.

#89190, undetermined death of 39-year-old female, August 31, 1989.

#89196, undetermined death of 2-month-old female, September 8, 1989.

#89203, natural death of 31-year-old female, September 15, 1989.

#89224, accidental death of 7-year-old male, October 16, 1989.

#89252, accidental death of 37-year-old female, November 17, 1989.

#89262, accidental death of 65-year-old male, November 29, 1989.

#89266, natural death of 24-year-old female, December 3, 1989.

#89269, suicide of 44-year-old female, December 6, 1989.

#90013, suicide of 14-year-old female, January 1, 1990.

#90016, accidental death of 40-year-old female, January 14, 1990.

#90025, undetermined death of 53-year-old male, January 31, 1990.

#90033, suicide of 30-year-old female, February 19, 1990.

#90044, homicide of 86-year-old female, February 27, 1990.

#90076, undetermined death of 43-year-old female, April 15, 1990.

#90080, suicide of 46-year-old female, April 23, 1990.

#90084, accidental death of 20-year-old female, April 29, 1990.

#90102, accidental death of 14-year-old male, May 24, 1990.

#90122, undetermined death of 35-year-old female, June 26, 1990.

#90129, suicide of 46-year-old female, July 4, 1990.

#90131, accidental death of 35-year-old male, July 7, 1990.

#90141, natural death of 32-year-old female, July 29, 1990.

#90152, homicide of 38-year-old female, August 14, 1990.

#90154, homicide of 51-year-old male, August 18, 1990.

#90176, suicide of 38-year-old female, September 20, 1990.

#90186, suicide of 32-year-old female, October 4, 1990.

#90200, accidental death of 37-year-old female, October 21, 1990.

#90215, accidental death of 27-year-old male, November 26, 1990.

#90220, accidental death of 37-year-old female, November 29, 1990.

#91011, homicide of 33-year-old female, January 18, 1991.

#91028, homicide of 64-year-old male, February 13, 1991.

#91036, homicide of 45-year-old male, February 27, 1991.

#91039, homicide of 57-year-old male, March 4, 1991.

#91057, homicide of 46-year-old male, March 28, 1991.

#91060, homicide of 36-year-old male, March 29, 1991.

#91075, suicide of 36-year-old female, April 16, 1991.

#91153, natural death of 37-year-old male, July 20, 1991.

#91154, homicide of 61-year-old male, July 22, 1991.

#91164, homicide of 44-year-old male, August 12, 1991.

#91185, suicide of 32-year-old female, September 26, 1991.

#91196, accidental death of 30-year-old female, October 8, 1991.

#91222, undetermined death of 40-year-old female, November 11, 1991.

#91232, natural death of 65-year-old male, November 23, 1991.

#91255, natural death of 15-year-old female, December 22, 1991.

#91263, accidental death of 41-year-old female, December 29, 1991.

#92006, homicide of 37-year-old female, January 5, 1992.

#92007, homicide of 40-year-old female, January 5, 1992.

#92037, suicide of 34-year-old female, February 9, 1992.

#92040, suicide of 25-year-old female, February 10, 1992.

#92041, homicide of 79-year-old female, February 11, 1992.

#92042, homicide of 77-year-old female, February 11, 1992.

#92045, accidental death of 40-year-old female, February 15, 1992.

#92061, accidental death of 38-year-old female, March 3, 1992.

#92072, suicide of 45-year-old male, March 13, 1992.

#92103, accidental death of 44-year-old male, April 25, 1992.

#92117, homicide of 57-year-old male, May 11, 1992.

#92133, suicide of 48-year-old female, June 6, 1992.

#92146, accidental death of 23-year-old female, June 27, 1992.

#92152, homicide of 46-year-old male, July 3, 1992.

#92158, accidental death of 32-year-old female, July 13, 1992.

#92188, homicide of 6-year-old male, August 23, 1992.

#92192, homicide of 30-year-old male, August 26, 1992.

#92212, suicide of 45-year-old female, September 23, 1992.

#92216, accidental death of 41-year-old female, October 4, 1992.

#92232, homicide of 46-year-old male, October 31, 1992.

#92246, suicide of 45-year-old female, November 16, 1992.

#92267, suicide of 45-year-old female, December 14, 1992.

#92273, accidental death of 35-year-old female, December 26, 1992.

#93027, suicide of 32-year-old male, January 28, 1992.

#93028, homicide of 3-year-old female, January 28, 1993.

#93061, homicide of 55-year-old female, March 10, 1993.

#93087, accidental death of 54-year-old male, April 11, 1993.

#93088, accidental death of 18-year-old female, April 11, 1993.

#93121, accidental death of 32-year-old male, June 12, 1993.

#93123, homicide of 92-year-old female, June 12, 1993.

#93145, accidental death of 21-year-old male, July 17, 1993.

#93146, accidental death of 27-year-old male, July 17, 1993.

#93203, accidental death of 35-year-old female, September 21, 1993.

#93216, homicide of 32-year-old female, September 28, 1993.

#93244, undetermined death of 45-year-old female, October 28, 1993.

#93264, suicide of 29-year-old female, December 3, 1993.

#93287, undetermined death of 37-year-old female, December 28, 1993.

#94005, suicide of 46-year-old female, January 4, 1994.

#94010, homicide of 42-year-old female, January 7, 1994.

#94011, homicide of unborn fetus, January 7, 1994.

#94045, suicide of 34-year-old female, February 6, 1994.

#94055, accidental death of 56-year-old male, February 18, 1994.

#94071, homicide of 30-year-old male, March 7, 1994.

#94073, accidental death of 44-year-old female, March 8, 1994.

#94092, suicide of 44-year-old female, April 6, 1994.

#94135, accidental death of 18-year-old female, June 1, 1994.

#94160, accidental death of 48-year-old male, June 27, 1994.

#94163, undetermined death of 46-year-old female, June 30, 1994.

#94180, undetermined death of 22-year-old male, July 21, 1994.

#94191, accidental death of 26-year-old female, August 4, 1994.

#94198, natural death of 41-year-old female, August 9, 1994.

#94277, suicide of 45-year-old female, November 5, 1994.

#94305, suicide of 46-year-old female, December 9, 1994.

#95012, undetermined death of 39-year-old female, January 16, 1995.

#95042, accidental death of 23-year-old female, February 22, 1995.

#95068, homicide of 21-year-old female, April 8, 1995.

#95069, homicide of 47-year-old female, April 9, 1995.

#95070, homicide of 20-year-old female, April 9, 1995.

#95071, homicide of 13-year-old male, April 9, 1995.

#95072, suicide of 25-year-old male, April 9, 1995.

#95077, accidental death of 16-year-old female, April 17, 1995.

#95078, accidental death of 44-year-old female, April 17, 1995.

#95098, undetermined death of 41-year-old female, May 10, 1995.

#95118, homicide of 71-year-old female, June 5, 1995.

#95119, suicide of 35-year-old female, June 5, 1995.

#95163, suicide of 48-year-old male, July 26, 1995.

#95167, homicide of 12-year-old male, July 29, 1995.

#95168, suicide of 45-year-old female, July 29, 1995.

#95176, natural death of 53-year-old male, August 9, 1995.

#95196, accidental death of 22-year-old female, September 5, 1995.

#95202, suicide of 40-year-old female, September 10, 1995.

#95219, accidental death of 16-year-old female, September 30, 1995.

#95221, suicide of 42-year-old female, October 1, 1995.

#96003, accidental death of 30-year-old female, January 4, 1996.

#96011, suicide of 18-year-old female, January 21, 1996.

#96014, suicide of 36-year-old female, January 23, 1996.

#96041, suicide of 90-year-old male, February 21, 1996.

#96042, homicide of 89-year-old female, February 21, 1996.

#96064, accidental death of 25-year-old female, March 23, 1996.

#96083, accidental death of 47-year-old male, April 12, 1996.

#96084, accidental death of 13-year-old female, April 12, 1996.

#96097, accidental death of 39-year-old female, April 29, 1996.

#96104, undetermined death of 33-year-old female, May 9, 1996.

#96120, suicide of 42-year-old female, May 28, 1996.

#97082, natural death of 22-year-old female, May 2, 1997.

#97090, accidental death of 25-year-old female, May 9, 1997.

#97099, suicide of 37-year-old female, May 22, 1997.

#97103, accidental death of 20-year-old female, May 23, 1997.

#97104, accidental death of 19-year-old female, May 25, 1997.

#97113, suicide of 34-year-old female, June 5, 1997.

#97119, undetermined death of 51-year-old male, June 15, 1997.

#97145, accidental death of 34-year-old female, July 15, 1997.

#97170, suicide of 41-year-old female, August 13, 1997.

#97195, suicide of 39-year-old female, September 22, 1997.

#97263, suicide of 33-year-old female, December 22, 1997.

#97264, accidental death of 36-year-old female, December 24, 1997.

#98002, undetermined death of 36-year-old female, January 2, 1998.

#98024, undetermined death of 52-year-old male, February 1, 1998.

#98027, accidental death of 42-year-old female, February 9, 1998.

#98032, accidental death of 44-year-old female, February 14, 1998.

#98045, accidental death of 33-year-old female, March 6, 1998.

#98075, accidental death of 43-year-old female, April 15, 1998.

#98087, suicide of 22-year-old female, April 24, 1998.

#98090, suicide of 29-year-old female, April 26, 1998.

#98151, suicide of 30-year-old female, July 7, 1998.

#98176, suicide of 34-year-old female, August 12, 1998.

#98196, suicide of 34-year-old female, September 18, 1998.

#98203, accidental death of 30-year-old male, September 26, 1998.

#98204, accidental death of 30-year-old male, September 26, 1998.

#98254, accidental death of 20-year-old male, December 11, 1998.

#98255, accidental death of 19-year-old female, December 11, 1998.

#98256, accidental death of 19-year-old male, December 11, 1998.

#99093, undetermined death of 40-year-old female, April 23, 1999.

#99098, accidental death of 27-year-old male, May 4, 1999.

#99104, homicide of 55-year-old male, May 14, 1999.

#99106, homicide of 39-year-old male, May 16, 1999.

#99112, natural death of 36-year-old female, May 31, 1999.

#99151, natural death of 24-year-old female, July 22, 1999.

#99152, natural death of 37-year-old female, July 23, 1999.

#99165, suicide of 40-year-old female, August 16, 1999.

#99173, accidental death of 16-year-old female, August 25, 1999.

#99181, accidental death of 17-year-old female, September 15, 1999.

#99190, accidental death of 29-year-old female, October 7, 1999.

#99197, accidental death of 47-year-old female, October 16, 1999.

#99240, homicide of 21-year-old male, December 23, 1999.

#00013, undetermined death of 42-year-old female, January 16, 2000.

#00014, natural death of female infant, January 17, 2000.

#00020, homicide of 28-year-old male, January 22, 2000.

#00027, undetermined death of 67-year-old female, February 1, 2000.

#00041, homicide of 37-year-old male, February 15, 2000.

#00049, natural death of 104-year-old female, February 26, 2000.

#00059, accidental death of 29-year-old male, March 13, 2000.

#00071, undetermined death of 14-year-old male, March 30, 2000.

#00098, undetermined death of 8-week-old male, April 28, 2000.

#00110, accidental death of 36-year-old male, May 4, 2000.

#00111, accidental death of 24-year-old female, May 4, 2000.

#00123, accidental death of 37-year-old female, May 21, 2000.

#00175, homicide of 45-year-old female, August 3, 2000.

#00176, homicide of 54-year-old male, August 3, 2000.

#00185, homicide of 20-year-old female, August 14, 2000.

#01010, undetermined death of 33-year-old female, January 6, 2001.

#01019, homicide of 35-year-old male, January 21, 2001.

#01028, accidental death of 32-year-old female, February 6, 2001.

#01038, homicide of 39-year-old female, February 17, 2001.

#01047, undetermined death of 32-year-old female, March 5, 2001.

#01068, suicide of 63-year-old male, April 3, 2001.

#01106, homicide of 24-year-old female, May 29, 2001.

#01134, suicide of 46-year-old female, June 30, 2001.

#01157, accidental death of 87-year-old female, August 4, 2001.

#01222, accidental death of 43-year-old female, October 27, 2001.

#01225, suicide of 72-year-old male, November 1, 2001.

#01240, homicide of 18-month-old male, November 13, 2001.

#01248, accidental death of 41-year-old female, November 23, 2001.

#01255, accidental death of 37-year-old female, December 3, 2001.

#01261, suicide of 25-year-old female, December 12, 2001.

#01268, suicide of 14-year-old female, December 17, 2001.

#02006, suicide of 37-year-old female, January 7, 2002.

#02011, accidental death of 86-year-old female, January 14, 2002.

#02019, homicide of 22-year-old female, January 18, 2002.

#02027, undetermined death of female infant, January 23, 2002.

#02039, homicide of 15-year-old male, February 11, 2002.

#02040, accidental death of 29-year-old female, February 12, 2002.

#02053, suicide of 36-year-old female, March 3, 2002.

#02074, suicide of 27-year-old male, March 22, 2002.

#02076, suicide of 32-year-old female, March 26, 2002.

#02078, accidental death of 27-year-old female, March 29, 2002.

#02084, homicide of 3-year-old female, April 8, 2002.

#02214, suicide of 49-year-old male, October 14, 2002.

#02205, homicide of 60-year-old female, October 23, 2002.

#02221, natural death of 29-year-old female, November 6, 2002.

#02226, homicide of 30-year-old male, November 14, 2002.

#02248, accidental death of 43-year-old male, December 18, 2002.

#03052, suicide of 37-year-old female, March 3, 2003.

#03096, suicide of 23-year-old female, April 26, 2003.

#03111, undetermined death of 30-year-old female, May 11, 2003.

#03181, accidental death of 33-year-old female, August 19, 2003.

#03182, accidental death of 52-year-old male, August 19, 2003.

#03183, accidental death of 47-year-old male, August 19, 2003.

#03222, suicide of 26-year-old female, October 26, 2003.

#03228, accidental death of 10-year-old female, November 7, 2003.

#03262, suicide of 52-year-old male, December 21, 2003.

#03263, accidental death of 69-year-old male, December 21, 2003.

#04046, accidental death of 35-year-old female, March 17, 2004.

#04054, accidental death of 26-year-old male, March 25, 2004.

#04081, homicide of 59-year-old male, May 5, 2004.

#04082, suicide of 55-year-old female, May 5, 2004.

#04145, accidental death of 23-year-old male, August 10, 2004.

#04148, accidental death of 22-year-old male, August 15, 2004.

#04169, accidental death of 23-year-old female, September 19, 2004.

#04203, undetermined death of 28-year-old female, November 13, 2004.

#04226, suicide of 27-year-old female, December 20, 2004.

#05032, suicide of 26-year-old female, February 18, 2005.

#05034, suicide of 33-year-old female, February 22, 2005.

#05094, suicide of 19-year-old female, May 6, 2005.

#05101, accidental death of 58-year-old male, May 20, 2005.

#05126, homicide of 25-year-old female, June 25, 2005.

#05135, suicide of 19-year-old female, July 7, 2005.

#05138, suicide of 41-year-old female, July 11, 2005.

#05154, suicide of 25-year-old female, August 10, 2005.

#05161, homicide of 29-year-old male, August 20, 2005.

#05210, suicide of 39-year-old female, October 14, 2008.

#05215, homicide of 22-year-old female, October 23, 2005.

#05224, undetermined death of 18-year-old male, November 12, 2005.

#05225, accidental death of 19-year-old male, November 12, 2005.

#06013, accidental death of 60-year-old male, January 14, 2006.

#06054, accidental death of 26-year-old female, March 11, 2006.

#06055, accidental death of 30-year-old female, March 11, 2006.

#06141, suicide of 29-year-old female, June 14, 2006.

#06196, homicide of 34-year-old male, September 12, 2006.

#06215, accidental death of 68-year-old male, October 15, 2006.

#06233, accidental death of 25-year-old female, October 29, 2006.

#06234, natural death of 43-year-old female, October 29, 2006.

#06244, undetermined death of 27-year-old female, November 26, 2006.

#06253, suicide of 37-year-old female, December 9, 2006.

#06265, homicide of 24-year-old female, December 19, 2006.

#07054, undetermined death of 61-year-old female, March 15, 2007.

#07064, suicide of 39-year-old female, April 4, 2007.

#07065, suicide of 33-year-old female, April 9, 2007.

#07076, homicide of 34-year-old male, April 24, 2007.

#07098, accidental death of 29-year-old female, May 24, 2007.

#07099, homicide of 26-year-old male, May 27, 2007.

#07205, accidental death of 26-year-old male, September 18, 2007.

#07214, undetermined death of 27-year-old female, September 27, 2007.

#07240, homicide of 56-year-old male, November 3, 2007.

#07242, accidental death of 46-year-old female, November 4, 2007.

#07252, suicide of 39-year-old female, November 18, 2007.

#07277, undetermined death of 36-year-old female, December 26, 2007.

#08011, natural death of 21-year-old female, January 11, 2008.

#08014, homicide of 26-year-old male, January 12, 2008.

#08017, suicide of 25-year-old female, January 13, 2008.

#08036, homicide of female, February 7, 2008.

#08037, natural death of 36-year-old female, February 9, 2008.

#08041, undetermined death of 45-year-old female, February 16, 2008.

#08043, accidental death of 4-year-old male, February 22, 2008.

#08051, suicide of 17-year-old male, February 29, 2008.

#08063, accidental death of 43-year-old male, March 18, 2008.

#08073, accidental death of 20-year-old female, April 14, 2008.

#08075, suicide of 23-year-old female, April 16, 2008.

#08080, undetermined death of female, April 28, 2008.

#08098, homicide of 25-year-old male, May 24, 2008.

#08119, suicide of 23-year-old female, June 25, 2008.

#08149, accidental death of 54-year-old male, August 7, 2008.

#08170, homicide of 44-year-old male, September 13, 2008.

#08182, suicide of 19-year-old female, October 3, 2008.

#08202, suicide of 29-year-old female, October 21, 2008.

#08210, undetermined death of 14-year-old female, October 31, 2008.

#08239, homicide of 33-year-old female, December 16, 2008.

#08241, homicide of 29-year-old male, December 16, 2008.

#09012, suicide of 20-year-old female, January 26, 2009.

#09033, accidental death of 41-year-old female, February 21, 2009.

#09066, homicide of 46-year-old female, April 18, 2009.

#09069, suicide of 20-year-old female, April 22, 2009.

#09077, homicide of 32-year-old man, April 28, 2009.

#09080, suicide of 28-year-old female, May 4, 2009.

#09085, suicide of 25-year-old female, May 12, 2009.

#09098, homicide of 9-year-old female, May 28, 2009.

#09107, natural death of 44-year-old female, June 11, 2009.

#09117, homicide of 29-year-old female, July 12, 2009.

#09121, undetermined death of 36-year-old female, July 22, 2009.

#09164, undetermined death of 27-year-old female, September 6, 2009.

#09166, accidental death of 25-year-old female, September 8, 2009.

#09170, suicide of 35-year-old female, September 11, 2009.

#09174, suicide of 28-year-old female, September 17, 2009.

#09178, natural death of 14-year-old female, September 21, 2008.

#09179, homicide of 75-year-old female, September 22, 2009.

#09216, suicide of 27-year-old female, November 5, 2009.

#09231, homicide of 22-year-old male, November 30, 2009.

#09237, suicide of 26-year-old female, December 8, 2009.

#09240, accidental death of 29-year-old female, December 11, 2009.

#10026, undetermined death of 42-year-old female, February 6, 2010.

#10037, suicide of 37-year-old female, February 16, 2010.

#10054, suicide of 14-year-old female, March 11, 2010.

#10056, homicide of 72-year-old female, March 15, 2010.

#10058, suicide of 25-year-old female, March 17, 2010.

#10059, accidental death of 17-year-old female, March 21, 2010.

#10062, suicide of 35-year-old female, March 23, 2010.

#10075, accidental death of 28-year-old female, April 9, 2010.

#10102, suicide of 24-year-old male, May 22, 2010.

#10153, homicide of 58-year-old female, July 17, 2010.

#10154, suicide of 81-year-old male, July 17, 2010.

#10162, homicide of 44-year-old male, July 26, 2010.

#10221, suicide of 32-year-old female, October 1, 2010.

#10223, suicide of 15-year-old female, October 2, 2010.

#10230, suicide of 13-year-old male, October 11, 2010.

Note: In some cases the date indicates when the deceased's body was found rather than the date of death.